waking energy

7 Timeless Practices Designed to Reboot Your Body and Unleash Your Potential

JENNIFER KRIES

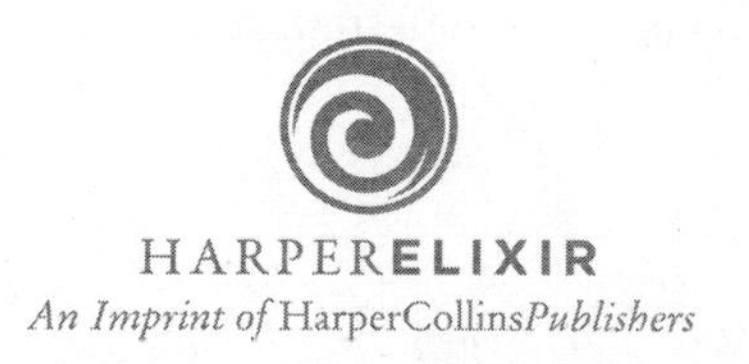

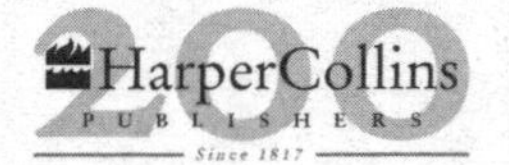

Photography by Chloe Crespi.
Meridian illustrations and Inner Smile illustrations courtesy of Lauri Nemetz.

Note: Ideally, all of the Inner Smile and Cosmic Healing Sounds should be performed seated.

This book is written as a source of information only. It is based on the research and observations of the author, who is not a medical doctor. The information contained in this book should by no means be considered a substitute for the advice of a qualified medical professional, who should always be consulted for any medical and health issues you may have. The author and publisher expressly disclaim responsibility for any adverse effects arising from the use or application of the information contained in this book.

FIRST EDITION

Designed by Bonni Leon-Berman

Library of Congress Cataloging-in-Publication Data is available upon request.

ISBN 978-0-06-236009-0

17 18 19 20 21 LSC 10 9 8 7 6 5 4 3 2 1

For my mother, Jane, who was and always will be Waking Energy

waking energy

ALSO BY JENNIFER KRIES

Jennifer Kries' Pilates Plus Method: The Unique Combination of Yoga, Dance, and Pilates

Contents

introduction

This book is really a love letter. It's my soul's autobiography—a weaving together of my personal discoveries, a tapestry of every healing movement that has changed and continues to transform my life—and the program I developed to share this gift with you.

As a professional ballet dancer, I spent years of my life treating my body like a performance tool, pushing myself past every conceivable physical limit. On stage, I was ethereal, powerful, magnetic. At times, I even felt superhuman. I cherished the thrill, the sheer elation that swelled inside me when the curtain went up, the honest sweat that soaked my costume from the exacting effort necessary to make the nearly impossible appear effortless. When I filled the stage with something beautiful, I was completely fulfilled. And when the last note sounded and everything went dark, I wanted more.

Dancing was the only thing that could magically take all the "stuff" inside—my brain's incessant chatter, the worry, the regret, the stress—and purify it, burn it all clean. Left in its place was a feeling of rebirth, an incredible lightness of being and a deep satisfaction in my soul.

And yet, right alongside this unutterable joy, I also felt incredible pain and anguish. Behind the velvet curtain, grueling, hours-long practices and bloody feet were the norm. The more it hurt, the more I suffered, the better, because it was a palpable sign that I was working hard toward my goal. This total dedication "at all costs" was reinforced by my ballet masters and mistresses (even ballet terminology speaks to domination). It seemed I was doomed, like Moira Shearer, a slave to the dance in the movie *The Red Shoes,* to love a profession that demanded I be its prisoner—trapped in front of the mirror for hours, day after day, my innocent, earnest young body constantly scrutinized through the warped and critical lens of my teachers. I can still hear the sharp echo of their voices: "Not strong enough," "Not fast enough," "Not thin enough," "Not pretty enough." In reality, I was all those things and more. But because I was fed by a constant stream of negative projections, it's no wonder I couldn't see it.

In spite of it all, I lived for it, because performing was my salvation and my greatest joy. As soon as I heard the magic words, "Places, please!" and felt the quiet beat before the stage lights went up—so bright they literally blinded me—none of it mattered. Not the packed theater, the critics, the hundreds of pairs of watchful eyes in front of me. No longer the dancer, I was the dance. I was the flow. I wasn't just in the zone; I was no longer of this world. The moment I stepped on stage, I had wings. I was a prisoner no more. I was beautiful. I was transcendent. I was free.

When I danced, gratitude rushed through the river of my soul, overflowing its banks, sweeping away any last trace of the pain. In those precious, ephemeral moments of bliss, every single cell in my body vibrated and pulsated with a transcendent joy. Even though I didn't know it at the time, I was tapping into my life force—the energy of creation, my essential aliveness. It was the energy of truth, passion, purpose, transcendence. I was harnessing it.

Words fall short in describing the insidious cycle that I willingly sacrificed myself to in dance—the descent into hell and then the payoff, the indescribable high, the out-of-body bliss I feel when I rose above the "mirror prison," when I escaped from the jealous, soul-crushing comments from teachers and peers. When I took flight, it all went away. I lost myself to the movement, that unspeakable ecstasy that I created with my body. Sometimes I barely recalled even hearing the applause when the curtain fell. And somehow it really didn't even matter, because I was already inhaling the sweet ethers from the upper stratosphere, floating higher than most humans could ever hope to fly.

Even now, I don't understand how to explain this deep, crazy love to someone who has never experienced this addictive sickness—the sensation of knowing that the moment I stepped on stage, I had wings. I was a prisoner no more. I was beautiful. I was transcendent. I was free.

To everyone who witnessed my lightning rise as a dancer, it seemed very clear that what I wanted most from life was to be a great artist. I too was convinced that what I wanted was to be Baryshnikov in a woman's body, with the same power and mind-blowing ability. But in truth, unbeknownst to me, quietly breathing and biding its time in a vault in the deepest reaches of my psyche was another truth: I was driven to achieve these heights to win adulation and love from a father who had always withheld it, because in spite of my worldly accomplishments, somewhere inside I believed that without his love and acceptance I was unlovable, anonymous, worthless.

All along, buried in a place that I couldn't access, I guarded an all-consuming desire to be loved—wholly loved—and accepted for who I was. I wanted to be loved for me. But I didn't know it then. Or if I did, I certainly couldn't admit it to myself. When you believe that you're not worthy of being loved, how can you admit to wanting something you feel you don't deserve? What I did know was that I yearned for the ability to heal the wounds I had sustained on the battlefield of my childhood, look past the poor choices I had made in partners, and find the kind of compassion and loving-kindness I yearned for and believed were out there for me.

This truth—that I hid an all-consuming desire to be loved—had me locked into a perpetual cycle of self-sacrifice and crushing disappointment, pushing me into undermining, self-sabotaging choices and leaving me depleted and drained. And I buried it so far inside my own psyche that it took a career-threatening injury—two of them actually, and later a nervous breakdown and near-suicidal depression—before I would begin to unravel the mystery I had so long denied, before I would embark on the journey to explore many paths to healing that would change my life.

I sustained my first significant injury while on tour in London and was forced to take a hiatus from dancing. It was there, while offstage, that I turned to Pilates for rehabilitation and also learned to teach it. So astounded by its miraculous effects in my recovery, I introduced it to public gym facilities back in the United States, eventually opening my own studio. An accomplished producer, Cal Pozo, discovered me there and asked me to cocreate and star in *The Method,* which became the first-ever Pilates video in the late 1990s. Though I had been teaching Pilates and yoga (and still actively performing) for years prior to the video's publication, its overnight global success marked the beginning of my career as a mind-body-spirit expert.

After my epiphany with Pilates and in answering the very real need to continue my own transformative mind-body journey, I delved headlong into the world of the ancient Eastern subtle healing arts. I traveled metaphorically thousands of miles, from China to India to Tibet, meeting with masters and studying with adepts (scholarly sages who transmitted many of the ancient practices contained in this book) who had dedicated their lives to uncovering the secret to living a life of peace and abundance. Through these ancient practices, I learned how to navigate life, turn my pain into beauty, and embrace a path to healing and being "awake"—to loving myself and finding my true power.

Just when I had myself convinced that I had turned every stone and cleared all the dark passageways of my psyche that prevented me from being all I could be, life tested me with another kind of trial. In January of 2014, after ending a relationship, I found myself suddenly single in a new city on the other coast. And just as I was starting to lick my wounds, my mother's cancer came back. Everything in my life seemed to explode and disappear all at once. This was a new kind of pain, not turned inward the way it had been with my depression, but like a maniacal driver, dragging me along on an open road for sport with my feet chained to the back of the car. When I lost my beloved mother that July, the pain was so intense that I found myself crumpled into the fetal position, sobbing and railing at the sky, not once, but many times.

I felt utterly helpless and alone, brought literally to my knees, and I wasn't sure that I could rise again. It was here, in my darkest hours, humbled beyond anything I'd ever known, that I circled back through my own history, integrating and falling in love again with the very same practices in this book that you too will soon experience. I tapped back into my essential aliveness, my life force. Every day, no matter how I felt, I dedicated myself to connecting with myself, to loving myself—to manifesting balance, strength, and radiance. I rose again. I thrived, both physically and emotionally, in ways that I wouldn't have thought possible. I reclaimed myself. And each element that now comprises *Waking Energy* reminded me how.

The writing of this book, which I began just as everything in my life fell apart, was divinely timed. When I first conceived it, it was wholly intended for you, but along the way it became my salvation once again. It not only became my journal, but a kind of memoir, my Zen koan, my daily ritual, my compass. Each time I sat down to write, I knew I was weaving the strongest fabric yet—a collection of teachings and wisdom that helped me to trust in my own strength again, to believe that I was held, supported, and nurtured, cradled in my own love for myself with the universe behind me. The hummingbirds and ravens who landed in the fountain outside my window every day became my companions, bearing me up on their wings. The messages of the ancients whispered on the wind, calling my soul to climb higher, to have faith, to hope.

The work and way of being contained on these pages not only restored me to myself, but helped me to give birth to a more authentic, brighter, self-loving, confident me, not once, but over and over again, every single day. And I lived every word I wrote in real time—my heartache, despair, anxiety, fear, loneliness—all answered by the magic of the practices, each day something different, another challenge, a new mountain to climb, and each time a new discovery that led me back to myself, my true essence, to beauty, love, strength, and radiance.

The Seven Ways I am sharing here are the very same ones that gave me my freedom. They are what healed, empowered, and liberated me. They helped to give me the precious ability to live into my soul's true purpose, living the examined life of a seeker, one that is dynamic, energizing, and joyful, one that honors the commitment to nurturing a strong body and a centered, conscious mind. And now I am sharing my hard-won secrets of empowerment with you.

Waking Energy is for anyone who feels overstressed, depleted, and anxious—and if you're a person living in the twenty-first century with a demanding schedule, multiple distractions, and endless demands, I am going to guess that's you. It's also for the person—and I am guessing this is you too—who recognizes a deep yearning within, whose inner voice wonders, "Is there more? Could I be more peaceful, more content, more whole?" The answer is yes, and Waking Energy is the way.

Informed by my personal experiences; my decades of expertise as a professional dancer, Pilates master instructor, and yogi; and my extensive study of myriad health and longevity modalities, Waking Energy uniquely integrates Western athleticism, Eastern philosophies, and ancient practices into one groundbreaking program.

This unique and timeless combination is a synthesis of techniques that is unsurpassed for cultivating balance, harmony, strength, grace, and energy. If you follow it faithfully, you will:

- Develop the body you've always dreamed of.
- Liberate the hidden power of your mind.

- Find the peace of mind you crave.
- Unleash focus and concentration, will and desire, as you come to appreciate yourself and your abilities for what feels like the first time.
- Transport yourself to a new level of awareness, where your physical accomplishments are reflections of your inner victories.
- Learn the tools to live your very best and longest life.

In nature there exists perfect balance: day and night, hot and cold, yang and yin. That same balance can exist in you, where all the boundless healing energy you will ever need is just waiting to be awakened. Once you learn how, you will gain access to all the energy you will need to live more instinctively; to live healthfully and longer, with less stress and greater vitality; to boost your metabolism and supercharge your immune system; to walk, think, work, reach, make love, and play with real zest, with true vim and vigor.

I'll teach you how to go deep inside your inner world, where you'll learn about the meridian and chakra systems and how to balance them in harmony—consciously energizing the powerful and intricate, sophisticated network of energy pathways. You'll awaken what the ancients called your "subtle body," the breathing, circulating network of energy fields and pathways that house your life force, your *chi,* where balance, true fitness, and energy await you.

You'll increase mental stamina and focus as you learn to calm and quiet the mind, cultivating your body's natural energy sources to find an unparalleled sense of peace and well-being in body, mind, and spirit. Every activity, from gardening to sex, will become more pleasurable when your body is so fit and so capable that you are able to feel good and just be in the moment!

Ultimately, Waking Energy will call you to truly *be* in your body and to honor it, just as it will move you to reclaim the natural rhythms of your life. You will feel that anything is possible and within your reach.

You will feel hopeful, positive, optimistic, empowered. You will feel more grounded and connected. From those times when you feel overwhelmed by life you will find relief. You will feel younger, more fluid, more flexible, and more patient, with deeper reserves and greater compassion—for yourself and others. You will discover that you have the power to transform a challenging emotional place into a refuge.

Waking Energy goes well beyond the realm of pure exercise. It is a way of life, one that will inspire you and grow with you, and one that will allow you to harness your full power, promise, and potential with life-changing results.

Waking Energy features seven distinct practices that can either stand alone as their own complete rituals or be combined to form a whole "flow." Whether you are a seasoned practitioner or new to the mind-body modalities featured in the Seven Ways, you'll experience an ideal platform of movement sequences for developing a proficient level of energy mastery that will empower, enliven, and enlighten you and engender true transformation in your health, spiritual richness, and longevity.

Part One of this book will explain the grounding philosophy behind the program and walk you through some important and fascinating information about energy and breath work, so that you'll come to experience it in an entirely new way through your own body and in the world around you. Part Two of the book is dedicated to the seven practices, each inviting you into a world all its own, where you'll explore its history, philosophy, physiology, and particular benefits. I'll offer clear, easy-to-follow, step-by-step instructions for movement sequences, specific breathing techniques, and directions for proper form and alignment (complete with photographs).

Once you are familiar with the seven practices that comprise Waking Energy, you will be encouraged to assess your mental, physical, and emotional state before each session and then choose each practice accordingly. The beautiful secret to this program is that it mirrors nature. Although each segment has a specific focus, each addresses all aspects of the body and mind. Each individual segment is a microcosm of the whole, just as we are individual microcosms of the world around us. You can do just one practice and feel confident that you have stimulated and activated all energy centers, conditioned your entire body, and balanced your whole being. Done together, they serve to complete a circle, bringing all the subtle energy systems into harmony and balance.

Waking Energy will meet you where you are—at any level of conditioning, fitness, health, or energy—and deliver exactly what you need to maximize your personal results. You will become so intimately familiar with each practice that you will learn how to customize it to suit the unique individual you are on any given day, allowing you to move synergistically with your own body's natural ebb and flow. With the new awareness that the practices give you, you'll be able to really tune in to your body. You can do as much or as little as you feel capable of. If you're anxious, it will calm you. If you're tired and depleted, it will nourish and invigorate you.

If you do the work, it works. It's that simple. There are no magic formulas, no special diets, no vision quests. All you have to do is start. And the most exciting part? The moment you begin, you will feel yourself coming alive again. You'll experience an instant energy boost. And once you see how invigorated you feel, how wonderful you look, Waking Energy will become as essential to you as eating and breathing. This regimen is so easy and accessible that it will stick where others may have failed or fallen by the wayside, and the benefits and inspiration will leave you eager to return to it over and over.

What's more, the effects of Waking Energy don't just stop at the close of a session. Whatever you have learned in any given segment, whether it is a new way to focus your breath, a technique to lengthen and strengthen a muscle, or a way to draw earth energy up through your body, you get to take it with you—the benefits are cumulative and lasting. Waking Energy is not just a set of exercises that you will engage in for a ten-minute, twenty-minute, or hour-long session, but a transformative state of mind and way of being that will improve all aspects of your life—your health, your outlook, your deepest, innermost self. Your progress will be mirrored back to you, your own true radiance reflected in the smiles and the twinkling eyes in others around you.

Know that the more time you invest in the program and the more you connect the power of the mind with that of the body, the more your spirit has cause to rejoice, the more ease and facility you will experience, and the more harmony and gratification you will bring into your life. As you practice and become more proficient with the work, you will be continually surprised and inspired by what you are capable of. You will find that when you harness your mind and befriend your body with clarity of intention and presence and with your conscious breath and movement, anything is possible.

You are so much more than you think you are. Your body and mind are a universe as complex, intricate, and infinite as the universe itself, a sacred channel for the limitless energy that surrounds you, charging you with the ability to transform yourself and the world around you.

We are all mystics. We simply need to be reminded of all that we're capable of and learn how to access the jewels that are already inside us. We need to remember that we have abundant magic at our very fingertips, and when we engage it, we invite infinite rewards.

Step onto this path and walk beside me. This is the path of the alchemist, where you will revel in the majesty and abundance of nature to reveal your own, where you will tap into your essential aliveness, where you will see nature's opposites reflected by your own contrasts, and where you will learn to love yourself wholly and unconditionally, cultivating so much love that you will be moved to share it with others.

We are all on the same journey. We are not separate from one another, as our thoughts would have us believe. What affects one of us affects us all. We all have the same desires in our hearts: to be loved, to be healthy, to be balanced, to be fulfilled, to find peace in our lives. Now, in this moment, in your very own living room or on your favorite patch of grass, you can awaken to the miracle and the majesty of who you really are. You are a shining light. You are Waking Energy.

A new world awaits where you can express yourself fully, freely, and celebrate who you really are, so that you can live life to the fullest, a world of "sacred fitness" for body, mind, and spirit, where you will become more conscious, more awake, and more alive.

Are you ready to awaken your life force, meet the energy of your existence, and unleash the fullness of your potential?

Are you ready to experience a deepening intimacy with yourself, at times becoming so at one with your body that you taste euphoria and experience an almost trancelike state in which you can merge with the energy universe that surrounds you and transcend your physical body?

Are you ready to feel your true power, and then go beyond—into a new world of physical vitality, boundless energy, and rising joy?

Are you ready to embark on your journey to the fountain of youth, to the center of you? Are you ready to awaken your life force and the powerful, healing energy inside you to shine with the radiance of a thousand stars?

Join me now. One of the most revolutionary, exciting, enlivening, energizing adventures of your life awaits you!

Welcome to Waking Energy!

part one

1

the way of ways

Say not, "I have found the truth," but rather, "I have found a truth." Say not, "I have found the path of the soul." Say rather, "I have met the soul walking upon my path." For the soul walks upon all paths. The soul walks not upon a line, neither does it grow like a reed. The soul unfolds itself, like a lotus of countless petals.

—Kahlil Gibran

I stood in the wings of the grand stage at London's Royal Festival Hall, on the South Bank of the River Thames, where in just a few hours I would perform for the queen. At eighteen, I was a gifted professional dancer who, having guested with a few internationally acclaimed companies, was by all accounts a star in the making. I had thrown myself into the rigors of ballet, practicing and perfecting my craft for grueling hours on end, becausc I loved it, and also because the moment I stepped on stage, I had wings. I was a prisoner no more. I was beautiful. I was transcendent. I was free.

Out in the world, I was accomplished, mature beyond my years, poised, articulate, reserved, and appropriately outgoing with everything under control. My inner life, however, was anything but what it appeared to be. At home, I was not okay. I was leading a double life.

Dance gave me an outlet, a way to escape my demons—my parents' acrimonious divorce a few years before and the stress of a volatile relationship I soon found myself in. I was as powerless to escape their clutches as I was powerful on the stage.

As the pain got worse in my personal life, so did my repressed rage. With nobody to speak with to process what I was experiencing, I started to become overwhelmed by my frustration and pain, though I wasn't entirely conscious of it then. I danced with more intensity, my deep-seated anger erupting through my movements, a force that daily required more and more energy to control and direct. Like a mutant weed, it was taking over, choking everything else inside. So on this fateful day of the royal performance, long past impatience and bigger than the container that restrained it, my anger, like a heat-seeking missile, was aimed at its target. My psyche had had enough, and my body found itself at its mercy.

Having quickly finished my sixth cup of strong British tea (I had just recently discovered caffeine), I was wired—like a rocket with enough firepower to blast the roof off the theater. I watched from the wings as the boys performed allegros, the big jumps, launching their bodies into the air, weightless. I felt the familiar pull to join them, to playfully compete with them as I so often did. I was blessed with something called exceptional *ballon,* meaning I could catch air very easily and gain nearly as much height as my male counterparts. I loved to soar through the air from the time I was a little girl, and I was always trying to fly higher.

Adorned in my usual attire—a jewel-toned leotard, black leg warmers over sheer pink tights, a pair of sweatpants fashioned into a shawl, and a well-worn pair of pointe shoes—with a light sweat glistening on my forehead, I took the stage for warm-up. I ran over to stage right to join two of my strongest male counterparts right after they started the short phrase that was preparation for a *grand sissone,* a jump where the legs went *ecarte,* splitting apart completely in midair, forming a 180-degree angle parallel with the floor.

Effortlessly, I launched my body into space, rising to a height equal to that of one of my friends and higher than that of the other. After this first flight, vibrating with an explosive energy that I could barely contain (not to mention the caffeine coursing through my veins), I prepared to repeat the jump stage left with the other two.

Charged with even greater intensity, I knew in advance that I was going to jump higher than both of them. With an "I'll show you" kind of attitude, I powered into the preparatory *plie* that propelled my body skyward. I used more sheer force than ever before. I went soaring into space, instantly transported with my legs split apart in midair and my ego riding on the rise of my body, gleefully aware of the other two bodies now slightly beneath mine. I ascended ever upward in a state of heavenly, floating bliss . . .

And then, two nanoseconds later, just as my top leg reached its maximum extension, a red-hot searing pain ricocheted through my left hip. I fell as if in slow motion toward the stage, crashing into a heap, writhing in agony. I lay in a crumpled pile, like a smoking aircraft fuselage, with flames lapping at my body. I moaned and rocked back and forth, holding my left leg, hot tears running down my cheeks, choking in my attempts to articulate what I was feeling to the boys who were kneeling down, huddled around me.

The team of osteopaths who examined me said that I had torn the tensor fasciae latae, a vital stabilizing muscle in the upper leg connected to the front of the hip bone, which assists primarily in forward locomotion. Sidelined and devastated, I watched as a girl who competed with me took the part I had worked so hard to secure. The doctors said it would be months before I would recover.

Confronted by my fragility, I felt a new kind of fear—the fear of losing something that I loved and made my life worth living. After my injury, my body no longer responded as it always had. Now even the most basic movements were painful, if not impossible. I had been catapulted from a false safety, a kind of naive and egotistical omnipotence in which I took my body for granted, into an abyss where I feared my body would be taken away from me, where I might never recover or dance again. I could not let that happen. It was a fate worse than death.

I was sufficiently incentivized to recover quickly and found my way to the Pilates Centre at the Pineapple Dance Studios on Langley Street in Covent Garden for rehabilitation. Involuntarily initiated suddenly into a harsh new reality, I had to learn patience, courage, determination, and hope. Surrounded by the warmth and support of the English team of osteopaths, I started to understand through each modicum of progress I made in my rehabilitation that positive encouragement went farther than the negative reinforcement I'd grown accustomed to in dance. I would need to be kind to my body if I wanted it to heal and perform again the way I wished. Through this poignant revelation, I found myself on a new path to being "awake," to loving myself and discovering my true power.

Pilates, which up to that point, had been my secret "bionic" weapon, suddenly became the thing that held the promise of healing. Helping me to rise from what I perceived to be a humiliating defeat, it empowered me beyond anything I had known before. It was no longer just a means of developing physical strength and power; it was *the* way to rehabilitate my body. Being a conscious participant in my healing and witnessing my own tangible advancement facilitated my recovery; the difference now was that I was aware of this miraculous process—I was the one healing myself. It was integral to finding faith and rebuilding my self-confidence. It was game-changing.

The Birth of Waking Energy

After following a new Pilates regimen and implementing the novel idea of being kind to myself, I defied the doctors' prognosis and within weeks

I was back on stage receiving accolades—a standing ovation for my final performance at Royal Festival Hall, a tribute for the queen.

Against all odds, I danced that final performance and danced it well. I knew I had to continue my Pilates journey when I returned home to the States, but it wasn't the only journey I would continue. I told myself that I would begin to unravel the mystery of my psychic unrest and the way it expressed itself through my body. I would continue to tirelessly explore the elusive dance of the psyche and the physical form, the sacred intersection of mind and body.

But, as they say, Rome wasn't built in a day. Rarely does a significant change happen overnight (especially in the domain of the mind). Even though I'd had a significant epiphany, my ego overwhelmed my inner wisdom, and I reverted to old ways of being. Intoxicated by the surge of power I experienced after making my comeback with the aid of Pilates, I continued to push myself and use my body as a machine more often than I was kind to it. This predictably resulted in another severe injury—this time, to my lower back—a few years later. Even though I continued dancing and my career flourished, I tolerated immense levels of pain each day. I moved through life feeling physically compromised, a constant, dull, nagging reminder that, contrary to appearances, all was not well and this physical and mental discomfort occupied way too much of my time and my focus—and drained my energy.

I believed, and this was confirmed by doctors, that the source of my acute back pain was pure overexertion, a legitimate physical injury; little did I know then that it was also and just as legitimately my body's way of finding a repository, a hiding place, for my psychic and emotional pain. It would take several more years of my continuing to push myself past acceptable limits and burying the pain, leading to a nervous breakdown and severe depression at twenty-one, before I would embark on the deep excavation that would lead to a profound and life-changing realization—that my physical pain had strong emotional roots and that there was no separation between my mind, my body, and my emotions.

Attempting to heal my chronic lower-back pain, I had tried everything—acupuncture, various massage techniques, chiropractic care, shamanistic healing, and others, and although these therapies helped, something inside me said that I needed to effect a sea change of my own, from within. So while I was in search of ways to heal my physical body, I concurrently and instinctively started to seek out practices that viewed the body as an integrated whole, where nothing was separate and everything was connected.

My journey continued with hatha yoga, but there too I continued to let my ego dominate, and instead of following my breath I would track how high my leg could go or how deeply I could coerce my body to twist into a pose. It wasn't until I discovered yin yoga, where I was forced again to slow down and *feel*, that I learned to leave my ego behind and came to truly understand that the mind–body connection was an undeniable truth. As difficult as this may be to believe, after just one two-hour yin yoga session, my back pain went away. It was *the* defining moment when I made the connection between the wisdom of the ancient practices that inform this book and the way to free my soul. The impact of the release I experienced, the depth of the emotional clearing throughout my body with this simple, but profound practice, and the new awareness I cultivated changed my life forever. I was finally free not just of the lower-back pain that plagued me. *I* was free.

With a new kind of inner fire ignited, I voraciously quested for more. I was determined to learn all that I could about healing my psyche and my body, and each step I took confirmed over and over again that the two were inextricably linked. It was as if my path had been preordained, because one magical discovery led seamlessly into the next.

After falling completely in love with yin yoga, I wanted to be able to teach it. I located intensive workshops that were perfectly timed with holidays. I found myself logging countless hours in study and reading voraciously into the wee hours. I traveled thousands of miles and frequented renowned wellness centers like Kripalu and Omega to study with some of the leaders in the field. The yin yoga and mindfulness meditation doyenne Sarah Powers not only led me to Jon Kabat-Zinn, molecular biologist and mindfulness pioneer, but also to some of my other cherished subtle-arts luminaries like Hiroshi Motoyama, famous for his modern scientific work on the meridian theory, and Taoist adept and qigong master Mantak Chia, whose work fascinated me, captured my imagination, and fed my soul. Serendipitously, while filming that first ever Pilates video, I met Gurmukh, the queen of kundalini yoga. They began my love affair with the ancient wisdom traditions, which continues to this very day.

Every investigative foray I embarked upon on in this healing journey was an attempt to solve the inscrutable mystery of how pain became vested in the body, a focused mission to finally heal my lower back and find fluidity and vibrancy in my body once again. But alongside this compelling need were an insatiable, burning curiosity and a primal suspicion that there was more, that we are far more capable than what we are led to believe. Each practice I explored and added to my arsenal was confirmation of my own inner strength and natural talents. I was finally able to free my life force, which was being misused, abused, and outright wasted because it was following an outmoded script, and show it a new route, a new way of being. By studying these ancient practices and integrating them into my life, my own ability to wake my energy grew, and I came closer and closer to wholeness, to glowing health and radiance, with every step I took.

My remarkable transformation forged along the journey through these practices has cultivated an extraordinary lifelong friendship—with myself. After what feels like a lifetime perfecting this life-force flow, of refining and perfecting the exercises into Waking Energy, I've developed a powerful combination of serenity, self-confidence, and self-love. When I look back at myself as the dancer on the grand stage at London's Royal Festival Hall all those years ago, I'm amazed at how much more buoyant and capable I feel now.

Waking Energy is a unique synergy of ancient teachings that fosters the connection of body, mind, and spirit, facilitates a heightened awareness of the self in the world through breath and movement, and results in an embodied awareness that sets the stage for miraculous transformation—for waking your energy. The seven practices all engender the creation of inner space, both physical and emotional, allowing the body to discharge held energy that can turn against it, to engage in a stunning process called somato-emotional releasing, where trapped energy (that's keeping old wounds alive and proliferating new stress and life-detracting thoughts) can be released and transformed into usable, life-enhancing energy.

In Waking Energy, I pay homage to the generations of disciplined seekers who paved the way and who, over thousands of years, pledged their lives to exploring the energy universe, dedicating themselves to creating a towering, veritably infinite library of work about how to bring consciousness to the mind and body in order to set the spirit free. The Taoist and yogic teachings you will soon discover will not only engage you and transform you physically, mentally, emotionally, energetically, and spiritually; they will help you to access your greatest potential and a feeling of oneness and inner peace.

I know, because I am living proof.

One for All

Tell me, what would it mean to you if you felt hopeful, invigorated, and alive again? What would it feel like if you were fully embodied, if you could stand tall, rooted and utterly confident in your own being? What would it mean if you saw yourself through loving, compassionate, appraising eyes?

I can answer that for you. It would mean everything. You would see yourself as an energy being, a being of light, at one with nature under canopies of emerald green trees, flying over whitecaps like a seagull celebrating its own wings.

What if I told you that you have the power to produce this state, those incredibly powerful effects, and the feelings that generate them whenever and wherever you wanted?

Waking Energy is about waking up to yourself, to life, to nature, to the world outside, and to the world within, so that you can enter this magical state of flow where you discover your essential aliveness and let it fly free—where you optimize, support, and nourish it. And the only thing standing between you and your essential aliveness, to opening this portal to a more enlightened way of being, to new ease and joy, is your very next conscious breath.

You will soon learn that the secret to waking your aliveness, your life force, is by consciously cultivating a mindful awareness of what you're doing and why you're doing it; by contacting, courting, respecting, and conserving it through "right action"; by using it wisely. It's a kind of embodied presence and attending to what is without trying to make it be any different than it already is—without spending your precious energy trying to change it.

The Waking Energy Way offers you a world of energy, and this is your pass, your golden ticket, to it. Welcome officially to the world that you can live in when you learn how to wake up the energy inside your own sacred vessel. And Waking Energy is one way for all. It is for everyone regardless of age, fitness, or capability. It will unite all aspects of your own amazing body, mind, and spirit, all aspects of who you are; it will unite the subtle body and the body you can see to nature and the world around you, to what lies beyond, and to what lies within—your own true nature, your timeless essence.

When you consciously wake up to yourself, to life, to nature, to the world, become aware and channel and nourish your essential inner life force, that becomes Waking Energy. When you learn how to waken and cultivate your energy so that your inner world matches your world outside, you will come to see that what is within is also without, and you will discover that you are a powerful agent of change.

The ancient Chinese philosophy of the Tao, which informs so much of

Waking Energy, is often referred to as the "Way of Ways," and although this book offers many different paths, they all converge into *the* way, the way to you. That's what separates Waking Energy from everything else—why it truly stands alone. All the practices you will encounter and explore demand total participation and yield consciousness, a deeper awareness of the self, others, and the world outside. Waking Energy is about giving yourself permission to express yourself fully, freely, consciously, to celebrate yourself and to live life to the fullest.

Waking Your Energy

We are beings of light. We are electric. We are energy itself. Right there inside us is more energy waiting to be awakened than we can ever imagine. Today's world has made us forget who we are. We are constantly looking for solutions outside ourselves—resorting to technology instead of turning inward. We have forgotten that everything we need to live our best lives, to wake our energy, is already here—inside us and around us in nature. Creating a balance between the fundamental cocreative energies of the universe within and without, the divine female and male energies, yin and yang, which make all of life possible, is the secret not only to waking your energy, but to improving your quality of life and longevity.

Waking Energy is a new way of being, a new way of breathing, of thinking, of seeing yourself and the world around you. It is an awakening. Waking Energy means waking up to who you truly are and to your greatest potential—to the world around you.

Waking our energy and enhancing our longevity depend upon balancing the dynamic and complex environment of modern life with a conscious awareness of nature and our primal needs. In spite of the seeming chaos and distractions that have become a hallmark of our modern lives, if we can refocus our minds so that we can make wise choices and invest our efforts in life-enhancing ways, we can simplify our lives and manifest vibrant health and energy. We do this through cultivating our energy—by becoming aware of and gaining access to a few key elements in our bodies, the immediate domain we have access to, that significantly impact the quality and length of our lives. Waking Energy is your introduction to the incredible importance of mental focus and not letting your emotions get the best of you—these are the first rules to longevity and peace, and they inform every practice in this book.

The Way of Nature

Close your eyes and think about someone who taxes your patience, someone you would rather not deal with if you had the choice. Or imagine how you feel sitting in traffic, trying to navigate a crowded shopping mall, spending hours in front of the computer, being late for an appointment, or hearing negative comments. Now consider how these scenarios affect your energy, how even the thought of them may drain you. They sap your very life force.

And now imagine what makes you happy. Envision someone or something you love very much, a beloved pet, a favorite memory, or a magnificent place in nature. Think about standing in the middle of the forest, under a canopy of towering redwoods, inhaling their intoxicating fragrance, or watching your feet slowly disappear in the sand as the tide rushes in and slowly slides out, the cool water on your legs, the taste of salt on your tongue. How do you feel *now*? Nature and living in harmony with her wakes your energy, empowers you, and makes you literally come alive again—reminding you of your own life force.

It follows, then, that one of the most powerful and immediate ways to tap into your own fountain of energy is to get out into the splendor of nature—to witness, experience, and *feel* the magnificence of creation. What is without is what is within. This is the fundamental principle, the overarching philosophy that informs the whole of Waking Energy. There is no separation within ourselves or between our inner world and the outer one—the great beyond. We are one with nature, with ourselves, with each other. Separation is an illusion. Just as our body is connected to our mind and our emotions, we are one with the air we breathe and the water we drink, inextricably connected to the world around us and everyone in it. Our personal ecosystem depends upon Mother Nature's. Waking your energy and fostering your longevity mean embracing these simple, all-pervasive truths.

By getting in touch with the world around you, by turning to nature, you can reveal and connect to your own energy. Everything that we need to be complete is within us right at this very moment. This idea is central to the Tao, the Chinese wisdom tradition meaning "the way," and complementary yogic philosophies like the Hindu *tantra,* meaning "to weave, stretch, and expand."

It all begins and ends with the energy of love, which is the energy that can help you create your own heaven on earth. Heaven on earth is a place where inner and outer support and mirror one another, where the earth supports us as we support it—where we develop an evolved consciousness that lets us know that as we are loving ourselves, our own ecosystem, we are loving the world we depend upon for our very survival. We need to serve and honor it, to live in harmony with nature and her myriad manifestations. We are the guardians of those riches. Here is your chance to rise to the occasion, both of loving yourself, so that you can cultivate true balance, wake your own energy, and generate the resources to look beyond, and of tending to the earth, the water, and the sky—the most essential prerequisite to living with integrity and balance.

At the core of Taoism is the teaching that the body needs love from the higher, conscious self both to survive and to nurture its own energy, which can then be shared. But we can't share the energy of love with true integrity until it flows beyond our own needs. The old adage, "To truly love another, you must first learn to love yourself," will take on literal meaning in each of the practices you will learn.

Another essential goal of Taoism is taking responsibility for the quality of our lives, especially by balancing our emotions and cultivating our inner calm, so that we refrain from giving our power and energy away by going to extremes. In the Waking Energy practices, the primary reason the movement sequences are so effective is that the body is treated as an integrated whole, like nature, which is also whole. As you stretch and breathe, you'll direct your energy in such a way that you can boost your calm and mental reserves and transcend negative unconscious emotional predispositions, helping you find a place of peace. In this way, you create a balance in your own personal ecosystem that influences every decision you make.

To do this, we need to dedicate ourselves to cultivating inner awareness, a kind of open-minded, open-hearted curiosity, that helps us to remember that we are all part of a bigger world than the one we inhabit on a daily basis. When we open to this broader awareness, we can tap into the energy from the world around us. When we engage in conscious movement practices that draw upon the limitless stores of energy in the fields of heaven and earth, we reconnect with ourselves, the planet, and the universe around us.

A sense of belonging arises in our own body—a reflection of our growing awareness of the unity and interconnectedness of all things in our world. As we start to observe nature and explore the same energies in our own bodies, we become more naturally attuned to the presence of life's opposites in others and feel more connected to one another. We start to shift from a Western perspective, in which we convince ourselves that the secret to living well and long is like an unfathomable mystery to be solved, something beyond what we actually see with our own eyes, to an Eastern approach, which has us look no farther than what is right in front of us.

The truth of what *is*, what we see reflected in our own bodies and in the world around us, then becomes a clear vision that we can integrate into our consciousness. We can start to cultivate essential awareness and aliveness—the energy we need to balance the two worlds. When we acquire the tools necessary to harness these universal energies and invite them to flow with our own, we become enlivened, excited, and empowered. We become more self-reliant and self-realized. We start to experience, to believe, and then to know that we have the power to heal ourselves and live our best lives. *This* is heaven on earth, and only we can create it—when we are present to what is.

If, through the cultivation of consciousness, you're able to maintain equanimity (at least most of the time), then you will have the internal capacity to make choices that serve you well. Feeding your spirit by making life-enhancing choices gives you more energy, so that then when life presents you with its inevitable challenges, you're better equipped to deal with them. By going the way of nature, you not only preserve and maintain your energy reserves, but in your best moments you can also supplement and reinforce preexisting stores. It becomes a kind of beautiful and self-sustaining domino effect.

When you align yourself with the universe and understand that you contain the universe within you, that you are one with it, you will start to feel truly whole. When you can align with what you feel, you can know your true needs and be independent and self-sufficient. When you see that your own body and mind are themselves fields of energy that reflect and interact with the larger fields of heaven and earth, and when you are living in alignment with your own instincts, everything just *feels* right.

Before you know it, you have returned to your own original, natural rhythms, you are living "the way," and you are on your way to becoming self-realized. Deep ease settles into your body, and you feel a sense of total well-being. You are able to surrender more easily, literally *to go with the flow* of the energies that surround you. When you can open to nature and receive her, you become more relaxed, and when you're relaxed, your body is open. Your muscles and nerves are at ease, soft, but ready, vital, and attuned. You become a conduit through which creative energies can flow more readily.

The Way of the World Unseen: The Subtle Body

From the time I was a little girl on the farm where I grew up in rural Pennsylvania, I was fascinated with the world unseen—the realm that lay beyond what my eyes could see. I felt connected to it, "at home" inside its invisible aqueous embrace. I was always either running through a field of broccoli flowers as high as my waist or lying on my back on one of the endless, green rolling hills that were my backyard, looking up at the sky. I would study the velvet brushes of color on a butterfly's wings or stand knee-deep in a stream, feeling the cold, slippery mosaic of a salamander's skin under my fingers as water bugs skimmed and skittered along. I would be utterly entranced, sometimes for hours at a time, under the sun, the sky, the oaks, the evergreens, my thoughts married to the wind. I was lost in a world where I was one with nature, marveling at her wonders.

Although we may be able to feast our eyes on a multitude of sights in nature that make us gasp in awe, there are many equally compelling sights that we will likely never see: deep space, the darkest ocean depths, and, as close as our next breath, the mysterious and magical hidden realm inside our own beautiful bodies. Within you, beneath your skin, in the places your breath travels in between your inhalations and exhalations, lies a flowing, circulating energy universe. This sacred matrix, containing an infinite network of the most intricate internal engineering, from your muscles to your tendons and bones, down to your fasciae, viscera, and the trillions of cells that comprise them, is actually a wondrous bioelectric web. This complex network of energy pathways is what is known as the "subtle body." And the energy intelligence that moves it all is your life force.

For millennia, the subtle body has been recognized by ancient traditions as the conduit through which the higher vibrational forces of the universe can flow into the physical body, catalyzing cellular growth and repair and expanding consciousness. Though the existence of this hidden domain has recently been established by science and medicine, when it comes to the actual workings of our own inner terrain, the world unseen inside our miraculous bodies, we are left mostly to rely on our feelings and imagination to navigate it. All the more reason why we are also so fortunate to live in a time when we can be the recipients of the gifts from earlier masters who dedicated their lives to confirming and exploring these innermost depths. Thanks to their work, we have resources to effect significant change in our bodies and our lives. Once you experience the dramatic shifts in the way you feel, you will be inspired to become a subtle energy apprentice, a budding "master" of your own inner world.

Sufis called the subtle body the "most sacred body" or the "true and genuine body"; to Taoists, it was the "diamond body." Tibetan Buddhists favorited the "light body" or "rainbow body," and for Kriya yogis, it was the "body of bliss." This world of invaluable riches is very much alive inside you right now, begging to be put to use. All you need to access it are your inherent gifts, your intuition, and your childlike wonder and free-flying imagination—your strongest allies in youth, which arose organically, as a natural expression of your nascent, sentient self. Soon you will see that "subtle energy" is anything but subtle, once you learn how to influence the way it moves and manifests itself in your body. Very simply, the subtle body is your passport to longevity. It is the place where you can wake your deepest font of energy.

Aside from creating balance through living in harmony with nature, making wise lifestyle choices (foods, practices, etc.), and trying to maintain as much emotional equanimity as we can, the way we integrate those things, the place where we can perform the inner alchemy that is responsible for waking our most prodigious stores of energy and promoting our longevity, is through the subtle body. It is here that we can cultivate the elixir of life from the marriage of yang and yin, the balance that results from all our practices. The subtle body is the place where we merge with nature and awaken the energy inside ourselves. We use both our physical body and our awakening consciousness to wake our energy, live long, and prosper.

By being present to and appreciating what you have, by acknowledging and honoring your body, your mind, and your emotions, you can tap into the elixir that is already in the body waiting to be discovered. You automatically gain entrance to a world where you have greater influence over the quality and length of life. Balancing yin and yang automatically means more energy, energy that you are able to allocate to accessing more still. The key to longevity is consciousness and moderation, which both lead to balance. On top of loving and nurturing your physical body, balance will help you learn how to manage your emotions and how to master your mind. That's in fact why all the practices I've featured in this book were originally developed—to help humans manage the mind and the emotions!

Working to establish a foundation of calm, peace, equanimity, and nonattachment that you can always access, working to establish a healthy relationship between your mind and your emotions, embracing a state of loving interdependence that fosters a positive, respectful, and cocreative independence, where the two parts are equally strong and in balance, is what to strive for. If you're going to strive for anything in life, this is the most important place to begin. And it's no small thing, may I add. It is this dedication to self, this utilizing your own body well that beautifies your life. This putting yourself to good use is something that makes you feel purposeful and inspired. And yes, this is what makes you eligible for energy cultivation, the act of becoming an energy worker, a practitioner in your own laboratory. Yes, this is what makes you best friend to your own subtle body and makes it dance with joy. It is by far one of the most powerful ways that you'll wake your energy.

A Rose by Any Other Name

Called *chi* in Chinese practices and *prana* in the Hindu yogic modalities, the life force is pure energy. It is universal source energy—the same energy that flows through heaven and earth and every living thing on the planet. The life force is the vital fuel that infuses the body's every system, organ, and cell with new life; it is responsible for feeding and maintaining the myriad functions of the human body; it is the catalyst and the reason for being that facilitates the body's perpetual cycles of assimilation and elimination, growth and renewal, from our first breath until our last.

Your life-force energy has been your constant companion, moving you and circulating inside you even before you took your first breath. It is in fact the force that made your life possible in the first place. And though it has been with you your whole life long, I would venture to say that it's not something you have been aware of before, or in quite this way. Through a paradigm shift that will make you aware of it and then through the techniques I will teach you, you will be able to actually meet it for the first time. In the world of energy, with a simple adjustment in what you believe is possible, a sizable shift in how you perceive your own power and your own innate talents as well as in how you see the world around you is destined to happen. If you can stay open and let yourself be surprised, temporarily trading your preconceived notions about what *is* for new ideas about what *could be*, you will not only expand the perimeters of what you believe is possible; your intention and action will make it so. You will have greater power, and new opportunities for energy expansion will continue to present themselves.

The electric currents that run through our own bodies and the frequencies and fields of energy that surround us—including magnetic fields and infrared radiation—all play a vital role in our physiological processes, right down to the cellular level. If it is the role of our circulatory system to move nutrients to our organs, tissues, and cells, then what moves the blood? The answer is bioelectricity—which is the energy that comes from the source—Mother Earth and the universe itself.

We and all other living things are formed and live in the earth's magnetic field, and our bodies also have a magnetic field of their own. Modern science (specifically Maxwell's equations and Faraday's law of induction) has shown that magnetic fields are generated and altered by one another and that they always affect one another. This means that the magnetic field of our body is always affected by the earth's field; in fact, they are aspects of the same force. Where there is one, there is also the other. There are negative and positive charges in the earth, and the same is true in our bodies. The human body is constructed of many different electrically conductive materials, which form a living circuit through which *bioelectricity* flows, circulating throughout the entire body, keeping the cells of the physical body alive.

If you think of your cells as tiny electric batteries, capable of storing electrical charges, then these trillions of baby batteries together form your human electromagnetic field. Electric energy is continuously being generated in the human body through biochemical reactions to food and air and circulated by the electromotive force generated within the body, particularly with movement. Bioelectric energy not only maintains life, but it is also responsible for increasing vitality, repairing physical damage, and restoring health. So it follows that if we can consciously connect to the primordial energies of heaven and earth, our own energy bodies become more stable and harmonious.

Taking this further, when we are injured or sick and our body's electrical circuits are affected, if we partner with others who are connecting to these same fields in their own bodies in a healthy way, the electrical fields from one human are capable of producing health improvements in another. Acupuncture, the insertion of needles into the body at strategic entrance points that connect to our energy pathways, and the method of healing known as "laying on of hands" are both especially powerful forms of subtle electrical stimulation that serve as examples of this process.

Waking Energy Anatomy: Your Inner Energy Architecture

Just as there are different names for the life force that flows through us, there are different interpretations of our inner energy architecture, though its functions and aims are the same. Each system is its own energy world, an interplay between subtle energy pathways, channels, and organs affecting all the body's systems, all the way down to our cells. The systems mirror one another in many ways, and at some strategic points share several common energy distribution and transformation centers. The traditions feature many of the same components with different names and associations, in keeping with each one's respective history, philosophy, and science. You'll discover that a central aspect of each of the practices is directing energy into the life-force center, the navel center, in one tradition called the Sea of Chi. It's here that some of the greatest energy transformation takes place, which is why the practices themselves were originally designed. Not only does keeping the life-force center awake and alive keep the organs well-nourished with fresh oxygen and blood; because it serves as a major energy distribution center supplying chi to the rest of the body through the meridian system, it means you are more awake and alive.

When you arrive at each of the practices in Part Two, you will naturally examine more closely how each of the wisdom traditions has designed this sacred inner space, each of their specific models for harnessing and cultivating your life force—for waking your energy. As you go deeper into your exploration of the practices, you will likely break into a smile when you start to see the many similarities and understand that the end goal is the same: partnering with the body to live your best life.

For all the qigong-inspired and inner-alchemy practices we will be learning, we are going to work with the subtle-energy anatomy based on the traditional Chinese medicine model, which incorporates energy pathways, called *meridians,* and storage and transformation centers, called *elixir fields*. For our yoga-inspired practices, including kundalini and the Tibetan Rites, we will be referring to the Hindu yogic tradition's system, in which energy pathways are called *nadis* and transformation centers are called *chakras*. All the practices in *Waking Energy* will follow one of these two templates, with the exception of Pilates, which does not ascribe to either specifically, but borrows from both and relies on stimulation of the lymphatic system, another subtle-energy system in the body, which will be described in detail. Once you draw universal energy in from nature through your body's portals, it commingles with your own and gets refined in these storage and transformation centers, producing more usable energy and creating balance and harmony in your own ecosystem.

We are comprised mostly of water, approximately 70 percent, which is conveniently infused with electro-conductive ions—among others, iron, magnesium, manganese, sodium, and potassium—so if your subtle body is a magical bioelectric web, then your physical body is the most perfect conductive environment for it. Water makes possible the interaction between your subtle body and the body you can see.

When you breathe, when you smile, when you kiss someone, when you dance, whenever you move, contracting and releasing the muscles of your internal oceanic self—your rushing rivers and your quiet streams—all of this pumps and propels subtle energy through a complex and intricate topography that is uniquely yours.

Imagine wearing a vast, simultaneously diaphanous and dense, internal compression garment—the matrix of your connective tissues. Woven throughout your body are *fasciae,* fibrous sheets and bands of collagen-based connective tissue beneath the skin that internally shape the body we know and inhabit. Fascia attaches, stabilizes, encloses, and separates our muscles, ligaments, tendons, bones, membranes (like the dura mater, the sheath surrounding the brain and spinal cord), internal organs, nerves, blood vessels, and lymphatic system. Like a body-wide net, varying in thickness and density depending upon the amounts of elastic fiber and fluid it contains based on the terrain of the body it encompasses, it essentially connects everything inside us.

Connective tissue not only is the common binding "thread" for all the systems in the body. It also houses an extraordinarily complex network of bioelectric intercommunication between all aspects of the body along our meridians and nadis, the subtle energy pathways that serve as the conduits for our life force, which charges, dialogues with, and nourishes everything along those paths. These energy channels in our bodies run through the connective tissues—particularly the stiff cartilage that links bones to other bones and muscles to bones. They not only do their part to conduct energy in this high-level electrical intercommunication, but, when properly stimulated with conscious movement, are capable of generating more. When challenged by conscious movement, such as our Waking Energy practices (especially yin yoga poses, which exert a great deal of targeted pressure on the fasciae), the fascia acts as a transformer for the energy pathways it houses, activating them as the tissue is stretched. As a result, energy grows exponentially and information flows more freely through the body.

The consistent and smooth flow of our chi through these pathways is essential for our well-being. When permitted to flow freely, our waking energy sets a positive, life-enhancing chemical chain of events in motion. Nerve signals from the body stimulate the brain to dampen pain by releasing natural "feel good" opiates, encouraging the natural sedation of the fight-or-flight response, which calms the central nervous system, lowering blood pressure and encouraging blood to flow optimally throughout the body, resulting in a panoply of physiological benefits.

Signals from the brain travel through the connective tissue, stimulating growth and repair processes in our cells and rehydrating the tissues and joints. The movement of muscles, the stretching of connective tissues, and the pressure exerted upon bone tissue in our Waking Energy practices generates bioelectrical activity in the meridians in much the same way that acupuncture needles do, literally waking our energy and helping us to keep our bodies humming vibrantly.

Dancing with Chi

Those who flow as life flows know they need no other force.

—Lao Tzu

You may think you can't "see" energy. Look around you. Watch a bird taking flight. Listen to a dog barking, the wind whistling through the trees, or chimes tinkling, animated by a strong breeze. This is life dancing with chi. The earth, the trees, the plants, the flowers, the sky and every star in heaven—they're all yours to reverently embrace with your breath, your intention, and your imagination for all that they offer you. They are all limitless stores of chi for you to channel into your body, inviting it to commingle with and supercharge your already exceptional innate power, which has been right there inside you all along.

Remember what it was to be a child playing on the playground, on the swings and in the sandbox, and tumbling down the side of a hill? This is how you will play today! You will be using your body to blissfully merge with nature, unreservedly jumping into the fray, more concerned with the thrill of the swoop and swell in your belly than you ever were about potentially skinning your knees as you leapt off the swing at its highest point. Now as a grown-up, with new skill sets and allegedly endowed with greater reserves of patience and focus, you have an advantage over your child self, mature talents that you will apply to your energy cultivation.

With them, you will connect to nature anew, giving yourself over to a new way of seeing the world as your energy playground. You will acknowledge, inhabit, and explore your very own beautiful body both as an energy vessel and the way back to your childlike knowing, instincts, and spirit. In the end, waking *your* energy is, more than anything, a returning to what you've always known how to do best—perhaps the most precious and elusive skill we humans possess—finding your innate joy, something that can only be experienced fully in the moment.

Be a child, and join the dance of life! Once you invite your imagination to take part in this new dance and acknowledge that energy is everywhere, you will be able to access it literally by summoning it—by placing your attention on wherever it is you want to invite the energy to flow. The Chinese say that chi follows *yi,* the "mind" or "intention," and "Where intention goes, energy flows." I hope for your sake that that expression will become a part of your life from this moment forward.

The primary reason that the Waking Energy practices are so powerful in making our energy "visible" to us is that every movement in the practices is done in tandem with a conscious breath, and it is breathing that serves as the major conduit for chi and its distribution throughout the body, facilitating the transport of freshly oxygenated blood through our entire circulatory system to enhance the lives of all the cells in our body—the process that literally creates the "juice," the elixir of life, that awakens our senses as we're doing it.

Your subtle energy will feel different from practice to practice. You may feel an overall sense of flow, a heightened awareness of energy circulating throughout your body, or relief, spaciousness, or lightness in your heart. You could feel an overall pulsating sensation or a more rising and empowering sensation with the more yang practices, such as after a kundalini sequence or following the Pilates mat work. Or you may experience the deep, grounding, and energized calm following even one yin pose. In the Love Thyself exercises in Awaken and Play specifically, you may feel anything ranging from a tingling sensation or buzzing in a specific body part to a sense of holding something fluffy, like a cotton ball or what you imagine a miniature cloud would feel like between your hands.

You may feel suddenly permeable or sense a pleasant warmth spreading all over your body; you may have a foreign, but curiously soothing gurgling sensation in your stomach or a new sense of openness or spaciousness in your body, particularly in areas where you typically hold tension. You may feel actual relief from pain. There may be a pulsing or magnetized feeling between your hands when they're rubbed together (charged) or heat coming from your hands when they are applied to the body to rub, massage, and stroke it.

Emotions also may begin rising up and out, from uncontrollable tears to laughter, deep peace, or pleasure. You may feel high, as if you have had a few glasses of great red wine, or sense radiance rising to the surface of your skin, like the pearly luminescence inside an oyster shell. You could feel a pervasive, warming bliss, or even ecstasy. Perhaps better than any other sensation you may experience, you may feel as though you are finally "coming home."

Another important aspect of dancing with chi is to become a witness to your own moods, patterns, and rhythms, to actually sense what happens inside your own body when you feel happy, or sad, or angry. What happens to your muscles when you feel shocked or upset by something? Do you feel muscular tension or, in the extreme, have a feeling of being trapped, of not having enough space inside your body? When we feel overwhelmed by stress or duress, the flow of chi slows and in some cases becomes stagnant. If you feel lethargic or depressed, your chi is likely deficient. What if you feel rage? That's a sign of excess chi.

The good news is that regardless of your mood or whether certain aspects of your body have too little or too much chi, in the world of traditional Chinese medicine, qigong, and all our Waking Energy practices—conscious movement is the grand equalizer. It is the "just right," the antidote to all the extremes in our lives, helping to literally balance every aspect of our being through our energy anatomy.

True Balance: The Dance of Yin and Yang

Let's listen to the sweet music of birds calling to one another as they begin their day, to the honking of the migrating geese flying in formation overhead. Inhale the smell of the earth, the fresh grass, and invigorating pine. Look at the ladybug that so neatly folded its delicate wings as it landed on that stargazer lily. Listen to the bees buzzing past on their way to pollinate the roses over the gentle slope ahead, and hear the grasses rustle with the activity of their denizens. Close your eyes and feel the energy of the morning—rising, expanding, warming, light, bright—*yang*. Later, as the sun sets, dappling light dances on the water, and the ducks dive down for dinner and surface, fluffing their feathers and then waddling up onto the bank to nest with the setting sun. As night falls, we are enveloped in quiet—a soft, diaphanous blanket of dark. Crickets chirping, morning doves cooing.

The nocturnal symphony has begun, the air cools and we find ourselves under a carpet of stars. Catching you breathless, the surprise of an owl's noiseless flight pulls your eyes down from its branch into the field below. The full moon rises like a big, happy pie over the horizon and illuminates the ground, only a few hours before a buzzing, bouncing, swaying, party, alive with activity, now an endless velvet throw of deep, silent purple-green. Close your eyes. Feel the enfolding, cooling, descending, dark, soft, quiet—*yin*. Night covers us, like a mother tucking her children in at bedtime, holding her finger up to her lips in a gesture of quiet, seducing us into deep rest and the inward sight of dreams—your whole body just melted with her. "*Shhhh . . .*" Did you feel it?

Heaven and earth, sun and moon, light and dark, hot and cold, dry and wet, hard and soft, above and below, and thinking and feeling are natural polarities and complementary opposites, expressions of *yin* and *yang*, the primordial feminine and masculine energies of the universe that manifest the relationships that inform all of life. Creating each other and never separating, they transform into each other in an endless cycle of life, death, and rebirth. Together they are what defines them individually. Everything inside and around us is made of these energies. Their interplay allows all things to come into being, and it is through cultivating a balance between them that we can manifest our own. Optimal balance of yin and yang allows our body's functions to operate at peak efficiency, resulting in untold benefits from vibrant health and energy, to significant weight loss and a return to youthful strength and vigor, to expressing our true nature—love, peace, and joy!

Through this sacred union of opposites in nature and in ourselves, we can create the fertile ground for our own transformation and evolution. Through the merging of our outer physical body (yang) and our inner energy body (yin), we have the marriage of great "minds." As you will come to see for yourself as you move through the practices, we have the potential to achieve our most vibrant health when we live in balance, yielding unfathomably limitless seas of energy.

Yin and Yang in the Body

The Waking Energy practices engage our body and mind and teach us to live proactively, helping us to cultivate a new kind of consciousness—movement that heats the body and then cools it, regulating the relationship between yin and yang within us that yields energy. When we move consciously in ways that moderate our inner energy "temperatures," we can balance and harmonize the body's energy systems, providing a powerful antidote to the effects of today's modern world. We do this by making time for "active" muscle-building, heart-strengthening exercise that creates heat and allocating an equal amount of time for "passive" body-opening recharging, for the still, deep, slow-moving stretches and conscious breathing that take us inside our bodies, into our emotional life where stress is stored, so that we can liberate chronic physical holding patterns and truly calm our minds.

Just as they are in nature, yin and yang in the body are in a constant state of flux, continuously subtly supporting, repairing, balancing, and transforming into one another. It's this constant transformation that is the basis for all change in the body's ecosystem, a give-and-take relationship that is the activity of life itself. Breathing is an example of this constant and unbroken flow—an inhalation always follows an exhalation until the end, our last breath.

Periods of work, high activity, output, and exertion are always followed by rest, recharging, and recovery. When we don't rest, when we don't breathe properly, when we don't honor our body and trust its wisdom, yin and yang become imbalanced. They argue, just as we do.

When we work excessively and don't take the time to rest or when we engage in intense, high-output workouts without ample recovery time, yin doesn't cool and nourish yang. Or when we don't move enough, when there isn't enough yang energy to warm and nourish our yin, then we can experience poor circulation and cold in our extremities and feel sluggish, lethargic, and depressed. Where one is deficient, the other is in excess, requiring a rebalancing that can be achieved by receiving energy-work treatment or through your own conscious energy cultivation—movement!

Sacred Geometry: Waking Energy in the Practices

The term "sacred geometry" is often used in kundalini yoga practices to describe the exact gestures and positions of our limbs that lend themselves to receiving and channeling energy to specific areas of the body to effect energy transformation. Certain shapes and positions allow the body to better funnel and transform energy, which facilitates subtle energy cultivation. Now that we know about the myriad energy pathways in our bodies, when we perform *asanas*, "poses," or *kriyas*, "exercises," with our arms and legs held at certain angles, we create spatial relationships that facilitate the flow of energy in and out of our bodies. Knowing this makes all the difference in the business of waking our energy. It is why we bring the body we can see and the subtle body together to create the magic they do when they are truly connected and working toward a mutual goal.

In all the practices you will learn, you won't just be moving, but connecting to source energy each and every time you lift an arm or a leg, and it's the awareness of this that wakes your energy and promotes your longevity. It's very simple: whenever you sit, stand, or lie on your back, stomach, or side, you will be partnering with source energy, swimming inside it. You will be using ancient Chinese and Indian energy templates to connect to the source, to harness universal energy to combine with your own via the energy portals and energy centers in your body.

To channel energy in the practices, sometimes you will fully extend your limbs like a young shoot reaching up toward the sun, actively collecting rays with your fingertips outstretched to their maximum capacity in a yang expression of rising energy. At other times you will be like the willow, with soft, relaxed limbs that are receptive, floating, inviting earth energy to flow in.

As we engage in conscious movement, the lines of energy running throughout our bodies become like tunnels filled with shooting rays of light that fill the space they flow through, nurturing everything in their path. Yes, we go through life moving our bodies, but we are often completely unaware of this rich dimension of energy assistance, this world of secrets that has the potential to change entirely how we move and how we think about how we move. When we add energy consciousness to our movement and precision to our form and alignment, the quality and content of the very actions our bodies perform take on new purpose and power. They become supercharged with this uniquely powerful combination of our awareness; our visualizations, which create perfect focus for the energy transportation; and our targeted breath, which escorts the energy wherever we need it to go. As a result, the simplest movements become light sabers of healing and transformation.

Just as water flows most efficiently through a straight hose, so it is with the energy that flows through our bodies. When our spine and limbs are well aligned, energy flows through them more efficiently and more energy becomes available, amplifying our efforts. When we consciously create our own lines of energy, we tone and relax our nervous system, increase our strength and endurance both in the poses and positions themselves and throughout the body as a whole, and create more space around our internal organs and in the outer body, decreasing the likelihood of injury due to muscular overextension.

Whenever you consciously partner with your body to establish the greatest integrity in your alignment, whether your body is meant to be flexed or soft, if you apply your attention to detail and effort and breathe into these lines of energy, your movements count more; they contribute more to your overall strength and health and become immediately more effective and transformative, affecting both your subtle and your physical body.

Whenever you move your body as a conscious, integrated whole, you instantly tap into more power than you ever imagined was available to you. It's not enough to simply assume a pose or a position in order to create change in the subtle and physical body. Any movement is good certainly, but it is *conscious movement* and *directing the breath and energy with your mind* that take it leagues beyond in the dimension of healing and transformation. Whenever you feel discomfort, a limitation or an impediment to your moving through an expanded range of motion, it means that energy is not flowing freely through this area. You need to use your mind to visualize your breath and energy literally moving into and through the area, massaging it, cajoling it to release and open. Wherever you focus your attention and your breath, as we established earlier, is where energy will go, connecting you more immediately and intimately with your life force and yourself.

From Balance Springs Bliss!

Contentment—a space devoid of worry and stress, where peace and equanimity reign. This is the beauty of yin and yang in balance. Yes, the euphoric highs in life are extraordinary and take us to places where we are so elated we can no longer feel our bodies, where we transcend time and space. But we also have lows, the deepest, darkest agonies that make us want to leave our bodies, the grief and longing that can leave us feeling numb, removed, asleep for a seeming eternity. What brings us into the moment, the very essence of our true nature? How do we travel to the epicenter of our essential aliveness, where we want to embrace ourselves, live inside our bodies, honor and cherish them, and kiss the earth that we have one; where we can see clearly and breathe the sweet, fresh air of yes; where we are attuned to what is with the energy of love, compassion, and presence? Balance.

Balance is bliss. It's a place where anything is possible, because you have the energy to make it so! When you start to discover the gifts you already have at your disposal—the abilities you naturally possess to establish it, inside and around you, you begin to create your own heaven on earth. When you align yourself with nature, you balance yin and yang, you enjoy vibrant health, and you wake boundless energy—energy to love yourself, to create, to play, to dream, to soar! And then, because you feel so good, you're happy to stick around longer.

Your body craves balance, and when you invest your efforts in your own good health, it rewards you by functioning beautifully. Balance can lead to longevity. It's an ever-evolving cycle of generosity and abundance. The more you give and invest, the more you love yourself, the more you are given, and the more is revealed to you. You have more energy to dive deeper, fly higher, and expand. As your ability to nurture and conserve your internal energy body increases, your outer body becomes more efficient, powerful, flexible, youthful. You have greater reserves of stamina and strength, and your mind becomes clear and calm.

You celebrate nature more, living in tune with her, showing your respect and gratitude for sustaining you. When you learn to heal yourself and experience the incredible life-changing benefits, you are moved to heal the world around you. With the new energy you cultivate and feelings of well-being you experience, you have more energy to devote to others. You have more patience and more love. You feel steady, strong, and bright. And your own energy reverberates around you, sending ripples radiating out into the world, lighting the spark of awareness and consciousness in everyone whose life you touch.

2

the breath of life

Imagine that you're driving along in your car with the radio on, calmly heading toward a favorite destination. Suddenly, your cell phone dings, signaling that a text message has come in, and even though you're not going to rummage through your bag to look for it because it's dangerous (not to mention illegal in some states), your pulse has already quickened. In this scientific experiment, Pavlov's bell has rung. In a way that would make Pavlov proud, you're jumping because the addictive part of your brain has been triggered and you're no longer as present as you were seconds before. Forget that you're operating a large piece of machinery where your safety—your very life, in fact—is at risk.

"Ding!" Another text! And wait, now what? The phone is actually ringing, which you feel compelled to answer, but you won't because you know better, right? Yet squelching that reflex to respond requires more energy than you might imagine, and you're suddenly feeling stressed, muttering under your breath about forgetting to turn off the ringer, *again*.

Our brains are so overwhelmed today by information overload—phone calls, messages, social media notifications, news reports, TV, Internet—

that we can't keep up with all the things we're supposed to tick off our endless to-do lists. Your car isn't out of gas, but you are. You feel exhausted and anxious. And you're in a really, really bad mood. Is it just me, or do you feel like shouting, "Stop the madness! I want to get off this merry-go-round and leave it all behind—the crush, the noise, the non-stop activity!"?

Let me remind you of something. You're in charge. All you need to do to make life-enhancing choices, like turning your cell phone off, is to stop and take a breath—a deep, complete, unhurried, full-body breath—and you'll have the clarity to create greater peace, not just in your car, but anywhere you choose.

When was the last time you took a deep breath? I'm going to bet that you just did. Notice that you suddenly feel refreshed, more awake, and more aware? The quickest way to wake your energy? Take a deep breath. It's the source for oxygen, which is the body's key element in producing energy.

Each time you respond to your phone, it targets the brain's pleasure and addiction center, the nucleus accumbens, flooding it with dopamine, which is then reinforced by the hippocampus, which makes sure you'll remember this feeling of instant gratification by laying down sweet memories of it inside your associated neural pathways. Then, within nanoseconds, the baton is passed to the amygdala, which ensures that you'll respond the same way the next time, creating its own conditioned response to this pleasing new chain of stimuli.

Today, whenever the phone beeps, we answer it. We sacrifice restorative moments of quiet and focus that contribute to our wellness and longevity for the checking of texts or the number of likes on our latest Facebook post. We're always looking outside ourselves for the boost. But the answer isn't out there, floating around in cyberspace. It's there inside you, right now. The answer is one deep breath. Your breath is the single most powerful tool you have to wake your energy, and you don't need special props or anyone else to help you.

Conscious breathing is how you can take charge of your life and your energy. The moment when your breath joins forces with your movement is when you can access the power of the universe and expand your energy-cultivation capabilities. Our breath isn't just our original energy engine and the central energy-delivery system; it's the engine of transformation and evolution in our lives. It's the vehicle for cultivating awareness. Ancient sages say, "When the mind is distracted, chi scatters." A passive existence is dangerous, because we waste so much of our precious life force, or chi, allowing ourselves to get pulled in different directions; but when we use our mind to direct our breath, every movement becomes our own. Every conscious moment becomes a waking-energy opportunity. Conscious breathing *is* Waking Energy.

The simple act of breathing starts the alchemical process of change within you. It's how you can travel deep inside, harmonizing the flow of energy throughout your entire body. If a journey of a thousand miles begins with a single step, then waking your energy begins with one deep breath.

Waking Energy Breathing Benefits

The powerful breathing techniques in the Waking Energy practices have been perfected over centuries. They facilitate the birth of healthy new cells, making us feel restored and rejuvenated. Cellular exchange, down to even the mitochondria, cannot occur if your breath does not join forces with your energy. When we *intentionally* direct our breath, we optimize this vital process, resulting in a windfall of benefits.

Breathing keeps our organs and blood supplied with oxygen, which is the very how and why of our health; because deep breathing massages the internal organs, it keeps the lower abdominal energy center awake and alive. It's the source of all the energy in your body and the means by which you can direct it. How we breathe determines how efficiently we are able to absorb energy from the universe as well as how well we assimilate chi from the nutrients we ingest.

Optimal digestion, for example, is facilitated by deep diaphragmatic breathing, which provides a kind of undulating massage that stimulates the internal organs of digestion. In order for the body to properly digest and assimilate food, our breathing must be relaxed and full, following a natural breathing into the belly, which promotes increased blood flow to the digestive tract and organs as well as facilitating the movements of the stomach and intestines to break down food and extract optimal nutrition from it.

The better you breathe, the more you activate your parasympathetic nervous system, which decreases the sympathetic stress response and gives your body the golden opportunity to recharge, regenerate, and heal. When you breathe deeply and smoothly, you call off the dogs of war, sending a clear message to the fight-or-flight branch of the sympathetic nervous system that it should go on vacation. Less stress also helps reduce the secretion of stress chemicals like adrenaline, cortisol, and norepinephrine. Damaging acid levels in the blood will naturally decline, reducing inflammation and your risk for diseases like cancer, which thrive in stress-induced, acid environments. When we highly oxygenate our blood, we alkalize it and make it more inhospitable to pathogens.

Every Breath You Take: A Sea Change

If you look beyond the physical components of breath—the oxygen, carbon dioxide, and other molecules that stream in and out with every inhalation and exhalation—inside each and every breath is your life force, your life expressing itself every moment.

Like the ocean's tide, a cycle of perpetual renewal, every breath you take is new. The ocean of air that swells inside you is called your *tidal volume,* the name for the normal volume of air displaced during a single cycle of inspiration and expiration that occurs without your applying any extra effort—about half a liter on average, a baseline that your body can flexibly alter to accommodate your activities.

Did you realize that you breathe up to 30,000 times in one day? And in the course of that day, your body will exchange 2,500 gallons of air with the world around you. You will breathe almost 8 million breaths each year, almost 265 million liters of air in a lifetime. If you live to be eighty, you'll breathe more than 600 million times! However, despite the prodigious volume of air we consume, only a very small proportion of it is actual oxygen that finds its way into our bloodstream. In normal, quiet breathing, we consume about a pint every minute or a little over 1,400 pints, or 175 gallons, of oxygen every day. Our body requires different amounts of oxygen for different activities, and luckily our breathing capacity can adjust very readily to our various pursuits, delivering varying amounts of oxygen to our body depending on what we're doing.

Most of us suffer from compromised breathing because we use just a fraction of our lung capacity. We've adapted to a limited sphere of breathing, and our breathing apparatus itself has atrophied. Because of this, our energy capacity has diminished. As a result, we are often living into just a small percentage of our potential. But there's good news. You can change this and rehabilitate your breath function simply by becoming aware of it. The average person breathes between twelve and twenty times per minute, but when you become more skilled in your breathing practices, consciously directing your breath, you can inhale the same volume of oxygen while breathing only five to eight times per minute.

The Eastern ancients understood the importance of breathing, studying it as a way to cultivate energy for vibrant health for thousands of years. With the breathing techniques you'll learn in the following practices, these health and longevity secrets can soon be yours. Your intention and awareness will strengthen your breathing and enhance your lung capacity, which means greater stamina and energy. The goal is to strengthen your respiratory muscles to become so proficient at breathing that your organs won't have to work as hard to pump blood through your body. This conservation results in the best reward—more energy for life!

Every breath is an opportunity to wake your body and your mind.

The breath itself becomes a force of change so significant that it becomes a sea change. All it requires is your conscious intention to manifest a whole new reality in which you feel energized, fully awake, and alive!

Conscious Breathing: The Engine of Transformation

Breath mastery for the ancients was foundational for waking their energy. The breath was a direct reflection of their "internal weather," the most accurate reading of their inner emotional lives. They knew better than anyone how emotions can get the better of us and our breathing and steal our energy. The practices they developed were all intended to avert energy theft—to quell distraction, balance the emotions, and calm the mind, so that they could cultivate energy without interruption to reach their ultimate goal, immortality.

When we let our minds get the better of us, we're actually blocking the flow of energy through our own bodies and compromising our own ability to absorb and integrate it fully. Our breathing becomes compromised by our emotions, the chief culprits in energy stagnation. They are energy enemies—thieves of the first order. To wake your energy and nurture it, you must first balance your emotional life, and you can do this by befriending your breath.

Think for a minute about the physiological symptoms you may experience when you're upset, anxious, or angry. Does your heart race, your stomach twist in knots, and your breathing become shallow, fast, and from the chest? These are the kinds of negative impacts emotions can have on your body's heart rate, digestive system, and nervous system. They play a powerful role in the chemicals that are released into the bloodstream. Our muscles react to these chemical cocktails, often leading to a kind of restriction that reduces our breathing efficiency—the musculoskeletal aspect of breathing, especially when we feel we are carrying the weight of the world on our shoulders.

Stress can lead to an actual restriction in the musculature of the breathing apparatus itself—the muscles of the shoulder girdle, the trapezius, and the neck. Our shoulders hunch forward, compromising inhalation, and rise up toward our ears, preventing proper exhalation. When we inhale, we engage the muscles of the diaphragm and the intercostals surrounding the rib cage. When we exhale, we relax the same muscles we use to inhale. When we feel excessively stressed, we can't relax the way nature intended, and our ability to thoroughly cleanse the lungs and fully dispose of accumulated stale air becomes compromised.

When we inhale, we aren't simply taking in oxygen; we're also taking in information and feelings from the outside world. When we exhale, we're not just cleansing our bodies of carbon dioxide, but releasing and discharging stagnant chi and all the thoughts, emotions, and tensions that contributed to it. In order to restore our breathing to its optimal functioning, we need to release ourselves from the mental and emotional burdens we carry (literally) on our shoulders, so that our body's systems can function optimally, reducing stress, and helping us breathe better. When we succeed, we can relax our shoulders, letting them fall into their natural, comfortable resting position where breathing becomes easier and more complete.

By going straight to the source, our breath, we can reconnect to ourselves and to the moment, to the realization that whatever is happening will change as soon as we allow it to.

Whole Body Breathing: Babies Know Best

If you want to know how to breathe well, return to your beginnings and look to nature. Babies and animals breathe naturally, knowingly, and effortlessly with their whole bodies. Starting deep in the belly, flowing up to the heart and further expanding the lungs, into the head, then back down to the feet—they breathe smoothly and deeply, from the belly first. Every inch of their bodies is affected by these waves of respiration. The other wonderful thing that children and animals do is that they act freely on their instincts without censoring them. To correct the oxygen–carbon dioxide ratio in the body when it's fallen out of balance, they will unabashedly draw in and absorb what they need from their environment, mouths wide open, yawning and sighing. There's a reason why movement scientists like Joseph Pilates studied animals: they are exemplary breathers and movers, utilizing their bodies with the utmost efficiency and effortless elegance.

We don't just lose our spontaneous and immediate connection to joy and laughter when we become adults; we also lose our ability to breathe naturally, deeply, and smoothly without thinking about it. We allow the quality of our breathing to be subsumed by distractions from the outside world—most of the time we use only about 50 percent of our lung capacity. When we emulate babies and animals, we breathe fully and completely, relaxing so that circulation operates at peak efficiency, and every part of our body is well supplied with ample energy.

When we're bored or tired, we tend to "underbreathe." If we haven't been moving for a while or have endured periods of stress during the day and our breath becomes shallow for extended periods of time, the body triggers a strong, spontaneous contraction of the diaphragm demanding that the body increase its oxygen supply. A yawn or a sigh is an outward expression of this little rescue mission, which also activates a physical counterpart to the sudden and spontaneous intake of air. Stretching or reaching the arms overhead creates more space for the lungs to expand and take in more air and thus more oxygen, making for easier, deeper breaths and new energy. In the world of energy cultivation, sighing, yawning, and stretching are signs to be welcomed and allowed their full expression. They're our body's attempt to regain balance, vigor, and interest, sending more oxygen to the brain.

Waking Energy Engine Anatomy

Did you know that starting around age thirty, our breathing tends to become more shallow? This happens mostly because, at this age, we tend to live in our heads more than in our bodies. Instead of naturally moving down deep into the lower belly, air moves higher into the mid-belly area, where there is less oxygen uptake. This means that insufficient oxygen reaches the brain and cognitive function slows, impacting memory and our ability to think clearly. The diaphragm doesn't get its proper workout, and the internal organs suffer because they miss their revitalizing massage. Without sufficient oxygen, we ultimately become fatigued and lethargic and more prone to health problems, including respiratory illnesses and even heart disease. Chi stagnates, the internal organs start to degenerate, and the cells of the body, no longer receiving ample oxygen, start to deteriorate at faster rates as well.

With natural breathing as your baseline, you can teach yourself to direct your breath anywhere you want to create vibrant health and energy. This "natural" breathing, or deep diaphragmatic breathing, starts in the belly and not only refocuses your energy in your lower abdominal energy center, but also assists you in building your lung capacity very quickly. When you consciously direct your breath into your body, making the most of your own natural resources, you revitalize it. You can send breath to places that are less accustomed to receiving that kind of care, such as your upper back, lower back, the sides of your ribs, and your neck. Sending fresh oxygen to injuries and chronically held tight places in the body can help them loosen and become more flexible and then actually involve or reinvolve them in the breathing dynamic to make your breathing more efficient.

For optimum health and energy awakening, breathing should be consistent, full, and rhythmic, using the diaphragm and ribs to fill and empty the lungs. The exchange of air in the lungs increases oxygen levels in the body, which strengthens cardiovascular and respiratory function, activates and optimizes digestion, stimulates and energizes the endocrine system, and reduces stress and anxiety. When toxins are properly eliminated, fresh air is brought in to replace stale air, mental clarity and concentration increase, your general outlook improves, and a sense of equilibrium is restored.

The Giving Trees: Everything Old Is New Again

It's nothing short of mind-blowing to consider that every breath we take contains millions of particles that have existed in our environment since the beginning of time. At some point, these particles have passed through other living things on planet earth. Each time we breathe, we inhale some of this timeless energy, and when we exhale, we make our own unique energy deposit, contributing to this grand cosmic swirl.

This important and intimate relationship, the one we conduct through our breathing with Mother Nature and her bounteous forests, is the most vital one we'll ever have, but most of us rarely acknowledge it. Every day and in each and every one of the Waking Energy practices, whenever we exhale, we are actually giving the planet an offering—something that we've borrowed from the atmosphere, utilized, and then returned—a part of ourselves, from our inner universe to the outer atmosphere, supplementing the fuel for our planet's plant life. We need the oxygen, a waste product of plant metabolism, and in return we donate our own, carbon dioxide, as nutrition for the plants, flowers, and trees that sustain us. Talk about a cocreative relationship!

Making the Most of Your Breathing Body: Ideal Posture and Focus

Learning how to control the breath is fundamental to waking your energy. The rhythm of the breath, energy, and the emotions are all inextricably linked, and when we reach a level of proficiency with our breathing, we can create exceptional internal harmony and health. You'll rely on two pillars of energy transformation: *establishing ideal posture* and *focusing your mind.*

When you establish optimal posture, every movement acts like a pump, disseminating energy throughout the body and helping you to cultivate even more. This doesn't just optimize your actual breathing apparatus; it gives your internal organs ample space to function at their best, properly suspended with integrity in their organic places that nature designed, where breath and energy can flow freely, nourishing everything it flows around and through.

Ideally, you want to establish a posture that makes you feel tall, rooted, and easy, so your chest is free to do its utmost in helping you to expand your breathing range and, hence, your waking-energy aptitude. Since the lungs are soft structures, they only occupy the room you make for them. You want to give them as well as the upper-body muscles and bones that house them an optimal environment to make breathing an effortless and complete exchange with the world around you, so that you can maximize your own energy-cultivation efforts. This happens when the shoulders are held open, back, and down to create the greatest expanse possible for every beautiful breath. Since you're delivering molecules of oxygen to your cells and expelling carbon dioxide, you want to be able to maximize your uptake and put some oomph behind the expiration, so that there is a complete cycle of cleansing as well. Complete breathing cycles help to counteract the buildup of toxins in the lungs caused by environmental pollutants and allergens.

Think for a minute about how your body reacts when you jump into the ocean and it's really cold water—how your shoulders rise up around your ears and your ribs expand beyond their normal range. It's all happening to accommodate the extra breath you need to signal to your sympathetic nervous system, which is responsible for your stress response, that all is well and that you will either soon adjust to the temperature or quickly make your way to the dock to sun yourself with the seagulls. Breathing is an automatic function controlled by the respiratory center, but it's also a musculoskeletal endeavor as well, and because of this, making sure your body is well aligned is integral to breathing optimally.

Even if we're not swimming with a Polar Bear Club, we tend to overwork the shoulders, raising them up, again to create the space needed to take a deep breath. This is often a sign of atrophy in the respiratory muscles, because even though the diaphragm is one of the primary organs responsible for respiration, it underfunctions in most people. Instead, the chest muscles are recruited to overperform, leading to bad breathing habits. You want to maximize your breathing apparatus, which literally connects you to your greatest energy source—the outside world—by strengthening it with deep diaphragmatic breaths. With a little patience and practice, the lungs, the diaphragm, the muscles of the abdomen, and the circulatory and lymph systems welcome the rigors of deep breathing.

Think of your whole body as a large, round, red, happy balloon that fully expands and naturally contracts with each breath. Like every inch of the balloon as it is inflated, you want to send your breath not just into the top and front of the chest and belly, but deep into the sides and back of the ribs themselves and into the uppermost and lowermost lobes of the lungs. When we inhale, we need to think of it as sending the breath down into our feet, into our deepest belly, then into the chest and up and into the head, and of course into every last inch of the body. When we exhale, we start by emptying through the feet, up into the legs, into the belly, using the abdominals to accentuate the contracting of the abdominal wall, helping the stale air to exit the chest and body completely, and finally visiting the head once again.

This is how you make each breath really count. When you're relaxed and breathing lower into the body, expanding the rib cage both laterally (side to side) and sagittally (front to back), you can really start to wake your energy, sending the breath down to nourish your primary energy centers. When you can do this, know that you've arrived at an exceptional starting point where breath and energy become one.

So what distinguishes deep, natural, optimal breathing from ordinary, everyday breathing? The diaphragm, the workhorse of the body's breathing mechanism. The deep, diaphragmatic breathing you'll perform in the practices will stretch and strengthen this resilient, flexible muscular membrane in addition to strengthening your abdominal muscles and invigorating your internal organs with a vital, age-defying massage.

The diaphragm sits beneath the lungs and above the organs of the abdomen, between the upper, or thoracic, and the lower, abdominal, cavities of the torso. It attaches at the base of the ribs, the spine, and the sternum. Breathing, formally called *ventilation,* consists of two phases, inspiration and expiration. Every time the lungs expand in a deep breath during inspiration, or inhalation, the diaphragm contracts, forming into a dome shape and descending into the abdomen. Because air always flows from a region of higher pressure to an area of lower pressure, it travels in through the body's conducting airways, the nostrils, throat, larynx, and trachea into the alveoli of the lungs, causing thoracic volume to increase and pressure to fall, drawing air into the lungs. The external intercostal muscles that run between the ribs pull the lungs up and outward, expanding the rib cage, further increasing this chest volume. Almost all the muscles in the upper part of your body, from the muscles in your upper neck, starting at the occiput, the base of the skull, and going all the way down to your lower back and sacrum, participate in the breathing process.

Each time you inhale, the muscles of the neck and shoulders help to lift the rib cage in order to accommodate the lung's expansion. During expiration, when the lungs contract in an exhalation, the diaphragm expands and rises into the chest cavity, and the external intercostal muscles relax, restoring the thoracic cavity to its original smaller volume and forcing air out of the lungs into the atmosphere.

When you arrive at the first Waking Energy practice, Awaken and Play, you'll have an opportunity to practice deep, diaphragmatic breathing and use it as the baseline for all the other breathing techniques you'll learn as you move through the Waking Energy Way.

Feeling Your Rhythms: Breathing in the Practices

How fortunate are we that nature gifted us with this most flexible and adaptable design? Breathing is unique when compared to the other functions of the body, because even though it operates automatically, it can also be consciously controlled. This ability gives us endless flexibility both physically and mentally in the way we live our lives—what we choose to do with our bodies and how much we're able to live life, how we experience life moment to moment.

There are as many different ways to breathe as there are to dance, each with its own rhythm, depth, beat, and style, each directly affecting your state of mind, your emotions, and the health of your body. In your Waking Energy adventure, your breath will be your most powerful ally, your faithful companion, and the most accurate compass as you navigate each modality along your way. The Waking Energy Way will help you to fully exploit the breath, taking an already brilliant design and supercharging it, amplifying its already prodigious power to heal, enliven, restore, and empower.

Your mind is naturally attracted to rhythm, and it's the rhythm, the speed and volume of the breath, that directly affects the body's inner energy flow. When we consciously alter our breath, we can catalyze dramatic changes that improve our body's overall function, resulting in virtually limitless stores of energy. Each of the breathing techniques you'll learn possesses its own unique dynamic, imbuing its paired modality with its integral power and having a profound influence over the kind of energy we want to elicit. Each has its own extraordinary merit and will help you to expand your breathing repertoire; you will learn to apply different techniques and integrate them to maximize the movements you do for each one.

Even the transitions within each breath are important and should be smooth and deliberate. The duration of each phase, from the pauses in between the breaths to the retention of oxygen to the exhalation, are just as important as the harmonious passage that connects them. The rhythmic beginning and ending of each breath is like a heartbeat that encourages the mind to stay focused and undistracted. Your breathing asserts a strong pull on your senses, and when they become totally absorbed in the sound and quality of it, it will yield greater energy—the most important byproduct of mindful, conscious breathing. Once you learn to move in tandem with your breath, it can become the most useful tool in your own growth.

In Chinese philosophy, there exist two complementary principles of the universe, yin and yang, that describe all things. The yin (the primordial feminine, receptive, passive) and yang (the primordial masculine, active, upward rising) ways of breathing that are central to the practices result in very different outcomes depending upon what type of effect you wish to have on your body. To achieve a specific kind of energy, you'll breathe in a way that moves in tandem with nature's cadence, mimicking the rhythms of day and night, so that you can balance and harmonize your subtle body by attuning it to the world outside.

In the morning, when you want to greet the day and raise your energy, you'll choose practices that either strike a yin–yang balance, like Awaken and Play, or that are more predominantly yang in character, like Unleash and Transform or Empower and Flow, which are characterized by an upward- and outward-reaching, pulsating breath that creates in internal heat that purifies and balances. In the evening, when you want to cool off and slow down, you'll draw your energy inward, quieting the breath to cultivate yin energy with the practices that feature a descending, softer, more luxurious breathing style to calm and ground your energies, ushering in a restful night's sleep.

What all the breathing techniques have in common is that they are the most direct route to cultivating consciousness, taking an involuntary act to new heights and making it the true engine of transformation—the most powerful means we have to proactively manipulate the way we move energy through our bodies, so our brightest inner light can shine.

Regardless of the style, the breath is the source of your stamina. As your lung capacity increases in each and every practice and you get stronger, you won't have to breathe as hard or use as much energy to execute the same movements. You'll have more energy in reserve. In becoming more aware of how your body works during the breathing process, you will learn to maximize your efforts when you inhale, exhale, and retain breath, and when you practice the more involved breathing techniques of the various modalities that comprise the Waking Energy flow.

Inhalation: Drawing Back the Bow

When you draw back the bow, you prepare to greet life!

Every time you inhale, you are starting a new moment in your life. Inhalation is the ultimate inspiration. It's the beginning and the most yang expression of the breath. In the practices, when you consciously direct your breath and inhale, you are embarking, venturing forth, gathering your life force. It's you filling up, preparing, surging, drawing back the bow.

The word "inhalation" was once synonymous with "inspiration," reminding us to acknowledge the ultimate link between breath and spirit. From the Latin *spirare,* "to breathe," the words "spirit," "respiration," and "inspiration" all share the same origin.

During inhalation, the chest expands and the lungs are filled with fresh air. But in the Waking Energy sense, inhalation also signals the intake of life force. The body's activity and creativity are generated through the act of inhalation. It is an act of receiving. When you inhale, you are actually collecting chi from the universe around you. When you consciously breathe in, every single breath becomes supercharged with your conscious intention, becoming so much more than a simple inhalation. The breath becomes a healing elixir. When you inhale, you are inviting energy to circulate and nourish your entire internal environment. But it's not just your lungs that breathe; your skin does too. You literally absorb chi through the skin, which is your largest organ of respiration and exchange with the world around you.

When you inhale, you are breathing with your entire body, the expanse of the protective canvas that envelops you, drawing in vital information and energy to fuel your every movement. From subtle to sweeping, from delicate to divinely expansive, your breath expresses itself through your upward, outward, rising action.

The Spaces in Between: The Power of Suspension

Like the space between two waves, where potential is made manifest, the space between the inhalation and the exhalation is where actions are born. In any of the practices you do, in your actual movements, if you attend to that moment between in the inhalation and the exhalation, in that pristine stillness you can gather your most powerful energy.

It's also in the space between the inhalation and the exhalation where true wisdom is born. In that space that seems to hang in the air, literally suspended for a seeming eternity, you can refine your intention, plan your attack, and enlist the power of your mind to assist you in hitting your mark when you're ready to let that arrow fly. After you've gathered all your resources to perform a specific action of your choosing, during the milliseconds preceding it is where your greatest power lies. It's there that you decide how the next moment will go, how this culmination of your efforts will flower. It's where patience and determination are born, the dynamic duo that truly can make anything and everything possible.

Exhalation: Letting the Arrow Fly

When you exhale, you're not simply emptying your lungs, but moving stagnant chi out of your body, making space for new chi, for more life force to enter in. In Waking Energy–speak, although it is the most yin expression of the action cycle you can participate in, you're stepping into your power in full bloom, literally expanding your chi like a shield of protection—your "guardian chi," the energy that literally protects your skin.

Your exhalation is the moment of culmination, a settling of action and affairs, the closing of the circle before the wheel turns again. In energy cultivation, when you exhale, it's a moment of full integration and absorption of that action as well as a complete letting go and surrender, an emptying. When we are empty, we are completely open, unfettered by the past, and not yet challenged by the future. It is a place of choice, and because of this, a place of great potential. It's a space where nothing but possibility exists, where you decide what you want to fill your own vessel with and usher in, not just in that next breath, but into your life.

Your exhalation is your effort fully flowering, the moment when your actions come into their fullest expression. It's a letting go—letting the arrow fly, a resolution of action, the ultimate yin expression, a total surrender to the steadiness of emptiness. When you exhale, you step into some of your fullest power. Exhalation is the ultimate surrender. In the Waking Energy practices, exhaling is a moment of clearing and letting go of what no longer serves you, so that you can be free to step into your future.

The exhalation is an opportunity to create more space inside, discharging stagnant chi, what's no longer useful, what's been standing in our way. When we release the breath, we move into the center of our sheer, unadulterated strength, the clear space that emerges after collecting new life force on the inhalation, after we've literally harnessed that energy and sent it out to blossom and explode! With a deep exhalation, we can do justice to our breath's flight, projecting it properly on its way—an arrow flying, a bicep curling, a javelin arcing, launching our body to soar in the air above, across the stage, over the ocean, across time.

Arriving: Letting the Breath Breathe You

When you take a seat on your meditation cushion, you give yourself the precious gift of quiet and stillness, the space and time to become a keen observer of the breath. In our busy world of cell phones and constant distractions, there are few pristine opportunities when you can observe your own breathing. These become moments that stand apart from time as we know it, because it's in those moments that you become so at one with your own breath that you learn what it means to let the breath *breathe you*.

When you let the breath breathe you, it is one of the deepest expressions of yin you can experience and also one of the most powerfully healing. It's yet another stellar example of how, once you acquire a new energy skill at any given juncture of your Waking Energy adventure, you can retrace your path, weaving it into the fabric of your own unique tapestry as you cycle back through it, bringing your new knowledge to bear upon everything you learn.

When you let the breath breathe you, it means there's no resistance, just total surrender to the fullest full-body breathing you can do, like the swell of the sea, billowing and softening with the currents as they flow in, around, and through you. When you experience it for the first time, you will have discovered the meaning behind every one of the ancient wisdom traditions you'll engage in here.

You'll come to know for yourself why the ancients designed their programs around the breath. With this whole-body breathing you can invite the mind to become so still that the body serves as a worthy accomplice, manifesting a quantum energy that moves so harmoniously and prodigiously through your subtle body that you can truly become one with nature. The very air that flows in and around you allows you to cultivate the deepest, most potent healing yin chi.

From Here to Eternity: The Subtle Body, the Body You Can See, and Beyond

We have a few "bridges" inside us. The duet of breath and energy forms the bridge between the body and mind. Water, the fluid content in our body, and the breath are the bridges between the subtle and physical bodies, and the breath itself is the bridge linking the subtle and the physical to the universe and beyond—it's what makes everything else possible.

Because of its simplicity, its purest, primal form, our breath facilitates the ability to access subtler realms. It is the conduit through which we move our intention, the engine behind the conscious breath, opening and activating our energy pathways, leading to the most perfect balance. Because of its own innate *tai chi* quality—the union of perfect opposites—our breath can help us to cultivate peace and calm in our external lives by honoring our body's vital need to move energy in and out. Conscious breath and movement help us create the life that we've imagined.

Intention and visualization are essential in waking your energy, but the magic carpet that will take you on the ride of your life, the unifying element that brings it all together, is the breath. It's the tool we use to effect each and every shift that occurs in the subtle body, bringing it ever closer to greater harmony and balance with the physical body, imbuing it with vibrant health and a radiance that shines for all to see. And it's what helps in our ultimate surrender, when we exhale for the last time—becoming the stuff of stars once again, cosmic dust, dissolving into chi and merging with all that is. Like yin and yang, where there is no beginning and no end, it's the bridge to the other side, how we enter the next life, the great world unseen.

But while we're still here, let's make the most of the time we have together.

Breathe! Quench your thirst. Drink from the cup of life! Breathe deeply, completely, fully, with your whole body. Feel it! Relish it, your most trusted Waking Energy accomplice, your most powerful link to nature, an intermediary between mind and body, and the bridge between the subtle body and the beautiful house you're renting in this life—your miraculous body, the body we honor and sculpt and strengthen and expand in the practices, the body that helps you to become all you were destined to be.

3

your waking energy journey

Would you have ever guessed that the palms of your hands and the crown of your head were really solar collectors—actual receiving disks for inviting star energy into your body? Or that the soles of your feet were pipelines for drawing the riches of the earth's energy up through your legs into the energy storehouses in your body? Or that each time you touch your tongue to the roof of your mouth and squeeze your perineum, you are completing a powerful energy circuit that instantly nourishes and supplements your life force and promotes your longevity? In Opening the Energy Gates in Awaken and Play we draw energy up from earth and down from heaven, and in the Sufist Grind from our kundalini practice we channel energy up from the earth through our perineum along the central channel to our higher centers. With each practice, even after just your first experience with it, you will start to immediately see how the universe itself becomes your playground.

Your entire body is an energy transformation station that invites, harnesses, cultivates, balances, and releases chi. There are specific sites in the geography of our bodies that we will use in our practices to engage energy; it is at these strategic points that chi can be channeled, regulated, and strengthened. We will distinguish these portals in each of the practices we do, which will help to deepen your understanding of energy cultivation and how to activate, balance, and utilize it.

The Age of Energy Interference

Not all the energy we absorb is revitalizing. The same forces of the universe that can infuse us with new power and life can also wreak havoc on our subtle body and disrupt our bodily functions. We are under constant assault from naturally occurring radiation, interstellar rays, and solar flares, which can adversely affect our central nervous system, brain activity, equilibrium, and our mental, emotional, and physical well-being.

Add to this environmental toxins, genetically engineered foods, mineral depletion in our soils, a reduced ozone layer, and the surplus of electromagnetic radiation from computers, cell phones, and other entertainment gadgets (of which we haven't yet even begun to understand the long-term or short-term adverse effects), and we have challenged ourselves in unprecedented ways with myriad sources of distraction and menaces to our health.

We have never been more stressed, and we have never been more disconnected both from ourselves and from one another. Our central nervous systems were not intended to handle such an overwhelming number of tasks, and as a result we are suffering from unprecedented levels of anxiety and various other afflictions and diseases. Left with little or no time to dedicate to our own selves, our bodies, and our energy—we are depleting ourselves. With each day that passes the increasing volume of electromagnetic frequencies produced by our various electrical and WiFi devices further destabilizes us, scrambling and disrupting our subtle bodies and interfering with our body-mind's self-healing mechanisms.

Moreover, with all our dependence on—I would argue, our addiction to—technology, we are also frittering away our energy by investing countless hours every day in activities that have no longevity and no legacy. The time we spend "posting" and "tweeting" is time we will never retrieve. The Internet is an extraordinary tool, but, abused, it is too often a gift that takes more than it gives. Ultimately all our devices pull us quite literally out of the present moment and can thus insidiously undermine the quality of our lives.

We are runners in a frenetic race to nowhere, and we are spending so much of our vital energy to do it. We are hurtling toward ever more energy-draining and attention-demanding multitasking that makes our brains atrophy. Instead of being our greatest ally, our minds run away with us, syphoning off precious energy in the process.

Many of the deleterious issues we're currently experiencing in the areas of health and psychology have evolved in reaction to our extreme energy exposure and output—a condition called "excess heat" in Chinese medicine. Some of the ailments and illnesses that are becoming more prevalent, from arthritis and osteoporosis to heart disease and cancer, are all terrible consequences of it. Like our beautiful planet, we are suffering from a microcosmic version of global warming. We need to literally "cool off." To regain our health and energy, we need balance. We need to generate more yin—the space that creates the energy for yang to refuel, to replenish what it needs to thrive.

The good news is that through the "energy cultivation" we perform in the Waking Energy practices we can significantly impact the quality and length of our lives. We may have a fighting chance to ward off the harmful effects of the extensive electromagnetic radiation from our modern inventions and conveniences as well as of our energy expenditure in attempting to keep up with the life they have created.

Waking Energy's uniquely balanced yin-and-yang flow is designed to counteract this excess heat and to balance yin and yang in our bodies, providing the soothing balm, the stillness, the cool and calm—the space and time in which to be reminded of what really matters most, our most precious asset: our mental and physical health. By moving stagnant energy out of the body and inviting new energy to enter in and strengthen the body's reserves and central nervous system, you will supercharge your immune system, improve your mood, enhance self-confidence, and increase your ability to greet life's challenges with equanimity as well as sculpt and shape a beautiful body.

Seven Ways to Awakening

So how do you wake your energy? It all starts with saying yes to yourself. That's what sets the stage. Then, by learning to embrace and revere nature, you cultivate an inner balance that radiates outwardly, positively impacting every aspect of your life. Once you start discovering and engaging your subtle body through conscious breath and movement, you'll really rev up the energy engines.

Once you learn to harness your own breath, these mindful exercises will help you to dislodge stuck or stagnant energy, energy that has forgotten how to move—the major energy culprit in our lives. Caused by everything from our history to lifestyle habits to emotional and physical duress, this stagnant energy literally steals precious life force. In the actual exercises you do, by consciously breathing and moving, you can access the energy within you and lubricate the passageways of your inner circuitry to mobilize, discharge, and transform that stuck energy into viable life-enhancing energy. That way, you initiate a maximum flow of stagnant energy out of the body and of new energy in, so that your body and mind can function optimally and, in so doing, you can reveal and reclaim your original self! You will have even more pure life-force energy to live your life now and realize your full potential.

Owing to this miraculous process, the work can spark the epiphany of a lifetime—that being true to yourself and allowing your hidden emotions the space to emerge are the keys to vibrant health. It's one thing to be aware of the benefits of the practices, but it's another thing altogether to experience what happens when you move consciously, when you intentionally unite your mind and your body. When you meet yourself where you are and learn to trust yourself, you come to know that everything you need to live your best life is already inside you. You suddenly recognize that those negative thoughts are just energy that needs to move, and you realize you have the power to transmute your emotional life. When this happens, the potency of the practices grows exponentially.

As you learn to cultivate your energy and revere it, hold it dear and view it as the precious commodity it is, you will become aware of your life-detracting habits—how you give your energy away. Once you start to develop this consciousness, you take your power back, and you get energized—instantly.

The seven practices that comprise Waking Energy follow a natural progression of seven steps from nature and the world outside to your inner world and true nature. The journey is meant to unfold holistically and organically. In the practices you will get to experience the dance of yin and yang for yourself as you learn to balance your own energy. You'll witness how each uniquely manifests itself and how it is expressed in the body as you learn the art of energy cultivation and mastery in each and every practice. You'll learn specifically how to open and energize the energy "portals" in your body, applying what is specific to each modality and then to each successive practice that comprises Waking Energy, thus maximizing your energy-cultivation skills. In order to do this, you'll learn a new language—the language of energy! Discover. Gather. Circulate. Purify. Direct. Conserve. Store. Transform. Dissolve. Transmit. Activate. Stimulate. Harmonize. Balance.

Regardless of the specific energy-cultivation names we assign to what we do in the practices, simply by moving with conscious intention, you'll be mobilizing the energy in your subtle body through each movement you do in each and every one of the practices. As you become better versed in this new vernacular, you'll naturally become more aware, more attuned to your body and its abilities, your own energy-waking potential. Learning the language of energy will help your energy-cultivating power grow exponentially.

Let me give you a sneak preview of each of them and the exciting work that awaits you:

PRACTICE ONE: Awaken and Play: Qigong

As day breaks, you'll begin with the yin-yang balance of qigong, Awaken and Play. Like a child again, you'll start to explore yourself and the world around you. After starting with Opening the Energy Gates, where you'll learn how to skillfully orchestrate the interplay between your body's own energy and the bounty of nature, the vast "energy fields" of heaven and earth you can use to calm and ground your energies and create balance inside, you'll move on to a sensual, playful, energy dance called Love Thyself, a self-massage in which you visit every single inch of your beautiful body. You'll move more slowly and have the opportunity to truly understand what it means to "discover the chi" (*qigong* means "energy mastery" or "direct the energy") and then how to move it through the stages of chi cultivation.

PRACTICE TWO: Unleash and Transform: Kundalini Yoga

Moving into late morning, you'll continue along the path with the driving yang pulse of the kundalini-inspired Unleash and Transform, where you will meet your inner commitment and fire. As you stoke it, pushing past the limits of the mind, you'll strengthen the lungs and the diaphragm, toning your entire body, and making your spine more flexible, simultaneously stimulating and balancing your chakra and endocrine systems.

PRACTICE THREE: Your Own Fountain of Youth: The Tibetan Rites

Then, rising to high noon with Your Own Fountain of Youth, the Tibetan Rites, you will spin with the earth herself, learning to tune your chakra system in another percussive, fiery, yang modality as it balances and harmonizes the chakra and vestibular system, increasing your overall dynamic strength, flexibility, and spatial power.

PRACTICE FOUR: Empower and Flow: Pilates

In the early afternoon, you'll progress to Empower and Flow, the Pilates practice, with its graceful, flowing yang pulse. It will help you to defy gravity and strengthen your "powerhouse"—the muscles of your trunk—with special emphasis on your abdominals and back, dramatically enhancing your overall muscular strength and stamina, flexibility, coordination and balance, and ease of movement as it activates your lymphatic system. You'll find your true core power as you "meet yourself on the mat."

PRACTICE FIVE: Go Deep, Open, and Energize: Yin Yoga

In the late afternoon, to bring your energies back down to earth, you'll Go Deep, Open, and Energize, with the yin yoga practice. You'll travel deep inside your inner landscape, recapturing youthful joint mobility and ease, as you soothe your mind, balance your meridian system, and experience the fruit of your labors—a slow-burning energized calm.

PRACTICE SIX: The Power of Love: Inner Smile and Cosmic Healing Sounds

As the day starts to quiet, moving toward dusk, you'll learn the true power of love. The inner alchemy practice Inner Smile and Cosmic Healing Sounds will help you to go deeper still into yin chi with the Power of Love practices, literally bringing a smile to your face as you are waking your energy, knowing how profound your quiet, yin energy-cultivation efforts are. (How could you not smile when you know your own smile is balancing and harmonizing the life of your organs and giving you more energy?)

PRACTICE SEVEN: Moving into Stillness: Meditation

Finally, as night falls, you'll move into the deepest expression of yin, Moving into Stillness, the meditation practice. Experiencing the fullest expansion and quiet like a night-blooming jasmine, the lotus itself, you'll learn the art of training the "monkey mind" (which jumps about, chatters, and refuses to stay focused) to cultivate mindful introspection and detachment from outside distractions. Breath by breath, as you create your own tranquility and peace of mind, inner contentment rises to bring a sweet glow on your face and a softness to your skin, an outward radiance of your highest nature revealed in perfect stillness and quiet before you begin again the following morning.

The practices also follow a corresponding emotional journey of seven ways:

Yes Leads the Way: It all begins with a decision to say yes to yourself and to the adventure ahead. Everything we do in life starts with a decision, an agreement we make with ourselves to perform an action. The Waking Energy Way starts the same way—with a commitment to be to open, present, engaged, and willing. When you make a decision to do something good for yourself, that in and of itself is empowering and life-enhancing. It wakes your energy. It makes everything else possible. So your journey here begins with "yes."

The Way of Nature: When you say yes to yourself, you are in fact also saying yes to nature, since you are one with her. When you open yourself to nature, you automatically connect with her flow and attune yourself to her rhythms, which match and strengthen your own.

The Way of the World Unseen: By becoming familiar with and engaging your subtle body, you'll start to see your body as an energy transformer, accessing the multiple "portals" in your body through which you can draw energy into your body from nature and the universe to capitalize on your own energy potential, waking even more energy.

The Way of Mindful Movement: You will learn specific movement principles in each practice that will help you to increase your energy capacity exponentially. You'll come to discover that the conscious breath is the most important thing. The breath will become your compass, helping you to move your body in new ways and unlocking your physical and emotional transformation.

The Way to You: Prepare to meet a "new you." You will meet yourself for the first time in this new way. It will be a conscious, intentional encounter, an act of some of the highest love there is, one in which you meet your every aspect. You will become your own advocate for the longing in your heart, making the purposeful decision to embark on a journey of conscious self-exploration that will lead to a real awakening. You'll open your eyes to the splendor, the magnificence, the joy, and the radiance of who you really are. Then, when you fall in love with yourself, this new awareness will offer even more immune-boosting energy generated from your own happiness. This only grows through the magic of the practices when you see and feel the incredible and immediate results in your body and mind.

The Way to Trust: Your body really does know best, and you will learn to trust its wisdom. It's your mind that can intercede and override your instincts. You'll learn to return to your most feeling, intuitive self through the journey of the practices and learn to partner with your body in order to wake your energy and realize your greatest self. Your body is a wondrous creation, deserving of joyful, sensual exploration, and it is yours to lovingly exploit and nurture. When your body is well fed, properly exercised, and given good direction and fulfilling tasks to perform, your body loves you and wants to serve you. It wants to be utilized and optimized in the spirit of reverence and sensitivity to limits—always in moderation and with a kind of "effortless effort," so that when the hour of need draws nigh, you are ready to rise to the occasion with energy to spare. When you commit yourself to energizing your body by giving it the loving attention it deserves, you'll command its loyalty forever.

The Way to Love: In keeping with the philosophy of the Tao, your cup will run over. You will literally fall in love with yourself and the world—bringing yourself into the energy of love and inspiring yourself to manifest it, which is the purest, most potent, and powerful energy we as humans can know—fuel for evolution, fostering self-realization and greater consciousness and possibility in your life.

The Journey of the Practices

Each practice is a world unto itself with its own language and unique qualities that will offer you something different each and every time you perform it. You will come to discover that each is inextricably connected to all the others, and that each builds on the others, sharing key elements in common. As you become more proficient with each one, you can apply these new skills as you move through the overall flow of Waking Energy. As you proceed along the path and circle back to revisit the practices, more and more will be revealed at every turn.

The degree of consciousness with which you approach your body, the levels of discipline and desire you have to achieve results, and the potency of the practices themselves all combine to promote the very mindfulness, inner and outer strength, and calm that will support your overall health and longevity and, of course, maximize your levels of everyday energy.

The practices are arranged in such a way that either following each one individually, or alternating or combining a yang practice with a yin, or moving through one after the other according to the flow they are presented in will automatically balance your energies. For example, kundalini and Pilates, like vinyasa yoga, are all yang modalities—heating, muscular, high-energy endeavors. Compared to those, the moment-to-moment demand in the yin practices, like Inner Smile, is very different, less physically rigorous, and can give you an incredible lightness of being, an ease and a fluidity that can only arise when space is created from within.

There is also a very specific rhythm, timbre, and texture in each of the practices. Qigong: Awaken and Play, for example, has a slower, softer, more introspective rhythm, allowing you the opportunity to play with finding and engaging chi. In some ways its diametric opposite, kundalini, moves quickly but asks you to trust that with every movement you are moving prana, channeling it up the spine, stoking the inner fire for your subtle body to do its good work.

Each modality offers its own unique contribution to the waking of subtle energy in your body. Pilates, for example, wakes it up by teaching you to perform movements using the *principle of opposition,* employing a simple law of physics to defy gravity, and *effortless effort,* learning to recruit only those muscles that are required to perform a task, while relaxing the rest of your body by breathing consciously and conserving your energy. You'll stimulate your lymphatic system and create unmatched core strength where the life force is centered as well as enhance overall muscular and spinal flexibility.

The Waking Energy Way will be your guide as you evolve—a lifelong companion. Even if you only did this practice at the beginner level for the rest of your days, it would improve your overall health and longevity significantly. However, I believe you'll be seduced and sufficiently inspired to aim higher and look forward hungrily to the next installment of Waking Energy.

Like the dawning of a new day, each successive practice here will offer you endless discovery at every turn, with every nuanced movement, every gesture, every breath, every tear, and every smile. As you become more adept at managing different commands in your body, you'll feel such a sense of accomplishment and curiosity that it will push you forward to new goals and discoveries. You may find yourself waking up in the morning feeling inspired and excitedly asking, "What does *today* have in store for me?"

Getting Started

To begin, I'd like to invite you to attend a private weeklong intensive "retreat" much like what you would participate in at an exclusive wellness center. You'll experience each of the practices one after the other on seven successive days, until you've completed the cycle of the seven practices.

In each of the following chapters, you'll be introduced one by one to the seven practices, learn a bit about their history and benefits, and then follow step-by-step instructions for incorporating them into your routine. For the first week, you'll follow each practice faithfully and consistently one at a time for seven days.

I recommend keeping a personal "practice journal," so you can log your progress and record your feelings and impressions after each day of practice. By recording how you feel physically, mentally, and emotionally both before and after your practice, what exercises speak to you, and what you notice about your energy, you'll develop your own energy expertise. You'll come to know that any kind of movement is good—the body appreciates it. But the radical difference between general movement and Waking Energy is that with Waking Energy you are consciously exploring, making a conscious decision to embark upon a purposeful expedition into the state your body is in and what it needs. With a new sentient awareness, an embodied presence, you are "looking under the hood" each day.

Let's be honest. It's not easy to stay within the lines. I have always had a hard time walking the path of a labyrinth (as you'll discover in the last chapter, on meditation, but even though you may be tempted, don't go hunting for it yet!). However, it is structure that provides us with the greatest foundation and affords the most creativity and the most expansive freedoms. Though you may be tempted to stray from the plan, in order to truly become your own energy master you'll want to be as faithful from the onset as possible. Quelling your rebellious tendencies and giving in to a sense of discipline are essential to the efficacy of the practice.

To *really* get to know the energy character of each modality in the Waking Energy Way, to truly deepen your practice and increase your proficiency, after the first "seven-day sampler," where you do the first practice on the first day, the second practice on the second day, and so on, you will return to the beginning and dedicate a full seven days to each separate modality. This means that you'll be practicing each modality in the Waking Energy Way for a full week, adding up to a full seven weeks.

Because the body and mind have a special affinity for ritual and respond in remarkably brilliant and immediate ways to this kind of consistent practice and exposure to new stimuli, this method is especially effective. During each week of study with each particular practice, you will continue to take stock of how you feel before, during, and after and journal about your experience. As you become well versed in each practice, you will become intimately familiar with your own energy anatomy. Having journaled about the effects of each and how they made you feel, you will then be equipped to know how to match each practice to what your body needs on any given day—customizing the program to suit the needs of your life. In this way, you'll be able to dance between the yin and yang energies, truly understanding how they work together as an integrated whole, and you'll really start to tune into what your body needs and be able to deliver it. For example, if you've had a stressful day, a yin yoga practice would be just the thing to send you off to a restful night's sleep. On the other hand, if you've been stuck at your desk for hours feeling mounting frustration, then a yang practice like kundalini or Pilates would be the answer to revitalize and calm you.

At the end of the seven weeks, you'll again make your return on the grand circle of the Tao and repeat the first week, in which you did the seven practices on seven successive days, one on each day, and see how you have improved. Like a true apprentice to Taoist adepts, you'll explore each modality thoroughly, channeling the ancient wisdom and ways of being and applying yourself to fully embracing, learning, and integrating this precious knowledge.

After week eight, once you're familiar with each component of the Waking Energy Way and you have a good understanding of its history, philosophy, and purpose as well as the yin and yang qualities of each, it will be time for you to establish your own practice. Here you can finally enjoy the feeling of autonomy in practice and fly solo, free to explore the practices on your own, again either individually in greater depth, or follow the menu of combination workouts I have designed to provide you with the most ideal balance of yin and yang energies in each and every workout you choose.

Making It Your Own

At the end of the nine-week program, you'll be equipped to take all that you've learned thus far and truly flow with nature, alternating yin and yang practices each day of the week, becoming your own energy master and creating energy balance in your own world—inner and outer. The Waking Energy Way is intended for you and your own unique, beautiful self and body. You can begin exactly where you are and take the practices at your own pace and level. In fact, that's the very point of the journey, to explore and experiment with freedom so as to create the best approach that works for you.

I've provided a nine-week sample program to get you started, but once you become aware of your own waking-energy abilities, you will be in awe of what you can do. You'll be inspired to play, to experiment, to get to know yourself, your body, and your needs even better. Once you understand how befriending your body can offer you an instant payoff in energy, in the way you feel and look, you'll have an entirely new perception of yourself. You'll understand in no uncertain terms that depending upon the kind of conscious movement you engage in, you can have significant influence over the quality of your thoughts and start to feel a self-reliance and self-gratitude you've never felt before. It can manifest on the spot. And it all starts with you becoming your own energy master by learning the practices so well you start to design the program that helps you to create the balance in your life that wakes your energy and changes your life.

Meeting Yourself for the First Time: The Way to Love

As you go the way of life, you will see a great chasm. Jump. It is not as wide as you think.

—Joseph Campbell

If you knew yourself the way the people in your life—your closest friends and loved ones—know you, you might actually really like yourself.

In fact, you might discover that you're so amazing, even you start to feel jealous of yourself.

It can happen in your next breath. Or with a smile—your own—as you gaze at your reflection in a mirror. Reconnecting with your body, your mind, and your heart and introducing them to one another can happen in an instant, or it can happen over a lifetime. It all comes down to a choice, to one single decision—one you consciously make or one that life makes for you. When you choose to take that first step and decide to make that virgin encounter a loving one, you awaken your power—you wake up the true energy inside you.

We meet ourselves over and over again during the course of our lifetime—through challenge and triumph, relationships, and love and loss. Each time, we discover more of ourselves and what we're really made of. But this meeting of yourself I speak of is unique. It's no small, casual get-together. It's a conscious, intentional encounter, an act of some of the highest love there is—one where you meet your every aspect. It's epic. Meeting yourself for the first time means heeding the call. It means becoming your own advocate for the longing in your heart. It means making the purposeful decision to embark on a journey of conscious self-exploration that can lead to a real awakening, opening your eyes to the splendor, the magnificence, the joy, and the radiance of who you really are.

Having lived a certain number of years on the planet, you likely already have a strong sense of who you think you are. You may think that you already live your life in an examined way, that you feel connected, or that you even possess a relatively keen awareness of yourself. That's a beautiful thing; it means that you are starting with a clear advantage, and you should feel great about it. But even if you feel as though you "met yourself" a long time ago and know yourself well, there is an entire dimension of existence that stands apart from this general knowing of oneself, a kind of chamber of secrets that can lead you to your own truth—your own best self.

Yes, this meeting I speak of will be different from any kind of awareness of or connection to yourself you currently have. Acknowledging yourself, being aware of yourself as a magnificent wonder of nature, a unique miracle, a feeling self who deserves your love and attention is another story altogether. Within each one of us, there is a longing, searching, seeking self—call it your heart or your soul. It's all the motivation you need to begin this new quest to truly meet yourself for the first time.

It's hard to put into words the immensity of the joy that will spring up inside you once you get to know yourself in a whole new way and come to realize that you are alive in an energy playground of endless possibilities! Energy mastery is an infinite journey. Joy and inspiration spring from knowing that you have the capability to harness the energy that exists in this magical realm and that you can become an eternal student right here, right now.

Let the journey of the practices return your childlike sense of wonder and curiosity, unfettered joy, ease, and a new kind of unself-conscious expression with which you can explore your energy anatomy—the entire world of your subtle body, which is invisible to the naked eye. Like the cosmos itself, the world around you—seen and unseen—offers an infinite variety of experiences to sample and savor. Great satisfaction and joy come from knowing that you yourself have the capability to harness the energy of this infinite realm. You have the opportunity to learn that you're so much more than you believe you are right here, right now.

You are about to unlock some of the most essential secrets to your longevity, such as discovering how to live your best life, tapping into the flow, the bliss, the power, and the beauty of being present to what is with no distractions, living into your essential aliveness, and finding what every human being seeks, hungers for, and quests after: peace and joy.

It is the gift of Waking Energy.

part two

4

awaken and play: qigong

In 1999, after I produced and choreographed two critically acclaimed dance theater shows at Lincoln Center and simultaneously opened my first large-scale Pilates and yoga studio in Manhattan's West Village at a time when I was trying to navigate an extremely challenging personal relationship, simply waking up in the morning felt like an act of courage. My back pain became so debilitating that on a bad day I couldn't even bend down to tie my own shoes.

One day, after leaving a yoga class early on the verge of tears because I couldn't take it anymore, I decided to take myself to one of my favorite haunts downtown that always made me feel better—East West Books on Fifth Avenue in Greenwich Village. After paging through books about foods and herbs to replenish my energy, I spotted one that looked as if it had been misplaced on the shelf. Wedged between *Eat Right for Your Type* and *Healing with Whole Foods* was Mantak Chia's *Awaken Healing Energy Through the Tao.* I opened to the introduction, and my life has never been the same.

Some people get starstruck when they meet celebrities. For me, it happened when I met Mantak Chia for the first time. After years of studying his prolific writings, the time had come to finally experience his teachings in the flesh. When I saw that he was on tour in the United States in 2007, I immediately registered for his weeklong intensive workshop "Awaken Healing Energy and Transform Chi," held in the Blue Ridge Mountains at a former ashram outside of Asheville, North Carolina.

It's hard to describe just how captivating Master Chia was, sitting up there on the stage with his feet firmly grounded into the floor, certainly already channeling earth energy up through the Bubbling Spring Points on his feet. Holding court like the sun itself, he radiated bright coronal rays out into the enormous, churchlike space, all the way up to the cathedral ceilings. When he laughed, it was infectious. He had his own gravitational pull. Everyone laughed right along with Master Chia, happily getting swept up in the current of his energy. Although he had a very easygoing, seasoned, and grounding presence, his spontaneous, unchecked laughter and the mischief in his eyes made him seem like a child!

I did quick calculations in my head. He was born in 1944. Here we were in 2007. He was sixty-one years old? How could that be? He didn't look a day over forty and had not a single gray hair on his head. I couldn't stop beaming, smiling to the point of erupting with schoolgirl giddiness just from feeling his grounded ease and observing his agelessness, this incredible radiance. He clearly embodied his lifelong practice and projected an energy that was like truth itself.

Historically, qigong has been a movement school dominated by men. For thousands of years, it was a kind of mysterious, esoteric secret society imbued with the tacit air of "invitation only," whose members were men in long black tunics, loose-fitting pants, and soft, black slippers, with their hair pulled back in pigtails. It is reported that they never spoke a word and were able to make themselves and inanimate objects levitate—most likely because they'd conserved their "talking chi" to such a degree that lifting heavy objects with their eyes was standard fare. Qigong, and the softer martial arts in general, although remarkably effective in creating vibrant wellness and slowing the aging process, were never particularly inviting disciplines for women. As far as energy mastery was concerned, only a minority of women ever felt welcomed into the chamber of secrets.

True to form, this weeklong workshop was attended predominantly by men. I was one of only five women there, out of about sixty-plus people. Nonetheless, this did not deter me in my personal quest to learn more. With the promise of superhuman skills within arm's reach, visions of flying over rooftops and leveling marauding groups of ten men at a time, my youthful warrior-goddess fantasies were set aflame. I wanted to be one of the few, the proud, and the brave, to be shown the way to do the covert work performed by the few martial arts heroines and female mystics before me and gain access to the precious secrets of qigong, especially *because* it was not something most women did. So aside from my deep admiration for Mantak Chia, the fact that the tradition said I was supposed to be shut out drew me to it even more.

One of the first to introduce energy cultivation to the West in the late 1970s, Mantak Chia was a world-renowned Taoist adept whose pioneering efforts in the United States brought qigong to the masses. A veritable fountain of qigong history and teachings, he was there generously sharing the gifts that he himself had inherited from older masters. Just being in his presence was a thrill. I was enraptured from the moment he began to the moment of our good-bye. I was so moved, I did something I had never done—like a nervous teenager or a groupie, I asked him to autograph my notebook, which I cherish to this day.

Ticket to Ride

Mantak Chia was my passport to the energy universe. In his workshop, I was taken on an extraordinary journey from the sublime to the ridiculous, along with my peers. We were the fortunate recipients of the wisdom of the ages, secrets passed down from his masters, who were themselves part of a legacy spanning thousands of years. I sat there reveling in the privilege as if I was living Lao Tzu's wise words in real time, holding me in a deeply familiar and comforting hypnotic embrace.

Then something shocking happened. Just when Master Chia was engaged in a profound message about cultivating deep listening, honing the ability to tune in to the voices of our organs and our body's inner wisdom, and the incredible benefits of being present and using the mind in the most focused way, he asked this powerful question: "If you can't hear yourself, how are you going to hear other people?" Seconds later, he belched loudly, right in the middle of his presentation. He then started talking about how we each have a "delete" key in our brain and how vital it is to the preservation of our energy to be able to let go of anger and obsessive thought. Suddenly he let out another great big burp, followed by joyful laughter. The crowd of sixty-plus people sat in stunned silence for five seconds and then started laughing right along with him. As the giggles grew into full-blown, sidesplitting laughter, Master Chia, obviously very pleased with himself, said happily, "See, it worked! All of that love chased out the evil wind!"

Master Chia wanted us to know that this combination of release and laughter is not only proof of our energy-cultivation efforts and one of the most immediate ways to move stagnant chi out of the body, but one of the most underrated healing processes known to humankind. He urged us to greet our natural functions with openness, acceptance, and even pleasure, the way children do, advocating that many of the world's troubles would abate if we'd only find it in our hearts to accept ourselves and others for exactly who we are. He then advocated burping as often as we needed to, especially when practicing qigong, as it was proof positive that we were successful in moving our life-force energy, our chi, powerfully through our bodies and using it to heal.

The second unforgettable memory I have of Mantak Chia was when he demonstrated the immense power of "connecting to source," or rooting deeply in earth energy. He wanted to show that when people are plugged into the earth's center, not even an incredible force can shake them. To prove this point, he surveyed the crowd and chose the biggest, strongest, youngest men he could find. He was sixty-one at the time, and everyone he invited on stage was easily thirty years, if not forty years, his junior.

As the first man came up on stage, Master Chia stood there like a live monument, with a big smile on his face, and commanded, "Push me!" And push him the guy did, with every ounce of strength he had. Master Chia didn't budge or flinch. The audience just smiled in bated anticipation, whispers rippling through the crowd.

Then Master Chia told the first guy to stay, and he invited two more men up. The three men pushed him with all their might, while the rest of us were all holding our collective breath as we watched. The man on the end slipped from his extreme effort—his legs slid out from under him and he fell to the floor, utterly bewildered. We all gasped with our hands covering our mouths.

Master Chia didn't stop there. He invited two more men up on stage. We were all barely breathing in expectation as we thought, *Surely this is it! There's no way he can withstand this kind of manpower!* The five lumberjacks he'd invited up were now breaking a sweat and getting red in the face, as Master Chia calmly stood there in Horse Stance, an immovable oak, like Annapurna, the majestic peak high in the Himalayas. One by one, he invited men up on stage to push him off his center, and one by one they fell, powerless to match his impossibly quiet, rooted, solid presence.

And then, without warning, he "unplugged" from his root, and all the men tumbled into a pile with Master Chia somehow, miraculously, at the top of the heap. Perhaps you have to be a bit of a trickster when you are an adept—you can't study so intensively without learning to balance it with comedy.

Welcome to Awaken and Play

Awaken and Play was certainly inspired by Master Chia's forays, particularly the "play" aspect, and you will find that if you can allow yourself to give over to play, you too will experience the freedom and life-force awakening that he did. Nothing shows you the path to yourself or your place in nature and the universe as well as qigong does. It is one of the most potent outlets and vehicles for catharsis you likely have ever experienced. A treasure trove of riches, this is the practice that started it all for me, and the one that inspired the name of this book.

With the Awaken and Play practice, you'll greet yourself and say, "Hello, body!" In the process, you'll cultivate an entirely new love for yourself as well as a newfound respect and appreciation for energy in the world around you. Awaken and Play takes you back to your innocent beginnings of boundless energy and unfettered joy. Let it be a return to the source wisdom you came into the world with as a child.

With Awaken and Play, the Waking Energy Way comes to life. It begins here. In this sacred flow, qigong represents the energy of morning. The sun is now rising over the dew-covered fields of your internal landscape, and you're about to learn how to capture and cultivate this precious nectar. Birds are singing for you as you embark on a journey filled at every turn with surprises. It is just as the ancient Chinese sage Lao Tzu said: "A journey of a thousand miles begins with one step." Your first step will be to align your being with your breath. With the breath, a veritable river of energy will start to move inside you—and in this chapter you'll learn how to consciously direct this flow.

Your body is a miracle, a gift, a wonderland, a sacred temple. It is your soul's temporal playground, a cosmos in miniature. Your body is a powerful vehicle for healing and empowerment that already naturally possesses the intuitive knowledge of what to do to restore your innocence and zest for life, once it is presented with the right tools.

Welcome to Wonderland!

the awaken and play practice

TIME OF DAY: Morning or evening

QUALITY: Yin and yang

SUBTLE ENERGY: Opens, stimulates, and harmonizes meridians and related organ systems.

BENEFITS: Activates life-force centers, optimizes all physical systems, creates smooth skin, improves endocrine and metabolic health, and strengthens the body overall.

The Practice

Opening the Gates

- Standing Meditation
- Opening the Energy Gates
- Meeting the Chi
- Collecting the Chi
- Swimming in the Sea of Chi

Love Thyself

- Shake It Up to Wake It Up
- Ringing the Temple Gong
- Upper Torso Rounds
- Hip Circles
- Celestial Shampoo
- Waking the Roots
- Eyebrow Press
- Jaw Massage
- Ear Love
- Wind-Palace Massage
- Arm Clap and Brush
- Tiger-Claws Thymus Tap
- True Mind Treasure
- Riding the Roller Coaster
- Making Nice
- Door-of-Life Love Tap
- Hindquarter Love Tap
- Hip Love
- Up and Down the Jing Channels
- Blossoming Open
- Wing-Tip Flex
- Goddess Breaths

Before You Begin

Before we discuss the exercises, let's go over some essential qigong elements that will help to maximize your practice. First of all, I'd like to suggest that whenever possible, you find a beautiful spot outdoors to

energy centers

Sea of Chi: Also called the Lower Elixir Field, the Sea of Chi is located two inches below the navel on the front of your body. It houses your prenatal chi and is the original furnace of all energy-cultivation efforts, the most vital center where all roads lead for good health and longevity.

Door of Life: Also called the Gate of Destiny or *ming men,* the Door of life is located between the third and fourth lumbar vertebrae of the spine, just beneath and between the kidneys, directly opposite the navel center. This energy center is associated with three powerful meridian points; two connect to the Conception Vessel, which is the primary meridian that runs through the front of the body and is related to reproduction, and one connects to the Governing Vessel, the meridian that runs through the back and governs something called *wei chi,* or protective chi. The Door of Life is a pivotal stop along the microcosmic orbit route (the circuit through which energy encircles our torso and mimics the shape of an embryo). It's essential in the nurturing of one of our most important energy sources in our body, prenatal chi.

Middle Earth: Also known as the Middle Elixir Field or the Crimson Palace, Middle Earth is located at the level of the heart and corresponds to the solar plexus and thymus gland.

Roof of the Mouth: Located just behind the two top front teeth (the *que qiao* point), the Roof of the Mouth is also called the Switching Point. Touching the tip of the tongue to this spot completes the circuit of energy between the two main meridian channels in the body, the Conception Vessel and the Governing Vessel. When you become more practiced in the movements, you can apply this as an extra challenge and means of cultivating energy.

Crystal Palace: The Crystal Palace, or Upper Elixir Field, is the region of the brain in the middle of the skull that holds the pineal gland and the pituitary gland.

practice, so that you can be in direct contact with nature. I also recommend wearing comfortable shoes and loose-fitting clothing made from soft natural fibers, such as cotton or hemp, as these best conduct the flow of chi.

Your body is a world unto itself with landmarks that can be mapped. These places on your body, which you're already familiar with, will take on new meaning for you once you begin to practice qigong. Qigong is like the armoire in C. S. Lewis's book *The Lion, the Witch and the Wardrobe,* a portal to a fantastical world of endless possibility and magic. It is so much more than you can see! As you explore your body anew, you may feel as if you've been issued special 3-D glasses—or even 4-D glasses—with which to perceive this array of energy portals that were masquerading as the body parts you thought you knew. Qigong is your "wardrobe door." Open it, go inside, and play; discover, embrace, and thrill over every new dimension of power and energy and love and peace you unleash. It is your portal to the other side, to higher states, to other dimensions, to the liberation of the spirit, the joy, and the equanimity that are your birthright, your true and immortal essence, and the greatest energy you have ever experienced.

In Awaken and Play, perhaps more than any other modality in the book, I am going to ask you to call upon your childlike wonder and curiosity and your rich imagination, which you perhaps haven't permitted to run free or dance passionately through you in a long time. Now is your golden opportunity to return to that feeling of freedom and creativity in your own being. I am going to ask you to actively participate in bringing your most fertile, wild, playful, and rich imagination to the fore. And I am going to ask you not simply to allow your creative visualization juices to flow, but to summon them!

The Essentials of Awaken and Play

Sun Ssu-mo (581–618), dubbed the "King of Medicine" during the Tang dynasty, wrote:

> "The Tao of nurturing life requires that one keep oneself as fluid and flexible as possible. One should not stay still for too long,

energy portals

Bubbling Spring Points: Your feet are incredibly important in waking your energy. They are the first point of contact between your body and the earth. The primary entrance points in your feet, called the Bubbling Spring Points, are located just beneath the metatarsals on each foot. Their presence makes your feet function like electrical plugs to recharge your chi. Each of your toes also serves as an entrance and exit point for drawing chi in and releasing stagnant chi into the earth for recycling. Zen Buddhist master Thich Nhat Hanh's words come to mind, "Walk as if you are kissing the earth with your feet." When you assume the Waking Energy Stance, visualize these energy portals opening and drawing in bounteous yin energy that is channeled up through your legs into your Lower Elixir Field and Door of Life.

The Root: The Root is located in the perineum, the small flat area of flesh located between the genitals and the anus. When I consider the Root and how I engage it in this series, I like to think of the doors on the Starship Enterprise, the sound of the hydraulic press and quality of movement when the doors open and close. Learning how to work with this all-important portal is very much the same, squeezing and releasing in tandem with your breath and intention.

Receiving Disks: The power to direct your energy and heal lies in your hands. *Laogong* points, located in the middle of each of your palms, are key entrance points for energy, and whenever you direct your hands toward heaven or earth, you draw chi into your body through these points in your hands. Like your toes, your fingers are also considered entrance and exit points for energy. By rubbing, gently pinching, and pulling them, as you will learn in Awaken and Play, you open and activate them, preparing them to perform energy exchange with your environment. You can also use your hands to direct healing chi into your body by placing your hands wherever your body needs more attention and energy flow.

Crown: If you were a marionette, the place where your string would go on the very top center of your head is the Crown, which is the central entrance point for receiving heaven energy.

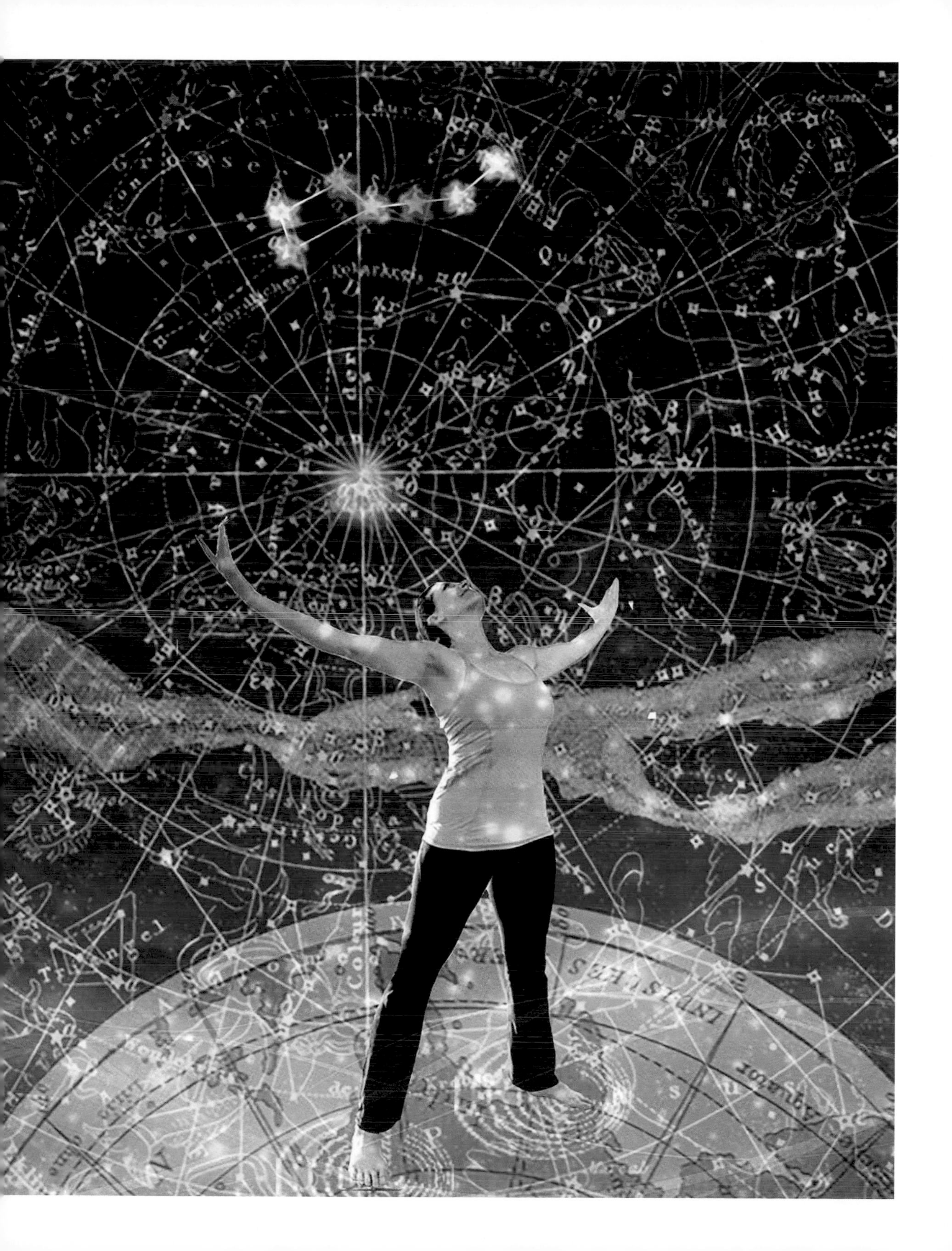

Qigong

Standing Meditation

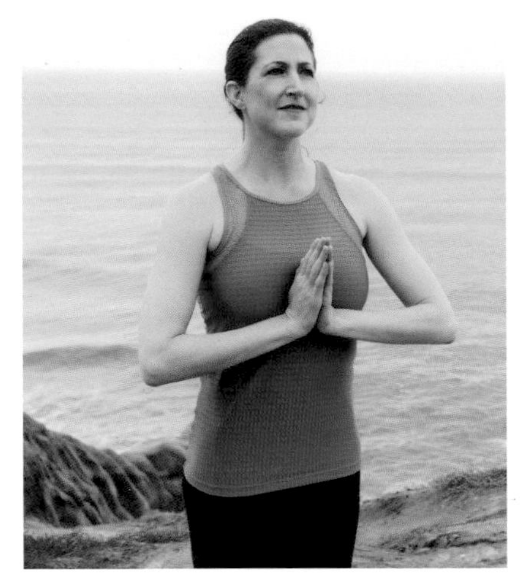

Opening the Energy Gates

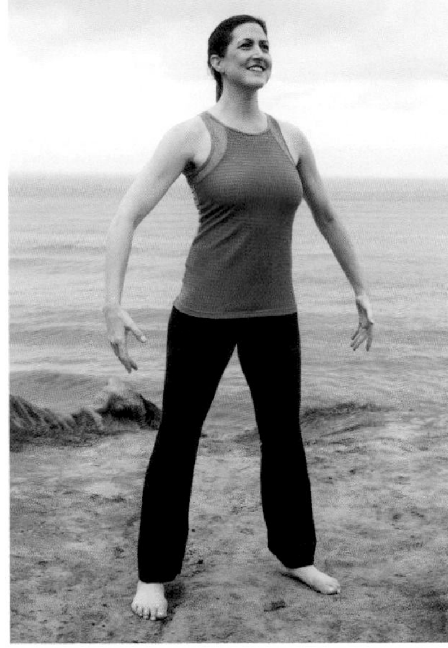

Meeting the Chi

Collecting the Chi

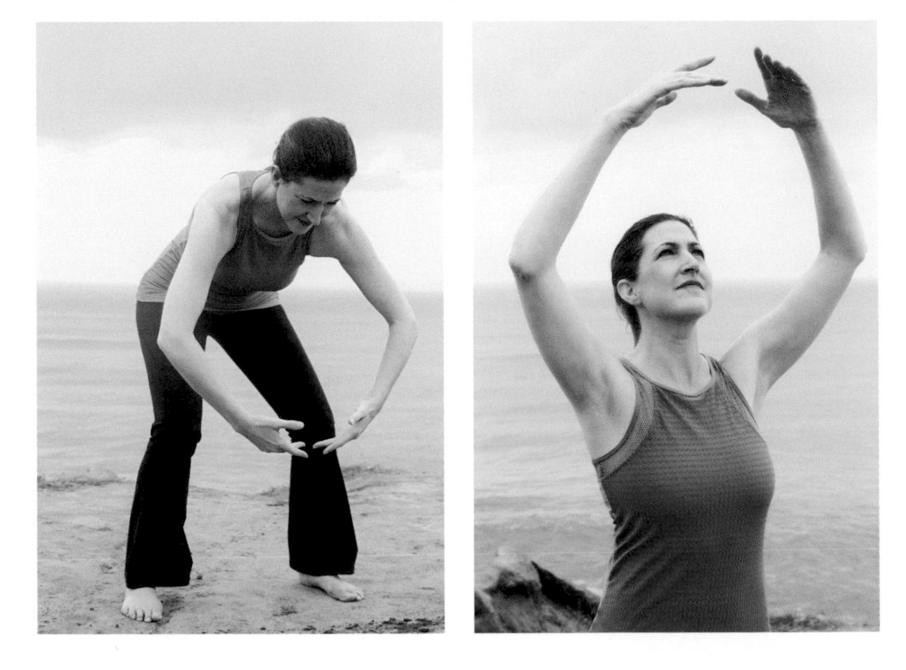

Shake It Up to Wake It Up

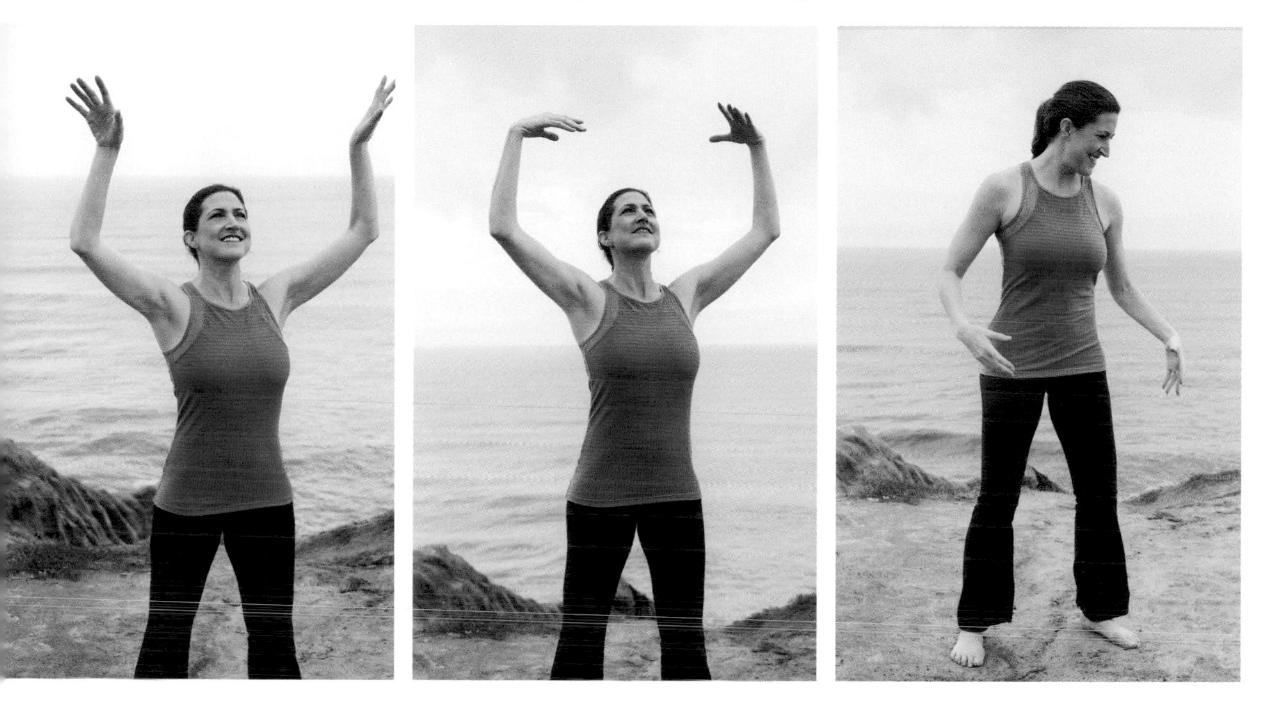

Ringing the Temple Gong

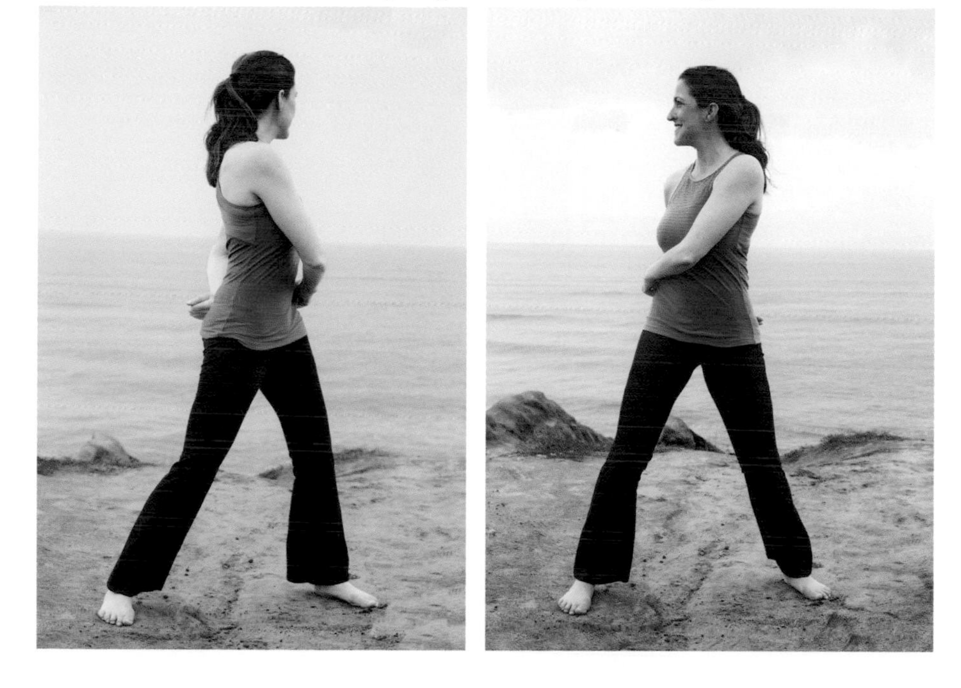

Swimming in the Sea of Chi

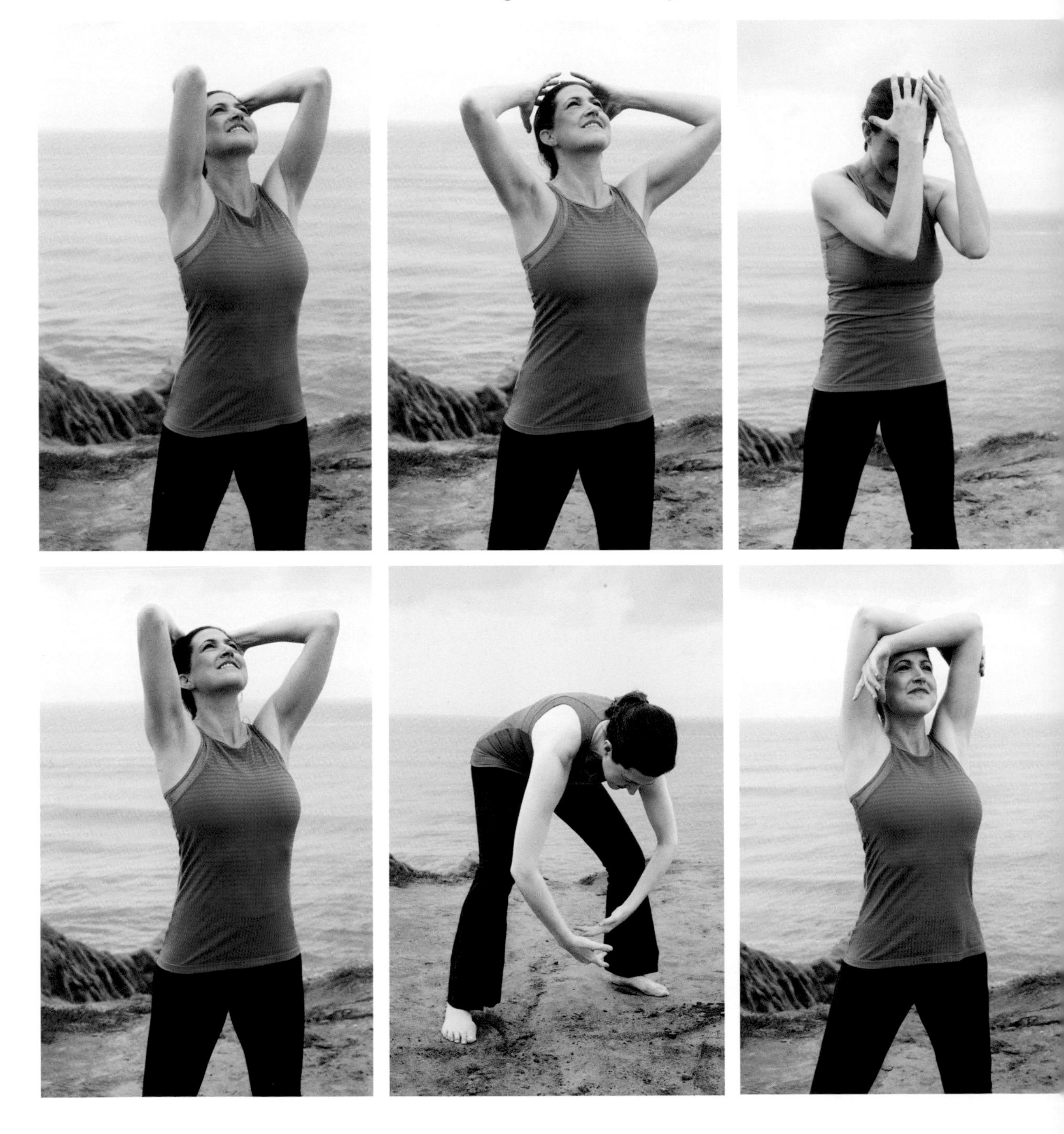

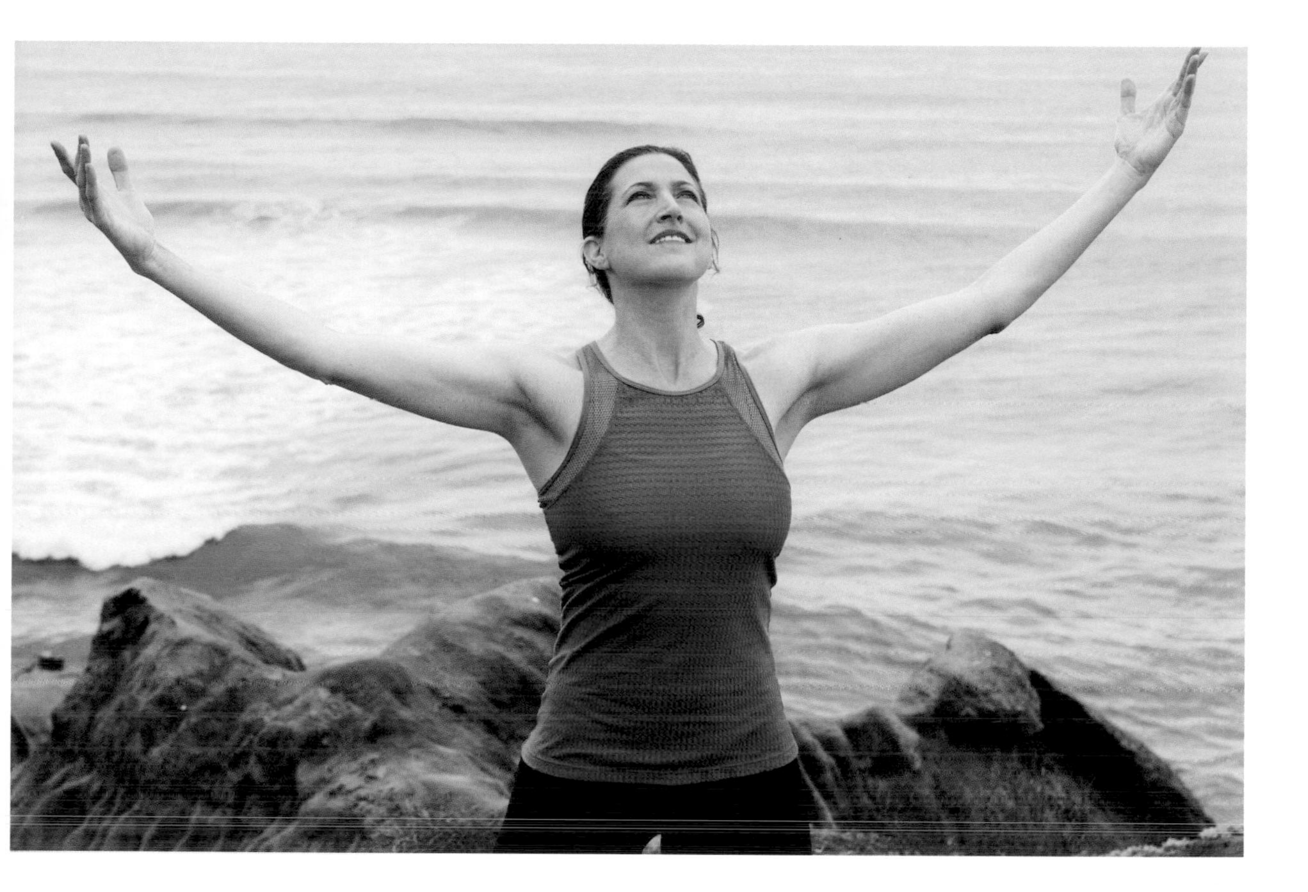

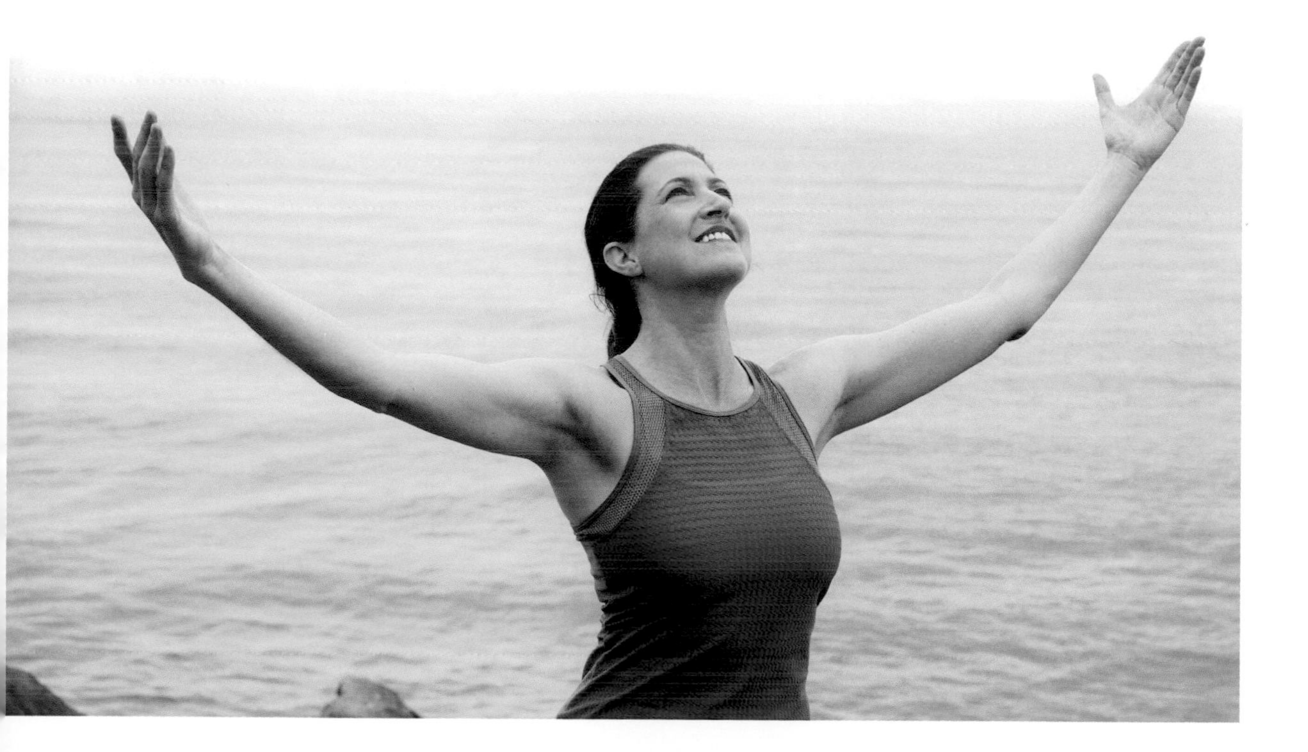

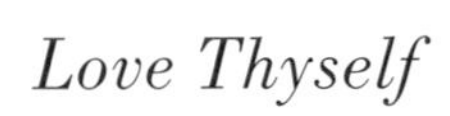

Love Thyself

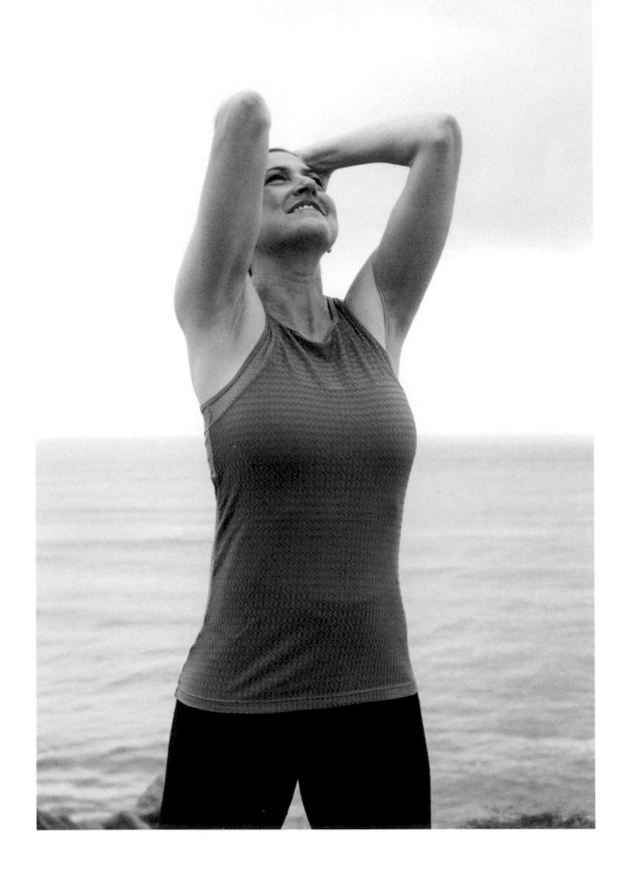

Hip Circles

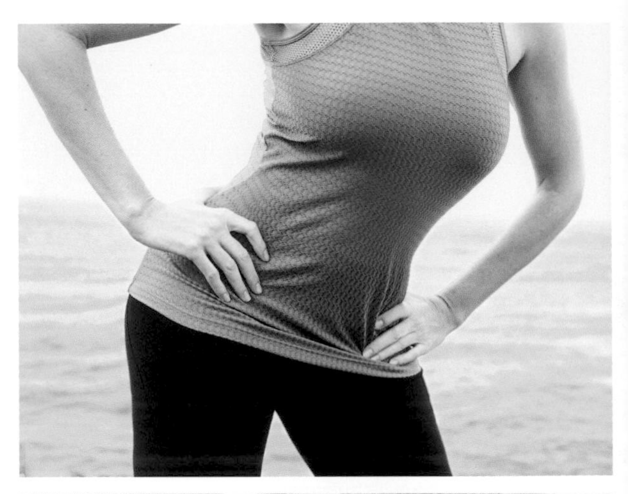

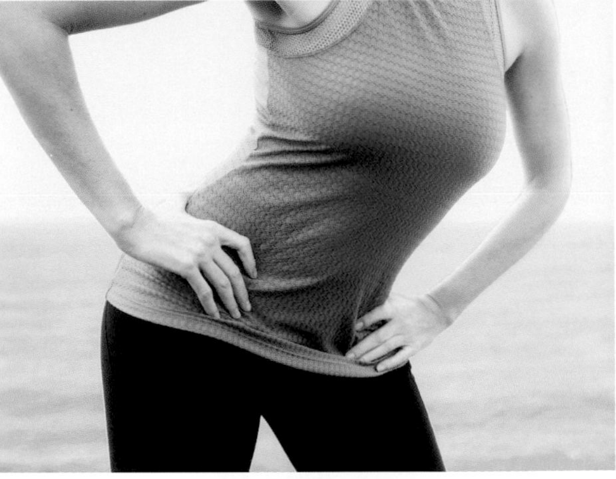

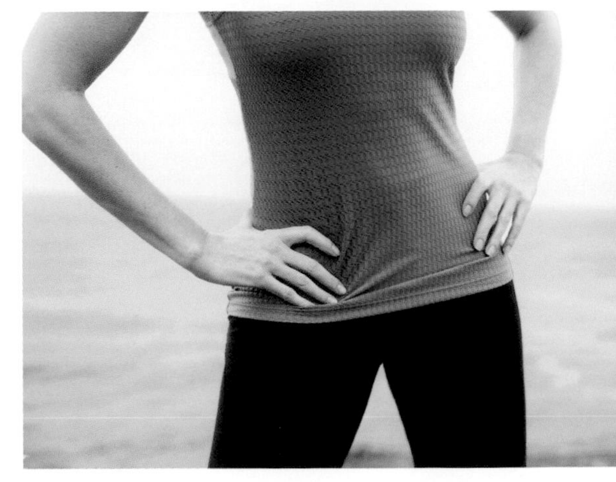

Upper Torso Rounds

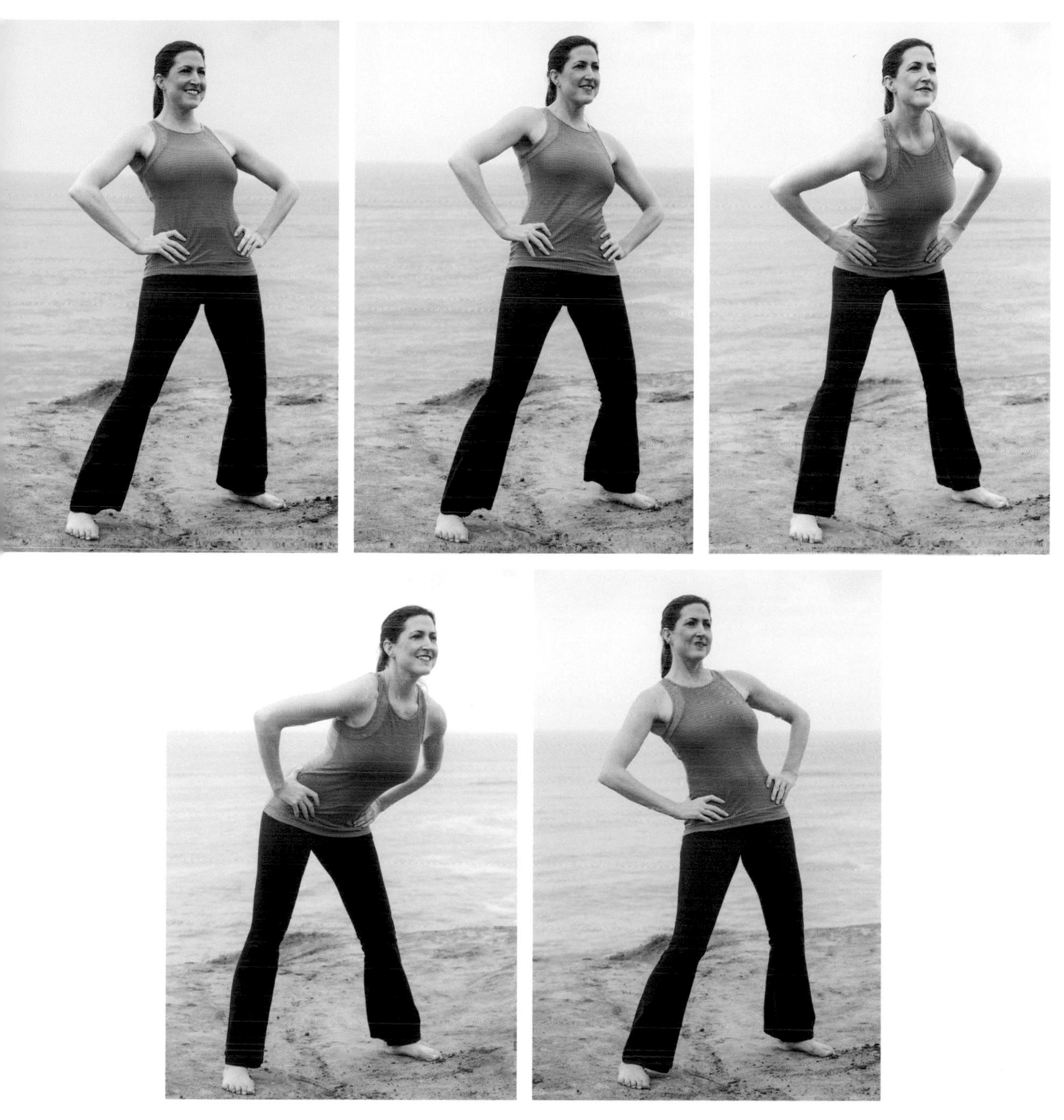

Celestial Shampoo

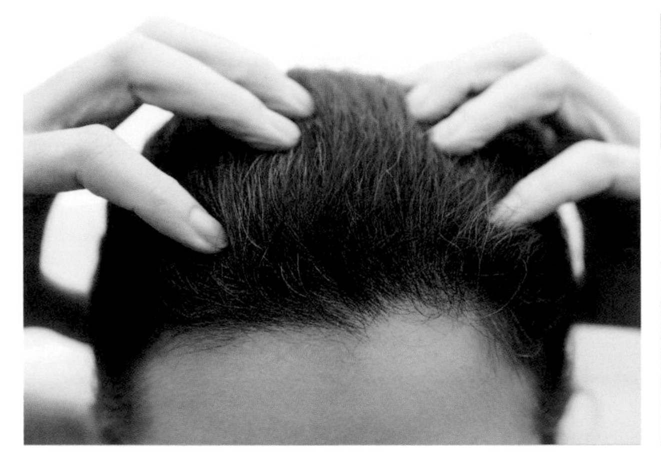

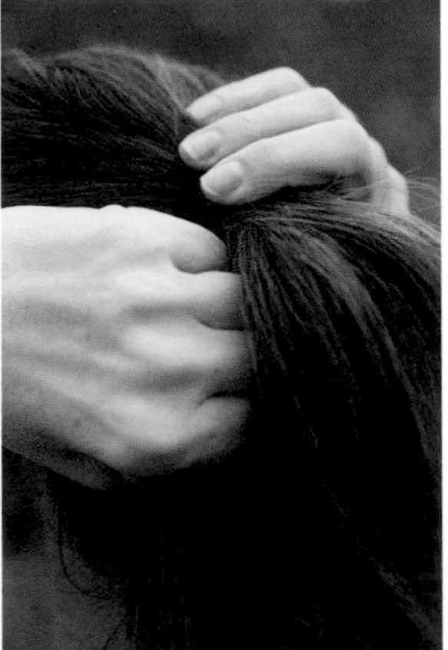

Eyebrow Press

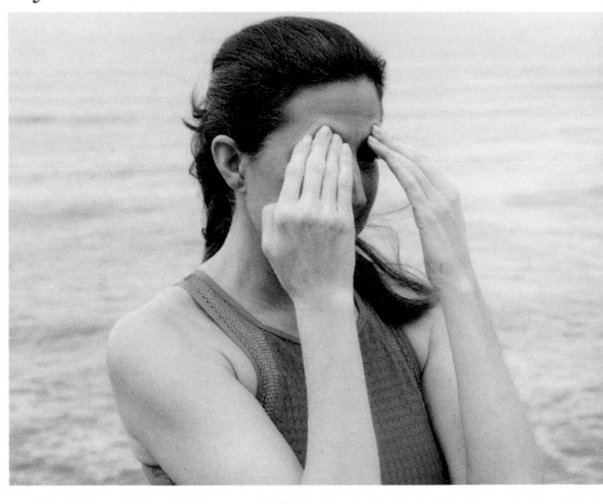

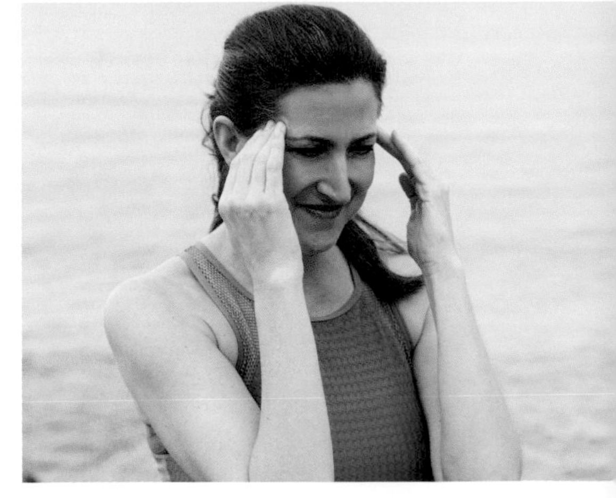

Waking the Roots

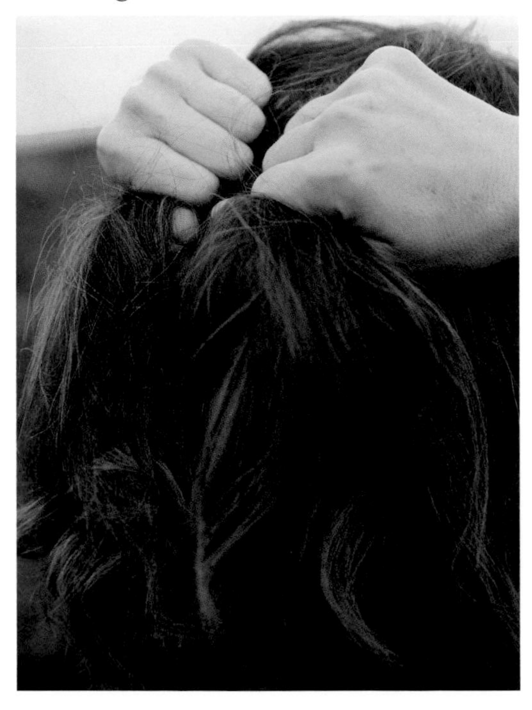

Jaw Massage

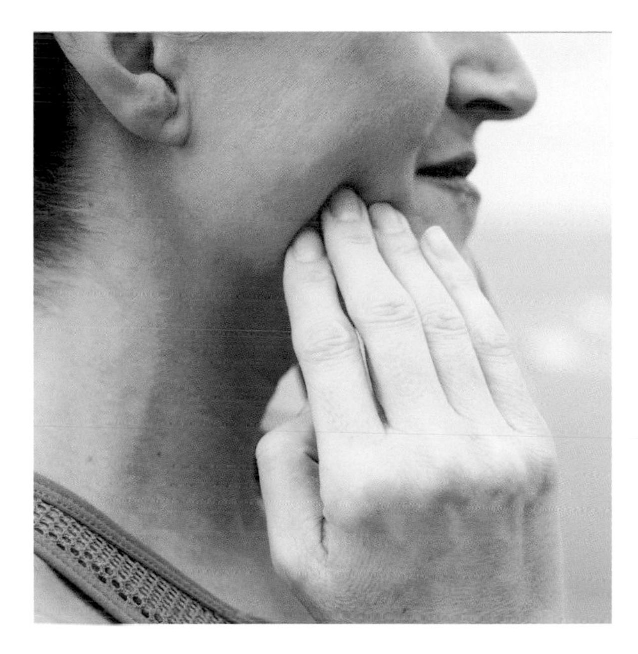

Wind-Palace Massage

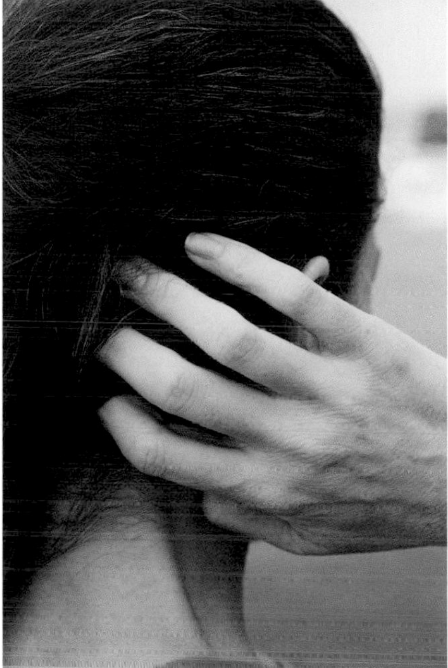

Ear Love

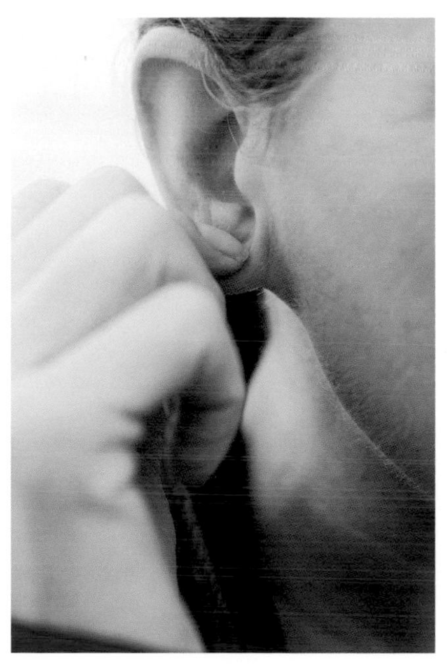

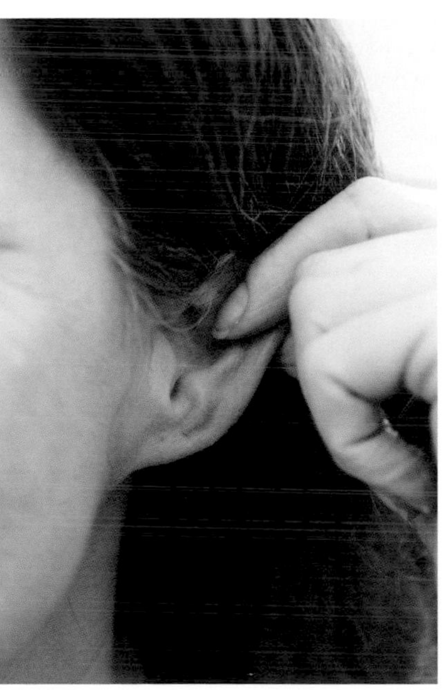

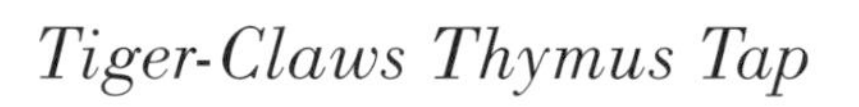

Tiger-Claws Thymus Tap

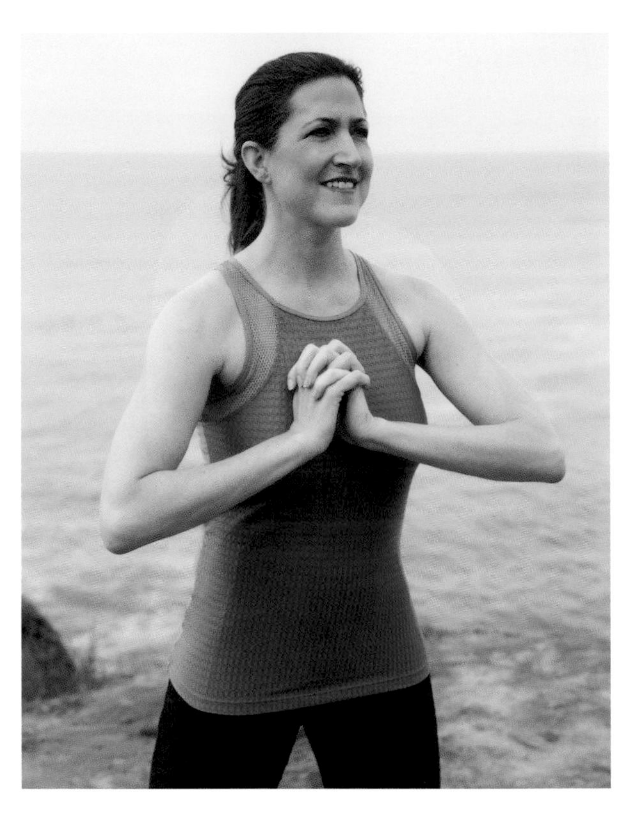

True Mind Treasure

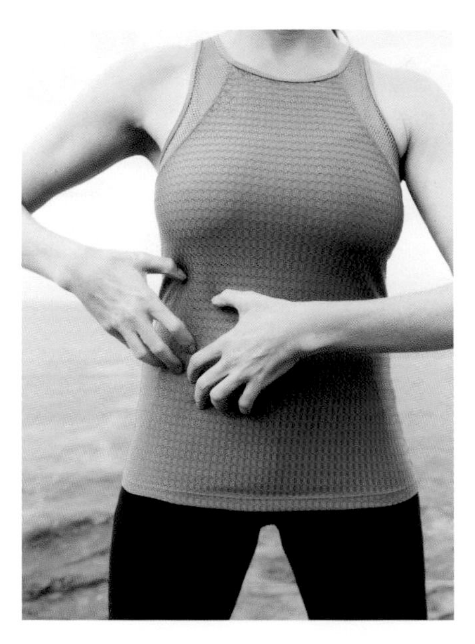

Riding the Roller Coaster

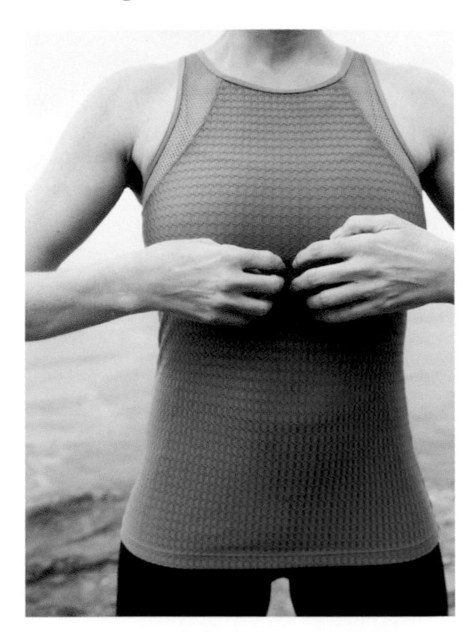

Arm Clap and Brush

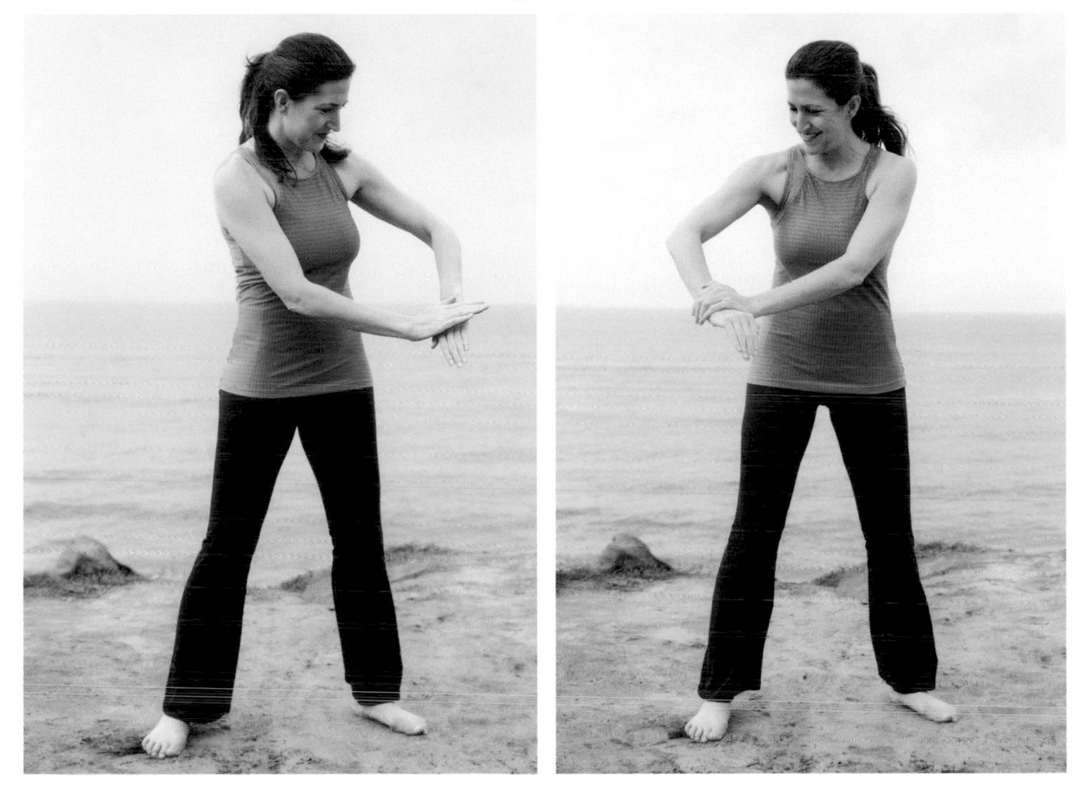

Door-of-Life Love Tap

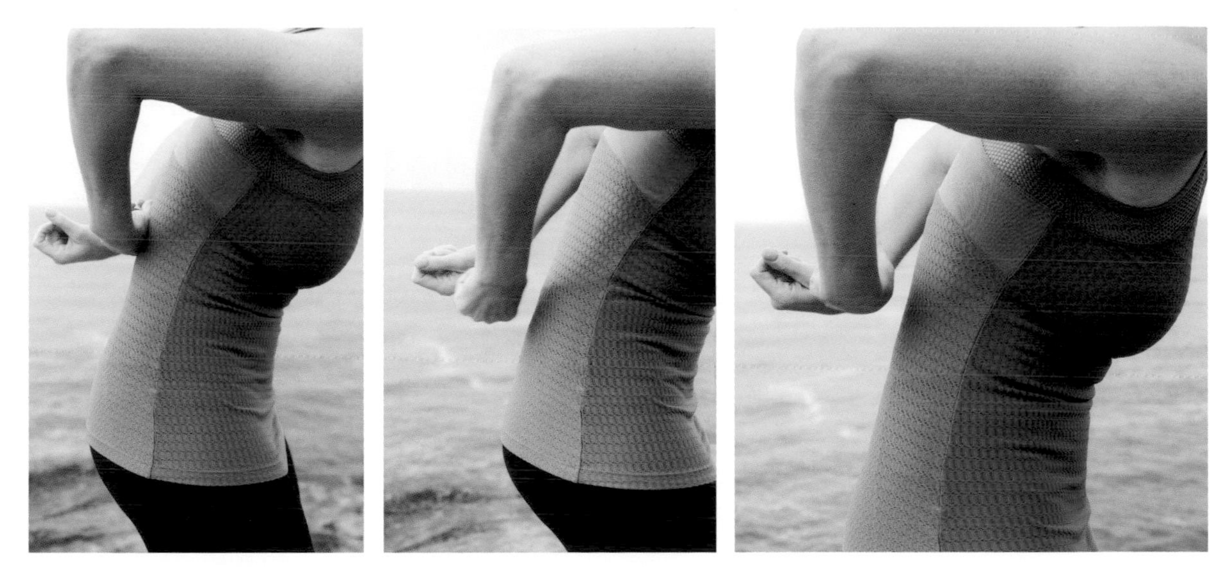

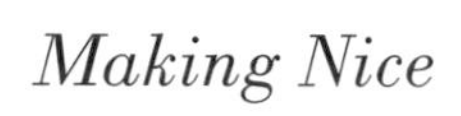

Making Nice

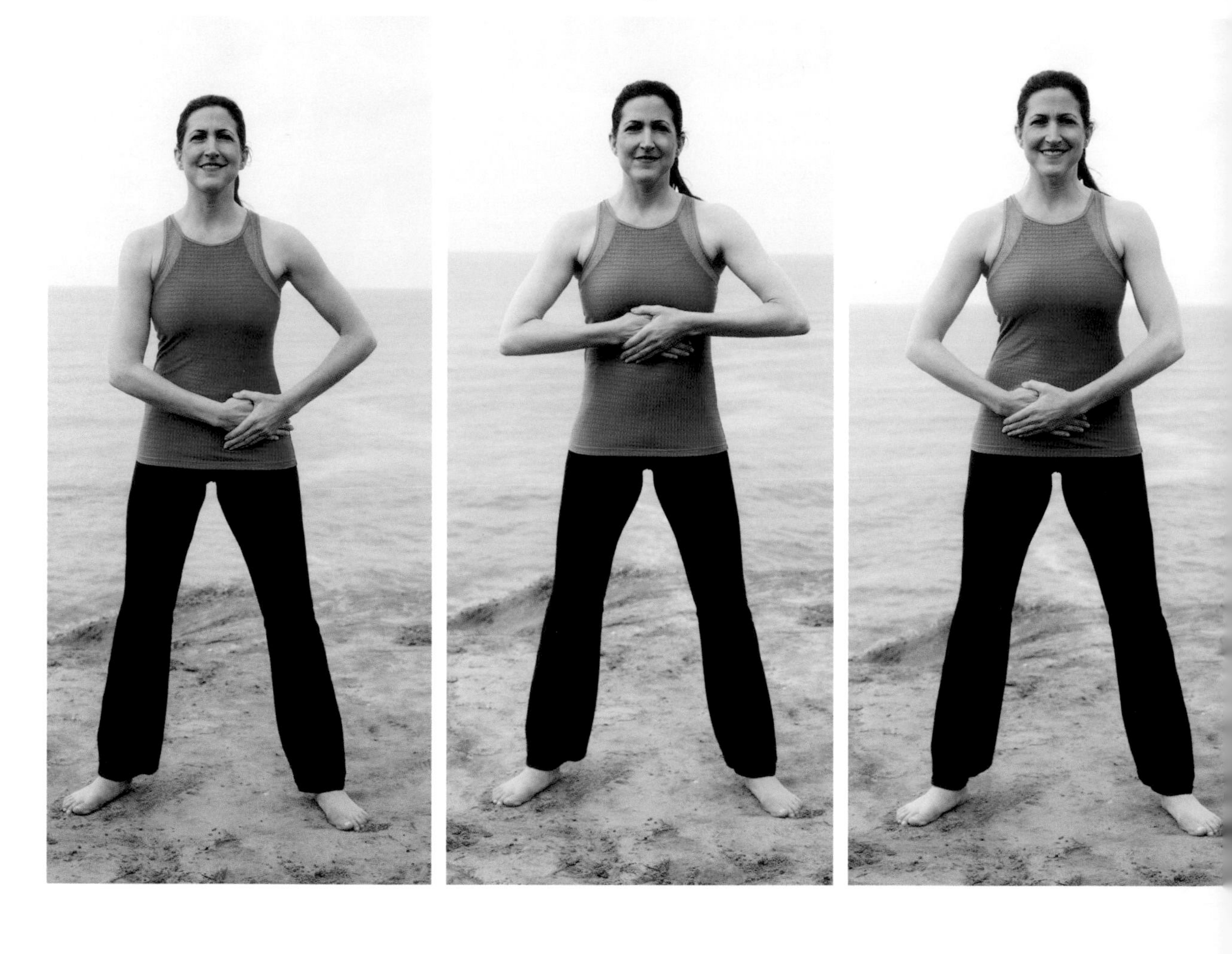

Hindquarter Love Tap

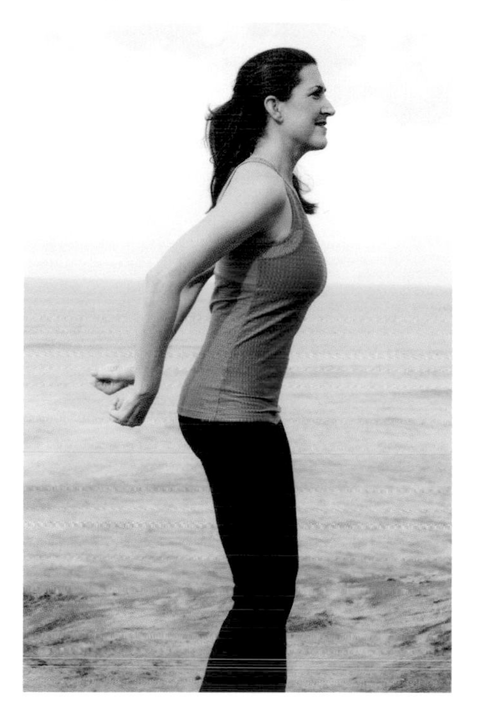

Wing-Tip Flex

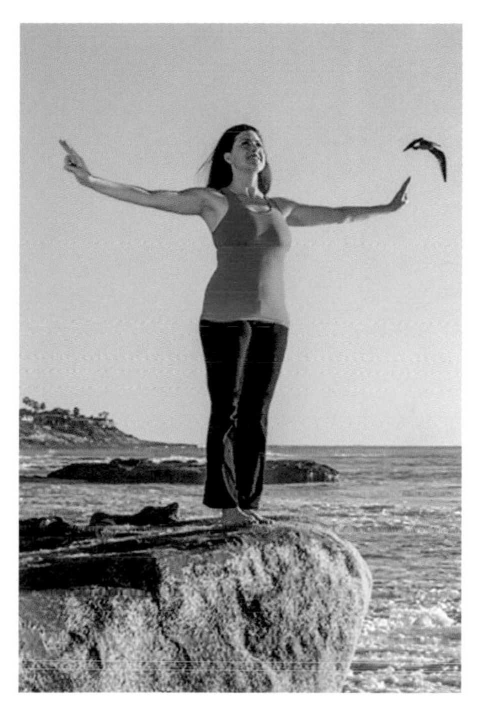

Hip Love

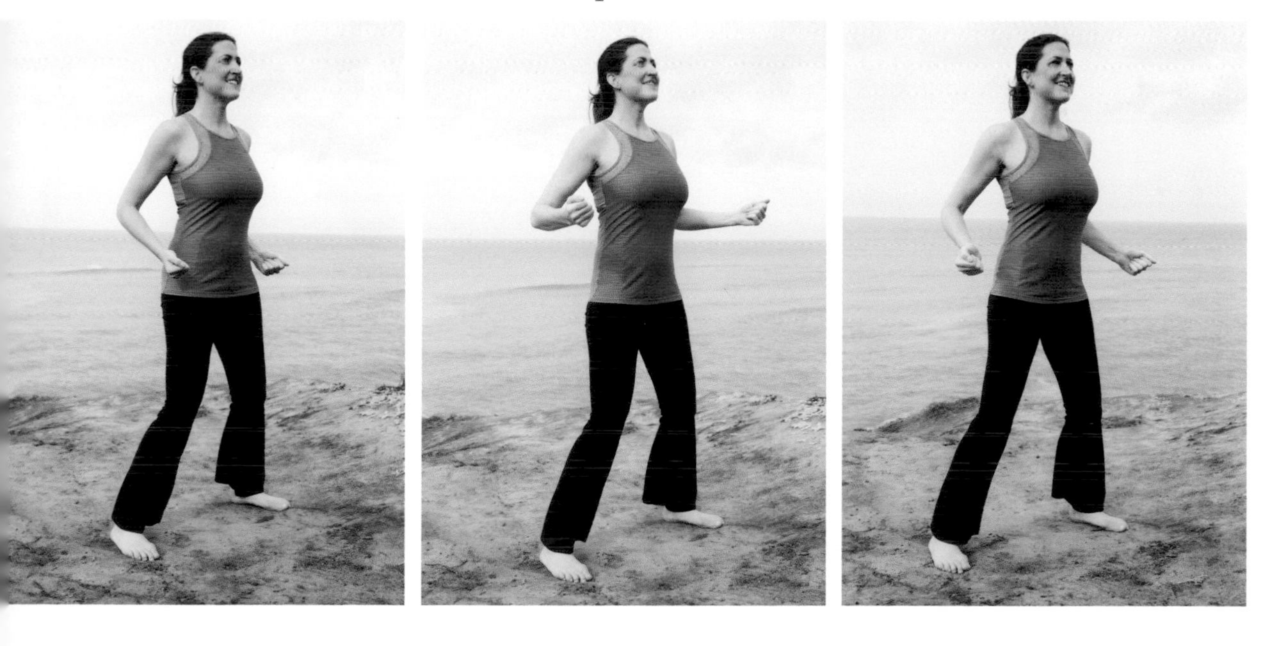

Up and Down the Jing Channels

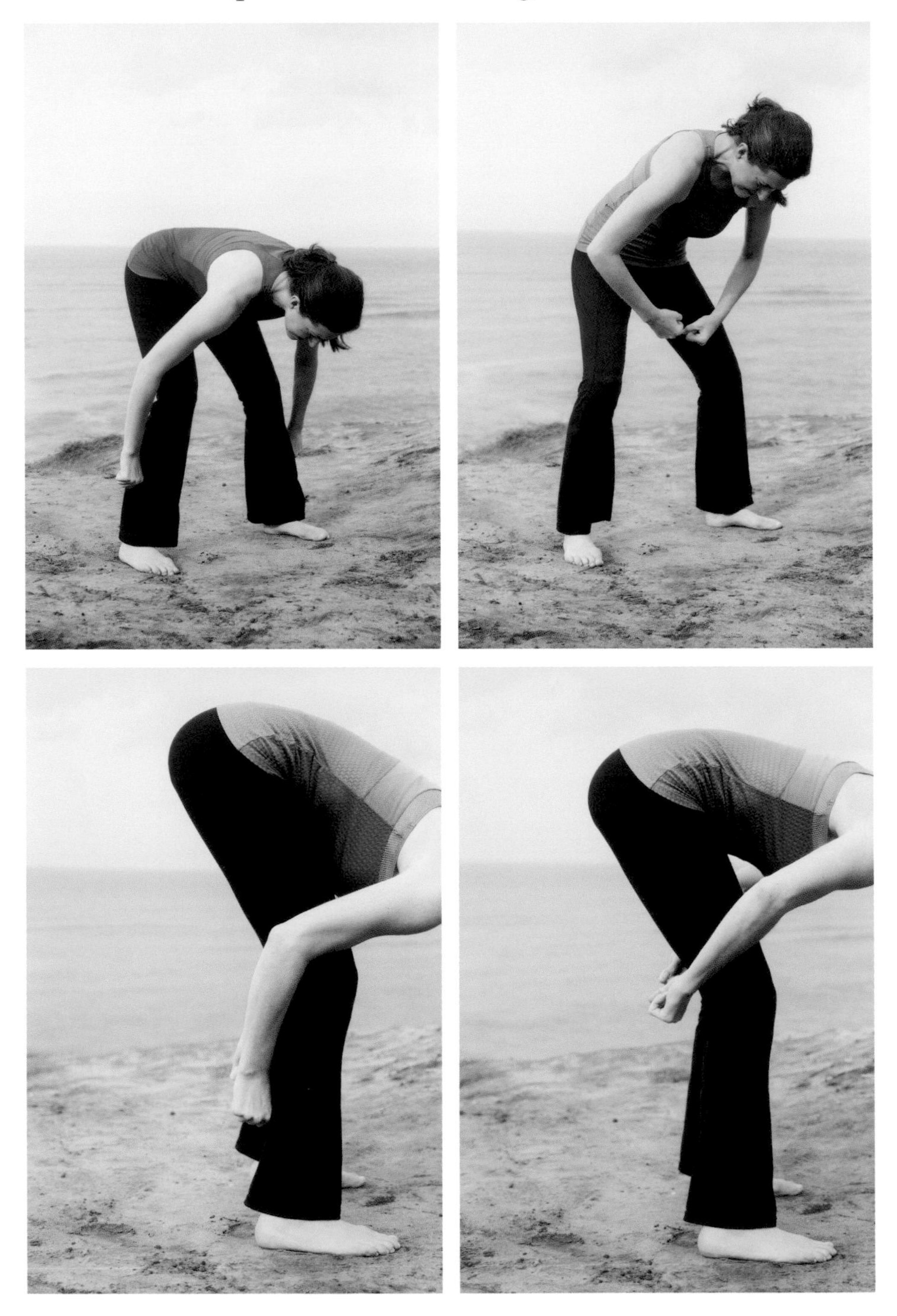

Blossoming Open

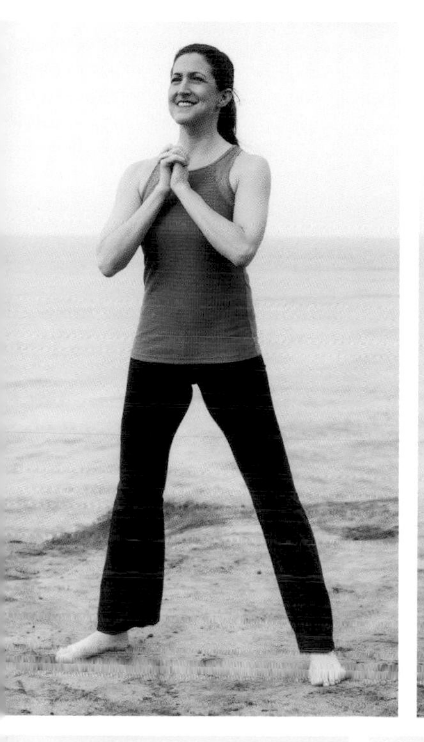

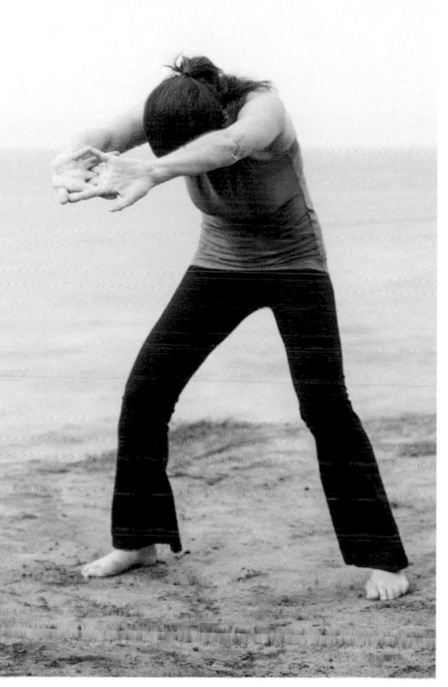

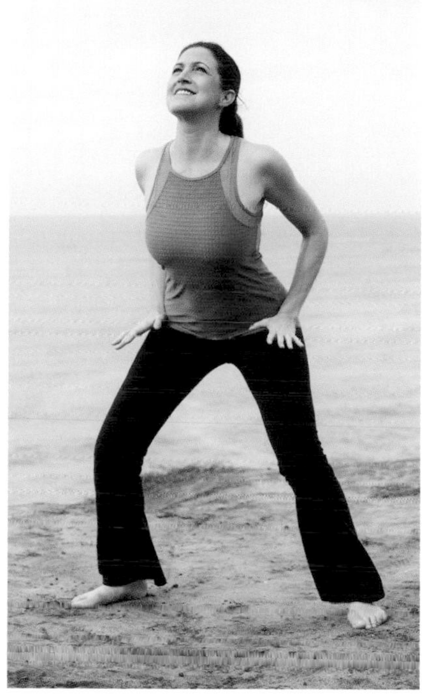

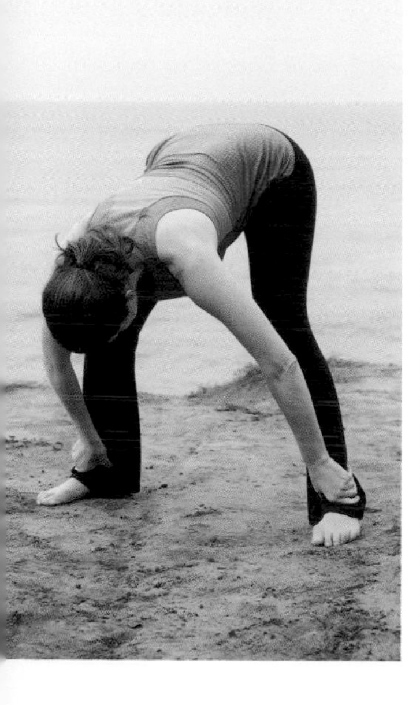

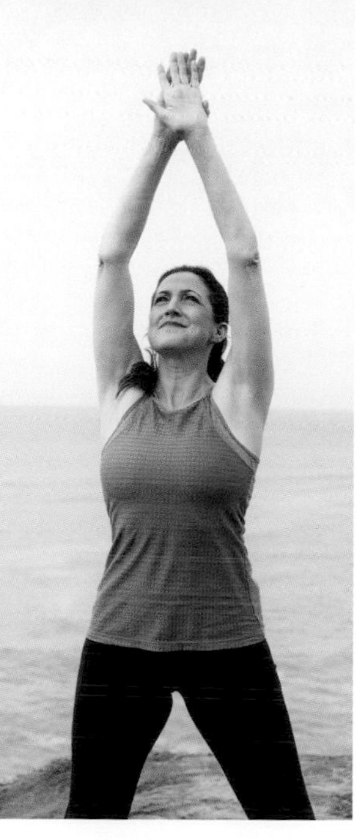

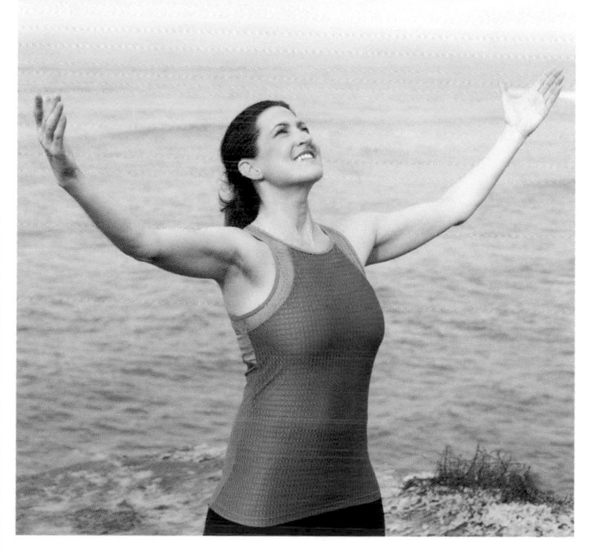

Goddess Breaths

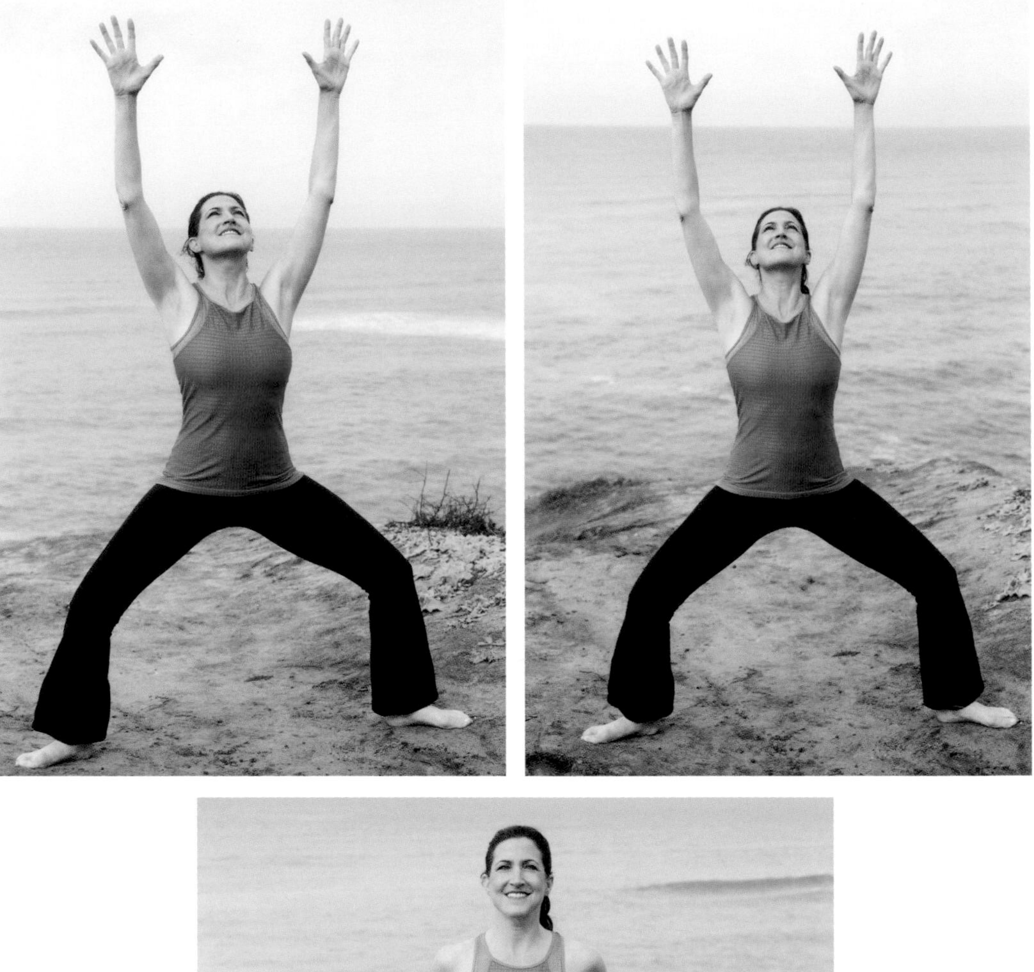

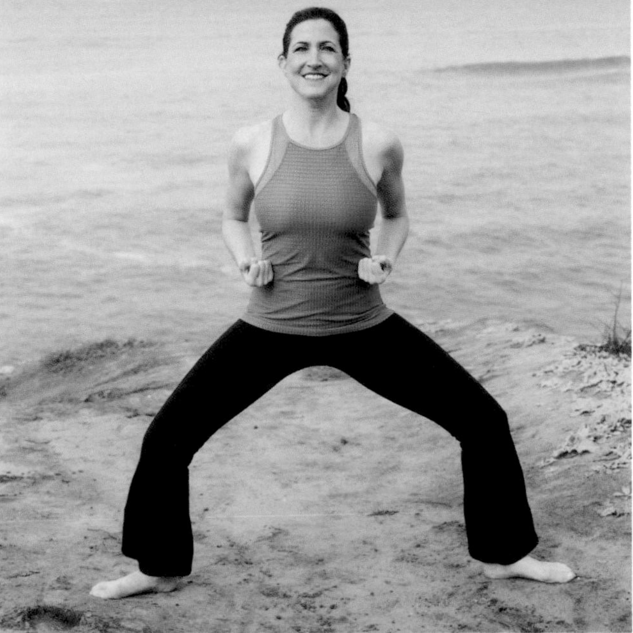

> nor should one exhaust oneself by trying to perform impossible tasks. One should learn how to exercise from nature by observing the fact that flowing water never stagnates and a busy door with active hinges never rusts or rots. Why? Because they exercise themselves perpetually and are almost always moving."

We too need to move if we want our bodies to be healthy and function optimally. Qigong gives us the opportunity to move like flowing water without interruption. During the following exercise sequences, you'll flow from one exercise to the next, pausing between them only to take conscious breaths that make you aware of the energy you are liberating and harvesting with your movements. Every movement should be done as if you were a river, flowing ceaselessly with a sweeping consciousness around each and every "rock" and becoming ever more aware of the miracles of nature that surround you and feed you.

With every exercise you do, focus your energy on keeping your feet open to receive chi from the earth and on keeping your crown open to receive chi from heaven. The idea is to continuously circulate chi through the microcosmic orbit, so that it then gets amply distributed throughout the rest of your body using your breath.

Perform the majority of the standing exercises at a moderate pace with deliberate movement and quiet intention. Do your best to respect your body by honoring it as it is rather than pushing it past comfortable limits. See if you can catch yourself when you've allowed your breath to become shallow or your muscles to tense up, and respond by breathing and softening. Use minimal effort. This is important, because you want your body to be as relaxed as possible in order to receive and transmit the energy you are cultivating and harvesting within your body. Just as we do in our lives, energy flows more smoothly and willingly without stress or opposition.

Unless otherwise specified in the instructions, throughout the practice concentrate on balancing, rooting, and focusing on your energy portals. The exceptions will be clearly marked. In general, move reverently, like a curious child who is enchanted at the prospect of discovering new grown-up worlds. Go at a slow, almost languid pace. Try pretending that you are in a library, fully aware of your every movement, careful, deliberate, in full possession of your balance, completely cognizant of your spatial awareness and placement, so that you move like a cat, gracefully and quietly, so you don't make any sudden moves that would disturb your surroundings.

In Opening the Gates, where you'll greet the utter splendor of the energy universe, you should carry yourself regally and with an air of utter reverence, as if you were a queen or a king meeting fellow royalty. Move at a pace that is moderate, reverent, and especially mindful, so that you are fully present and dedicating yourself completely to the moment.

As you progress into Love Thyself, know that it also has its own rhythm and pace, which is like that of a river flowing from beginning to end. For the most part, it never stops. The transitions between exercises matter; flow through these gracefully without interruption. You will want to move with quiet and at times playful control, allowing your bones to lead the movements, rather than your muscles, which is actually harder than you might think, but oh so worth it.

For each of the exercises, I'll specify what the preferred quality of movement is and what rhythm and speed to employ, so that you'll be able to execute the movement with the greatest confidence and ease. Just as important, give yourself permission to be free, joyful, sloppy. Go crazy!

In the warm-up sequence, Opening the Gates, and in the Love Thyself exercises such as Hip Circles, Tiger-Claws Thymus Tap, and Celestial Shampoo, your movements can be more playful, more spontaneous, more individual than elsewhere. These are the sequences that should carry your energetic signature, so be sure to make them your own. Allow them to serve as true outlets for self-expression and the free exploration of your body. The goal is to release old, stagnant chi and usher in new chi in the way only you can. Love Thyself in particular is meant to be a conduit through which you learn how to let go and act like a child again, unself-conscious, joyful, and *free*.

When you start circulating energy into certain areas of the body, such as your stomach, you may find them particularly and unexpectedly sensitive. You may even feel nauseous or dizzy when you perform certain movements. If this is true for you, rely on your breath to help you regain your equilibrium, and slow things down. Take a break to have a sip of water or even end your session. Resume only if you're ready. Do whatever you need to feel better, calmer, and more in control and settled before beginning again, but do *start again*.

Note: When you are first learning the practice, there may be times when you don't feel perfectly balanced as you attempt certain movements. This is completely natural and okay. Everyone starts somewhere. Maintain a sense of play and good humor—laugh about your difficulties! The laughter will generate beneficial chi. Resist getting attached to perfection. What we all need today is less stress and greater ease in every aspect of our lives. Know that with practice you'll get stronger and hold your balance better. You may start out as a clumsy sapling, but before you know it you'll be a solidly rooted oak tree. Give yourself permission to feel free when you're moving, like the wind dancing over hill and dale and through the trees. Sometimes, just as in life, the wind is a gentle breeze; other times, flower pots get knocked over!

Breathing

Breathing is the most powerful agent of alchemy we possess, a conduit for true transformation. You'll need to learn a few different breathing patterns for the Awaken and Play series, which is composed of two sequences, Opening the Gates and Love Thyself. In the first sequence, a series of warm-up exercises, your breathing should be performed mostly through the nose. In Love Thyself, most of the exercises invite you to be freer, more playful, and more expressive in using the breath as a vehicle for energetic and emotional catharsis. For these exercises you'll inhale through your nose and exhale through your mouth to expel stagnant chi.

As a rule, in all your breathing throughout the practice, whether you breathe in through the nose or mouth, when you inhale, you'll first feel the breath traveling all the way down, circulating, and stimulating everything in its path (when you breathe correctly into your perineum and sexual organs, it feels like an expanding, somewhat delightful, spongy sensation), and then the breath moves all the way up to the throat area, where it feels as though it's blossoming like a flower. As you exhale, you will start with the lower belly, which gently pushes the air out, causing the lungs to empty naturally, and feel the air exiting from your center, from your solar plexus and then your lungs. Regardless of the style of breathing you are employing for any given exercise, your goal is to be as relaxed as possible, so that everything is conspiring with you to make your breath as powerful an elixir as possible.

Believe me when I tell you that as you're doing the love dance that is Love Thyself, you may tap into pockets of long-held tension or suddenly become aware of an intense sensation in a specific part of your body and instantly feel compelled to create a "way out" for the feelings you have. In these visceral and emotional moments, you'll want to exhale through the mouth—and perhaps even do a Horse Breath or two—in order to expel stagnation and release the frustration that inevitably occurs when the body has been ignored for some time.

As humans, we tend to regret what we have *not* done, rather than welcoming the idea that we are now being introduced to a new way of being and inviting it in with all the positive energy we can muster. That said, frustration will be rearing its head frequently when you first begin. Indulge yourself and release as much pent-up (stagnant) energy as you feel compelled to, and know that by virtue of this practice it will hopefully become something you experience less and less frequently.

Now on to one of the most effective breathing patterns for enhancing chi flow and creating more internal space, the Horse Breath.

Horse Breath

The Horse Breath is by far one of my most favorite things, and once you learn it, I believe the same will be true for you. It is a superlative means of moving stagnation and frustration out of the body. You will engage in the Horse Breath not only in your qigong practice, but in any other practice in Waking Energy when you feel the need; very soon, you'll start to incorporate it into your daily life too!

1. Inhale deeply, relaxing your jaw and mouth.
2. As you exhale, slightly part and soften your lips and send your exhalation with considerable force out through your lips so that they vibrate heartily, making a deep sound like a heavy sigh. The lips will ripple like waves when they crash on the shore. To get the most out of the release, allow the exhalation and vibration to be sloppy and full.

Qigong Hand Positions

For the most part, you will use your hands as charging disks, rubbing them together to activate them for chi transmission throughout the practice.

Fists: Make fists with your thumbs flush on the outside of your index fingers. You'll use your fists to tap and thump various places on your body to release stuck chi.

Heart Clasp: Bring your right hand to clasp your left with the left thumb looped over the right.

Tiger Claws Unite: Bring your hands together so that the fingers interlace with your right thumb crossing over your left.

Tiger Claws Open: Open your hands and form the fingers into large "cat" claws, a position you'll use to tap the head and stomach primarily.

Sword Finger Position: Raise your hands with palms facing you, and curl your ring and pinky fingers in toward your palms, holding them down with the thumbs while extending your index and middle fingers straight out.

Alignment

The first step in claiming your place and plugging into the energy universe is to maximize the efficiency of your body as energy transformer, which is aligning yourself with your purpose: being the best channel for chi cultivation that you can possibly be. You will do this first through establishing an alignment in your body that opens your energy pathways, improving your receptivity to fresh chi and your ability to transform and discharge stagnant chi. The ideal alignment is the Waking Energy Stance, which will be your default starting position throughout the Awaken and Play practice.

You'll want to claim the space you're moving through as your own—meaning sensing your own energy in space and feeling tall, worthy, and proud. Acknowledge your power as the presence you are in this moment. Give yourself a strong nod before you practice, knowing that qigong is a way to say yes to yourself. Then take this feeling and root yourself in your place in the world as an energetic being, activating and feeling the vibration, the internal hum, the magnetizing of your own bioelectric nature; you are standing like a strong pillar of truth between heaven and earth, in your corner of the world, right here, right now. Infuse yourself, your body, and your stance with the energy of self-love and open yourself to new possibilities.

The Waking Energy Stance will help you to develop your overall balance. The stance naturally strengthens the legs, which provide a sturdy base so that you can get centered and be ready to do the good work that lies ahead. With a strong stance, you'll feel fully supported by the earth, like a tall, magnificent tree, so when you root, make a point of sending your energy roots directly down into the earth, and allow those roots to spread out, like a stunning subterranean canopy, extending your power and reach far beyond your own feet and legs and body.

When you have your root and you are centered and balanced, your mind will be calmer, and your muscles will be at your disposal and completely under your command because of the influence of your mind and your intention. Being clear about your intention will facilitate the optimal functioning of your entire subtle energy system, urging energy to flow freely, effecting true change in your body and in your life. Investing in a relationship of trust with the earth and knowing that it "has" you when you decide to "drop down" into it is the very secret to keeping your muscles relaxed and maximizing chi cultivation. This will enable you to "push" an object with true power and incite meaningful chi circulation in the body. With the correct stance, you will come to fully embody yourself. Now to properly assume your stance, I want to invite you to inhabit your body.

Let's explore what the proper alignment looks and feels like.

Waking Energy Stance

The significance of your stance when doing qigong is vital to your success in balancing your chi. In the ideal stance, the three elixir fields in the body (Lower, Middle, and Upper) are aligned one above the other along the Conception Vessel and the Governing Vessel, which intersect the elixir fields and distribute chi throughout the subtle energy system.

1. To begin, stand tall, with your feet hip-width apart and in parallel alignment, with your toes pointing forward. Your head and neck are lengthening upward effortlessly. Your shoulders are open and relaxed, arms down by your sides. Soften your knees slightly. Make sure that both legs share your weight equally.
2. Tuck your pelvis ever so slightly and lightly bounce or pulse your legs so that you can feel how the knees almost become shock absorbers. It's like being on your very own mini-trampoline. Test the feeling now before you root into the earth, and when you first begin to learn the practice, feel free to perform this "test" as many times as you need to in order to feel it becoming second nature.

3. Focus your attention on your feet and open the Bubbling Spring Points to receive earth energy, drawing it up through the meridians in your legs to your kidneys and adrenals.

The Power to Heal Is in Your Hands

Shaking, thumping, tapping, rubbing, massaging—all the techniques in Love Thyself that you are about to learn to wake your energy—cultivate glowing good health and longevity. Taoist adepts have used these methods for thousands of years to stimulate energy flow in the body. These techniques restore health to blood cells even as they shake stagnation loose from the fabric of the body in much the same way that shaking out a rug on the porch shakes loose the dust and detritus caught in its fibers. The joints and tissues become more fluid and free, as trapped, stagnant chi is released and discharged from the body. The cleansing process is further enhanced when we bring our consciousness to transforming our negative emotions.

Just to be alive and thrive, to stave off and protect ourselves from the deleterious effects of the environment we live in as well as from ourselves, since our "thinking minds" and personalities create so much stress and duress for us, we have to tap, clap, thump, and shake. These techniques shake loose the negative byproducts of overthinking and overindulgence in food and drink, both of which manifest as stagnation. They balance and smooth the flow of chi in our bodies.

Manipulating chi in this manner is how you can offset the stress from being alive on this planet. The effort you invest will strengthen your body and your spirit, making you a more formidable opponent on the battlefield of life, capable of managing the challenges of living in today's modern world and succeeding in accomplishing your dreams. With the right tools, anything is possible.

You will find that the simplest qigong movements are the most powerful. They will equip you to surf the waves of our seemingly random universe and all the diverse challenges you can encounter as a human being, improving your overall health and your ability to rebound from life's twists and turns. The practices here serve like a kind of internal trampoline, giving you a defensive resilience that makes you anywhere from strong to virtually bulletproof depending upon how much of yourself you invest.

You have likely never touched yourself in the ways that you will be asked to touch yourself here. When was the last time you massaged your gums? Or bathed your eyes in pools of warming chi from your hands? Or tapped on your own pubic bone, or solar plexus for that matter? Or felt the irrepressible surge of pleasure that arose when you simply touched yourself in a way that wasn't done strictly for pragmatic purposes? Or should I ask, felt the pleasure that arose when you touched yourself in a way that yielded a surprise, like the warmth that rises to your cheeks when someone kisses you unexpectedly or you are taken utterly by surprise by a stranger's smile, a great handshake, or a hug?

Well, I have news for you. You can inspire and generate the very feelings of the amazing hug or the kiss, and more, inside your own being. That's what the energy dance Love Thyself is all about. You will get this feeling of pleasure when you caress your own body for the purpose of bringing it into greater balance and vitality and when you experience the unbounded, free-flowing movements that are the dance of love. In this sequence, you will also explore feeling whatever sensations are waiting for you inside your own body, as a lover you've not yet met would. Perhaps most important, by allowing yourself to receive the pleasurable sensations that you yourself generate by doing simple movements and by giving yourself nurturing attention and energy, you are soon going to discover what feeling good *is* in your own unique body. When you do, those feelings of pleasure and new energy will give birth to more. It's that miraculous, and that simple.

You will move like a river dancing over rocks, flowing effortlessly through the topography of your own body. You may do things that feel like self-pleasuring and you should allow yourself to enjoy all of it! Imagine your own laughter dancing over the map of your body and leaving amazing endorphins buzzing on your skin as it travels along. The extraordinary effects of qigong will feel like laughter on your skin.

The Practice

Opening the Gates

Our Awaken and Play practice officially begins with Opening the Gates, a sequence of exercises that invite you to become fully embodied, establishing your place in the energy universe and activating the dance of internal energies. You'll greet the chi of heaven and earth and invite this universal energy to combine with your own.

Unless otherwise specified, stand in Waking Energy Stance throughout this sequence. As with all the sequences in the practice, perform this one at a moderate pace, with deliberate movement and quiet intention.

Standing Meditation

The Standing Meditation is a sacred way to greet your subtle body and establish your place in the energy universe. Rooting deep into the earth and reaching high into the infinite cosmos above, you become a strong pillar of truth, vibrating between heaven and earth. This practice calms and centers the mind, preparing it for the work ahead and engendering feelings of self-awareness, self-worth, and belonging.

1. Start in the Waking Energy Stance and bring your palms together, fingers pointing up, in front of your heart.
2. Close your eyes and breathe deep gratitude into your heart. Imagine that your entire body is a beautiful flower. As you inhale, your breath

makes the flower blossom open. As you exhale, silently repeat, "I am letting go of what no longer serves my highest good. I am creating space for what is new."

3. Inhale again and set an intention for the practice you are about to do. I always say that when you set your intention, you are not only setting your intention for what you wish to manifest in this moment, but in your life. This can be anything you wish it to be. Breathe this intention into your heart and spirit and into every cell in your body.
4. Now seal your intention by bowing your head and bringing your fingertips up to meet your forehead, uniting head and heart.
5. As you exhale, return upright, slowly open your eyes, and lift your gaze to the horizon. Bring your hands down to rest over your Sea of Chi and allow the warmth from your hands to radiate into your belly.
6. Let your hands float down to your sides. Acknowledge the bounty that surrounds you as you embark on your voyage to create heaven on earth.

Opening the Energy Gates

Opening the Energy Gates inspires a childlike curiosity and innocence, sparking a feeling of newness and discovery in the mind that gives you a sense of purpose. It also awakens and nourishes the spirit, welcoming it home.

1. Visualize the Bubbling Spring Points in your feet as wide open to receive the nourishing yin energy of the earth.
2. Find a place in your visual field to softly focus on—a beautiful tree, a patch of green grass, or anything that catches your eye or inspires you—and use it as an anchor as your inner eye, or *yi,* joins you in ushering in new energy.
3. As you inhale, with your palms facing down, slowly raise your arms upward at your sides to just above the height of your waist. Imagine that you are opening your body to the chi that surrounds you, as if

you were opening the door to your castle to receive guests. Once your arms arrive at just above waist height, pause and "brighten" the position a little. This means feeling that the energy you are collecting is cushioning your arms, keeping them aloft without your effort and creating a floating sensation beneath your hands.

4. Now is the time for subtle feeling and imagining. As you lift your arms, feel that you are summoning the power of the earth and inviting it to enter your body and enliven it; imagine that you're inviting in the jewels of the energy universe around you, welcoming all good things into your life. This is a sacred moment: you are entering the "church of you" to light your innermost flame and call in the great spirits from all of time to bless and guide you.
5. As you exhale, lower your arms softly. Feel that the energy you ushered in as you lifted your arms is entering your body as your arms come down.
6. Repeat the movements. Inhale as you lift your arms and focus on the *laogong* points in the palms of your hands. Feel the chi of the earth rising into your hands and traveling down through the meridians in your arms to your Lower Elixir Field. At the same time, envision earth energy entering your body through the Bubbling Spring Points in your feet and traveling up through the meridian channels in your legs to recharge your kidneys and adrenal glands.

Meeting the Chi

Meeting the Chi acquaints you with the energy that you harness from outside that melds with your own inner chi, combining to form powerful healing energy you can play with and use to nourish your body.

1. Bring your hands a few inches in front of your Lower Elixir Field.
2. Rub your hands together vigorously for a few rounds of breath to charge them, opening your *laogong* points.

3. Separate your hands and feel the "buzz"—the chi you created that's vibrating between them. As you inhale, pull your hands slightly wider apart, creating a ball of energy between them. As you exhale, bring your hands back together, cushioning this soft, spongy, dynamic, subtle energy and allowing it to play between your hands.
4. Imagine that the chi ball you're holding between your hands is a small planet earth. Turn your hands, bringing your right above your left, cradling the chi ball and feeling that the energy between your hands is radiating into your Lower Elixir Field and infusing it with life.
5. Feeling a buoyant, spongy, cotton-ball, cloudlike subtle resistance between your hands, breathe into the delicate electrical sensation, this union of heaven and earth, this circulation of yin and yang energies. They've started their sacred conversation and made themselves available for powerful healing in your body.

Collecting the Chi

Collecting the Chi is one of the simplest, yet most powerful heaven-meets-earth exercises around. It brings earth yin chi and heaven yang chi into your subtle body, starting a harmonizing dance of universal chi. As you collect the energy you will use to heal and empower yourself, it imparts a sense of wholeness by rooting the body to the earth and underlining your purpose for being.

1. Bring your hands up to heart height, palms facing each other, and sense a chi ball vibrating between them.
2. Inhale as you expand your arms out to your sides, palms still facing toward one another.
3. As you exhale, bend your knees and slightly tilt your torso forward. Simultaneously use your arms to scoop yin chi from the earth into the embrace of your hands and arms.
4. Carrying the chi with you, bring your torso upright, still exhaling;

straighten your knees more—though not all the way—and bring your hands to chest height.

5. Inhale as you begin to open your arms and expand the chi outwardly.
6. When your hands have risen out to the sides of your waist and your elbows are softly bent, continue inhaling as you raise your arms upward to collect yang chi from heaven through your *laogong* points. Raise your gaze slightly as your arms lift to encircle your head, with your palms facing down toward your body.
7. Exhale as you draw yang chi down with your hands, bringing your palms about six inches above your head and then passing them in front of your face, beaming the chi from heaven into your third eye.
8. Let your hands continue to float down to the height of your heart, "washing" your face and upper body from a slight distance with the chi you've collected. Let your hands remain in front of your heart for a round of inhalation and exhalation, consciously drawing energy into your Upper Elixir Field.
9. Repeat the entire sequence of steps three times, consciously tuning in to the distinctive qualities of the yin energy of the earth and the yang energy of heaven.

Swimming in the Sea of Chi

Swimming in the Sea of Chi welcomes you into your own energy field, inviting you to dive into the bounteous universal chi that surrounds you, heightening your awareness and awakening your sense of gratitude for the chi you have gathered to cleanse and purify your aura, the energetic bubble that emanates from within you and extends up to seven feet around your body like the halo around a full moon. It helps you to relieve mental stress and renews clarity and focus. It imbues the spirit with calm, as it draws energy down to your feet, grounding you and making you feel settled and secure.

1. With your feet firmly rooted, place your attention on your Bubbling Spring Points, opening them wide and drawing chi up through your legs. Simultaneously, open your Crown wide to pull chi down through your Conception Vessel, the line of energy that runs down through the front of the body, to your Lower Elixir Field. Consciously breathe into your Bubbling Spring Points and your Crown for a few rounds of breath.
2. Now, without shifting your focus entirely, direct your attention to your Root and start to draw chi up through it into your Lower Elixir Field.
3. Direct the energy you're calling in from your Bubbling Spring Points, Crown, and Root to your hands.
4. Bring your hands together, palm to palm, and start to rub them vigorously to generate heat and bountiful new chi that you'll be able to "swim" in.
5. Rub the hands together with increasing intensity and focus, breathing naturally but deeply, and becoming ever more aware of the energy you're creating. Imagine that as you are rubbing your hands together you create a pool of pristine, healing, cleansing water. Continue also to place some attention on your Bubbling Spring Points, your Crown, and your Root.
6. Separate your hands by six inches. Feel a buzz in your palms again, becoming aware of the waking energy that you've summoned and focused. Think of the Dead Sea or of a highly mineralized, potently healing hot spring—your own sacred imaginary bathing reservoir. Picture the basin: perhaps it's fashioned of magnificent, glittering mosaic tiles or seashells, or smooth porcelain.
7. Now, dip your charged hands into your sacred bowl, scooping up handfuls of fresh, earth-infused energizing, healing, cleansing chi. Bring your hands closer together so that you can splash your face with the purifying waking-energy "water," and each time you do inhale deeply.

8. Caress your face with your hands and the water, as if you were rinsing off a soapy lather. After you splash your face, immediately bring your hands down from your face and head in a tossing-away motion, shaking out your hands at your sides. Exhale deeply through your mouth, letting out a deep, audible sigh of relief, knowing that your exhalation is also carrying the stagnant chi that was stuck in your head and face out and away from your body.
9. Now, in a kind of rhythmic dance with your hands dipping into your "pool of chi," continue scooping into the energy bowl and make larger, splashing motions, sweeping your hands up over your forehead and the top of your head and running them down the back of your head and over your shoulders. As you bring down your hands, shake off stagnant chi.
10. After you have done this three or four times, imagine your sacred basin has suddenly grown in size and you're now standing in a pool of chi that surrounds your upper body. Instead of dipping into a bowl, lower your arms toward your waist, and, with an upward sweeping motion, begin wrapping your hands and arms around your body. Hug yourself as you drag your hands up the sides of your torso as if you were taking off a shirt. As you perform this action, shift your focus from drawing earth chi upward to drawing heaven chi downward. Inhale as your head and eyes move upward with your arms until they are facing heaven—in essence, you are celebrating it. As you open your arms to heaven, you are consciously harnessing astral chi. Lift your gaze to smile up at the sun (whether you are actually outside or imagining it) and feel its soothing, penetrating warmth on your face and body.
11. After completing the "taking off the shirt" action, raise your arms to heaven, opening your chest and shoulders, and acknowledge the heaven chi. Consciously draw chi down from heaven.
12. In one grand gesture, throw your arms outward and down to your sides as if you are shaking water off your hands. What you're doing is shaking off stagnant chi and making room for new chi.

13. Repeat the "taking off your shirt" action, allowing the movement to morph into a larger, more involved physical action by deeply bending your knees and once again shifting your focus to drawing earth chi up into your body.
14. Now imagine that you're at the edge of an ocean, standing knee-deep in water. Bend your knees deeply and inhale as you bring your hands and arms together to scoop up the "ocean water" with your hands. This time, instead of hugging your body as your arms travel upward, cross your arms about six inches in front of you and create a kind of space for a globe, or orb, between your arms and your body. Once your arms reach the height of your upper torso, open your arms expansively once again to receive heaven chi. Very quickly thereafter, as you bring your arms down to begin doing that same action again, shake the hands off once while thinking, "I am letting go of what no longer serves me."
15. Repeat the entire series of steps nine times.

Love Thyself

Love Thyself is a reunion. The sequence is a dance of courtship with your most sacred, timeless self—inner and outer. Reminding you of how important you are to yourself, it will inspire you to cultivate the self-respect, reverence, appreciation, and awe for the miraculous being that you are, which you so rightly deserve. When you practice the self-massage sequence Love Thyself, you'll feel as if you're being introduced to a long-lost friend.

By allowing yourself to receive the pleasurable sensations that you yourself generate by doing simple movements and by giving yourself nurturing attention and energy, you are soon going to discover what feeling good *is* in your own unique body. When you do, those feelings of pleasure and new energy will give birth to more. It's that miraculous, and that simple.

Shake It Up to Wake It Up

Shake It Up to Wake It Up opens and lubricates the joints as it stimulates the lymphatic system, removing toxins from the body and yielding greater immediate energy and mental clarity.

The full-body shake we're about to do is like beating a dusty rug. Of course you're not a dusty rug, but believe me, there many things hidden in the tissues of your body that need to come loose! Shaking your body is an opportunity to shake out these hidden issues. Like a rug that receives multiple footsteps daily, your body receives and processes toxins and stressors as you move through your daily life. And if you've been in the world for a while, that's a lot of footsteps.

Letting everything you've experienced lie dormant can easily lead to energy stagnation. It's my guess that there is a good amount of stagnation inside your body that needs to be moved. As soon as you begin shaking, I promise you'll start to feel better and instantly feel your energy waking inside you. You are about to shake your entire body in a way you probably never have before. I have a sneaking suspicion that you're going to love it so much that you'll want to do it every day.

1. Start to softly bounce up and down, imagining that you have no muscles, only bones. Be as gentle as you can to start, so that you can master the sensation of moving without effort. The bounce you do should be on the low-key side to begin, so make your knees the shock absorbers of your bouncing action. As you bounce, allow your arms to relax and bobble up and down along with what the rest of your body is doing. Breathe naturally and deeply.
2. After ten to twenty seconds of bouncing, start to increase the scale of your bounce to include your whole body. Involve your hips, shifting weight back and forth from one foot to the other, and bring your arms overhead where you can shake them freely in the air, as if you were shaking excess water from just-washed hands. As you increase

the intensity of your total-body shake, maintain the effortless effort you established when you began and returned to your breath, making sure that you are exhaling now through your mouth—even letting out an audible sigh occasionally as you shake and bounce.

3. Now bring your hands down in front of your midsection and start an action that resembles a sloppy piano player, making your hands flop up and down from your wrists. Shake your hands from side to side as well, again as though you are shaking water off them.
4. Next, shift your focus to your hips. Bounce from side to side, swiveling your hips and leaning into each hip as if you're listening to a new song with a deliciously seductive, pulsating beat. Let your head move in the opposite direction from your hips, as if you were dancing a sexy Latin salsa or meringue. (If you don't know how to do a meringue, just make it up—think of the sultriest, sexiest dance you can!)
5. Now increase the hip action, so you're doing a more straightforward 1960s twist. Work your way through one pass of twisting in one direction and then go back the other way, all the while allowing your arms to move in a complementary way that feels natural and fun. Let your head go along with the action; and remember, the movement should feel easy, effortless, carefree, and inspired by your own rhythms, with no judgment or worrying about how it looks to the outside world. Care only about how it feels. Know that every shake, twist, and flick of your wrists is waking the energy inside you. You are removing blockages, facilitating detoxification, and ushering in some much-needed brand-new chi.
6. After you've really gotten going—your heart is beating faster inside your chest—and you've generated some good heat (sweating is a good thing!), come back to center and return to the up-and-down bouncing. Now transform the full bounce into a heel drop, where you rise very slightly up off your heels, lifting your arms up to the sky with long, loosely straightened elbows, and then, with very little effort, drop down into your heels, giving in to gravity with all your body

weight and allowing your arms to swing down in tandem with that motion. Do the heel drop with a coordinated arm swing nine times in total.

7. After you've completed the last heel drop, shake each leg separately, as if you were kicking something off your foot. Shake the leg out and down to kick whatever it is off. (And by the way, the "whatever it is" is actually stagnant chi!) Lift your right leg and give it one good, full-leg shake all the way down to your toes, and then immediately switch to your left leg and do the same thing. Allow your upper body and arms to naturally counterbalance the leg-shaking action.
8. After you have completed four sets of leg shaking, return to your Waking Energy Stance and maintain it as you breathe for a few rounds, and then get ready for Ringing the Temple Gong.

Ringing the Temple Gong

Ringing the Temple Gong opens the central channel, releasing and liberating held chi as it stretches the muscles surrounding the spine. It lubricates the spine itself, stimulating the nerve plexuses radiating from the spine. It relieves tension in the back, neck, and shoulders and unleashes powerful energy that is immediately distributed to the rest of the body. When you first begin doing this exercise, you may feel stiff, tight, or restricted, particularly in your spine, upper torso, shoulders, and neck. Although you may not be able to twist very much from side to side initially, as you continue to breathe and twist, you'll find that your spine starts to open up, so that you feel freer and experience a larger range of motion.

1. Start to gently turn your torso from side to side, initiating the movement from the waist, rather than the arms and shoulders. Your arms should be relaxed so they are almost limp.
2. Breathing smoothly and naturally, start to move rhythmically, gently twisting your body without effort as far as it will naturally go from

side to side, allowing your shoulders, arms, and hands to swing as a consequence of the movement that's being initiated by the torso.

3. Using the palms of your hands and your fists, let your hands naturally start to thump against your body. Target your hands so that the flat of your right hand comes to your upper left chest or rib cage as you turn your body to the left, while the back of your left hand forms into a fist and thumps against your lower back. Do the opposite when you twist to the right: let the palm of your left hand thump your right shoulder or rib cage while your right hand forms a fist and thumps your lower back. As you twist and thump your body, you are stimulating your lung chi, your Sea of Chi and Door of Life, and your kidney chi simultaneously.
4. As you continue twisting right and left, work your way down the body using the flats of both hands to thump and pat the middle of your torso, so that you are stimulating your liver, spleen, pancreas, and kidneys.
5. After a few rounds of breath, gradually increase the vigor of the movements overall, forming fists with both hands, and use your fists to thump your Door of Life, the lower back, and the sides of the hips.
6. As you continue to twist from side to side, lower your fists so that they're striking your buttocks. If you aren't able to twist that far yet, let one of your hands thump the Lower Elixir Field as the other thumps the buttocks. Each time one of your hands hits your body, it is like a love tap—aim to make each one count by directing your focus into your hands so that they transmit the energy you are generating in your central channel and distribute it to your Sea of Chi and your Door of Life, which are like central stations from which energy trains are being dispatched to each and every part of your body, near and far.
7. With every twist of your torso, aim to gently increase the torque of your body, and as you do, deepen your breath so that you facilitate greater opening in the spine, and start to look behind you each time you turn.
8. As you increase the range of motion in the twist, your arms will naturally start to swing with more vigor, a little higher, and the love

taps or thumps will also become more potent because the velocity of your body rotating around your spine will increase as well. Your fists hitting your body should feel good, like a teaser massage, an amuse bouche, or appetizer, promising delicious things to come.

Note: As you swing and increase your range of motion and speed up to a moderate pace, you may feel slightly dizzy. First of all, know that this is completely normal and not at all dangerous, even if it brings up some anxiety. However, if you feel dizzy, please stop and rest until you regain your equilibrium. Once you're feeling calmer and more grounded, feel free to start again—or simply move on to the next exercise. Trust that the more often you do this exercise, the stronger your vestibular (balance) system will become.

9. Once you've started moving into deeper twists and have established a healthy rhythm—not too fast and not too slow—and you feel as though you're twisting with less restriction than when you began, start to bend one knee and straighten the other as you twist from side to side. Move slightly more slowly to accommodate the transition to the straight-leg variation, which creates a stretch in the front of the thigh of the straight leg. As you deepen into the bent knee and straighten the opposite one, your pelvis and body should be in line with the straight leg, actively engaging the muscles in your straight leg to straighten it even more and, as you do, lean slightly back with your upper torso to create a kind of diagonal angle with your upper body.
10. Now, without pausing at all and making only the most minor adjustments, you're about to flow into the next exercise.

Upper Torso Rounds

Mobilizing the back, pelvis, and hip joints is achieved by doing Upper Torso Rounds. They improve digestion and elimination.

1. Place your hands on your hips. Straighten your legs slightly more than you would in Waking Energy Stance and start to rotate your upper torso (from the rib cage up) clockwise to the right, keeping your face forward, revolving around the stationary axis of your pelvis.
2. As you circle clockwise, breathe naturally and send your breath to areas that are calling out to you, those that feel restricted or uncomfortable. Send your breath to those places to open your energy pathways and remove the stagnant chi that's responsible for the restriction.
3. Deepen and extend the perimeter of the circle as you continue circling, according to what you feel you are capable of. Breathe more deeply when you encounter any sense of limitation in your attempts to move smoothly and seamlessly.
4. Perform a total of nine repetitions clockwise, and then reverse and circle counterclockwise nine more times.

Hip Circles

Hip Circles open and activate the Lower Elixir Field as they lubricate the hips and mobilize the musculature of the pelvis. They stimulate primal movement through the lower energy centers of the body, rooting you deeply into the earth.

1. Soften your knees and place your hands on your hips.
2. Start to circle your hips clockwise starting to your right—going right, back, left, forward—and as you do, send your breath into your hips and pelvis. Pretend that your hips are like a wide spatula, stirring peanut butter inside a jar. Move with that dynamic quality—at a moderate, meditative pace, so that you are circling the hips as smoothly and as thoroughly along the perimeter of your circle as possible, waking up your Root and stimulating the unobstructed flow of energy in your Lower Elixir Field.
3. Circle the hips nine times clockwise and then switch directions and

circle them nine times counterclockwise. As you do, place your attention on keeping your Bubbling Spring Points, Root, and Crown open to receive chi.

Celestial Shampoo

The Celestial Shampoo stimulates blood flow in the scalp, releases muscular tension from overthinking and stress, and calms the mind as it opens the Crystal Palace to receive heaven energy.

1. Rub your hands together vigorously, charging them with heaven and earth chi, to create the most divine celestial shampoo with the energy you've collected so far in the flow.
2. Take the precious nectar that you have in your hands and bring the palms of your hands onto your scalp to massage the hair on the top of your head.
3. Then using your fingertips, massage the chi into your scalp, as if your favorite hairdresser were treating you to the best shampoo massage of your life. Make sure you cover the entire expanse of your head, giving it all plenty of attention, coming down around your ears and going to the base of the skull as well as the top of your head.
4. As you massage your scalp, start having fun with Horse Breaths. Most of us allow negative thoughts to proliferate, so massage with the intention of chasing the ghosts out of the machine, so to speak. Use Horse Breaths to send them on their way, from your body-mind and into the earth, where they'll be transformed into energy for the plants, flowers, and trees. Do a Horse Breath whenever you feel inspired or compelled to do so.
5. Continue massaging your scalp until you feel complete. Then, holding your arms away from your body, give your hands a good shake to cast off stagnant chi and do another hearty Horse Breath for good measure before proceeding to the next exercise.

Waking the Roots

Waking the Roots, which immediately follows the Celestial Shampoo, stimulates blood flow into the scalp, clears the mind from excessive thought and multitasking, and calms the spirit.

1. Grab your hair by the roots in small fistfuls and, very gently but firmly, pull your hair away from your scalp. Do this all over your scalp to uproot the stagnant chi that has developed from excessive thought. As you move over your head with your hands, breathe in and out deeply and naturally, waking up the chi on your scalp and inside your brain. You are deliberately moving negative thoughts out to make way for new ideas and positive thoughts.
2. Holding your arms away from your body, shake your hands vigorously and do a nice big Horse Breath.

Eyebrow Press

An exercise that stimulates an important liver meridian point to relieve liver stagnation and headaches caused by stress or long hours staring at a computer screen is the Eyebrow Press.

1. Rub your hands together vigorously to charge them. Then place your thumbs underneath your jaw on either side of your face to serve as an anchor and bring your index fingers up to press into the inner upper crests of your eyebrows, right by the bridge of your nose.
2. Press and drag your index and then middle fingers progressively along the arches of your eyebrows, stroking outward toward your temples, allowing your ring fingers to naturally join in the completion of the sweeping motion.
3. Then allow your pinky fingers to extend freely on their own away from the face and serve as entrance points for chi, as you use your index,

middle, and ring fingers on both hands to massage small, very gentle circles on your temples. Breathe deeply.

4. Start again and do a total of three passes over the eyebrows followed by circles on the temples. Then continue to the next exercise without pausing.

Jaw Massage

Be prepared to discover some surprisingly sensitive spots doing the Jaw Massage. Like the nasal area, the jaw area is loaded with tension and stuck chi. Think of all the "heavy lifting" your mouth does—how hard your jaw works at chewing, talking, and helping make facial expressions. Speaking of expressions, the jaw is also a reservoir for unexpressed feelings, particularly feelings of stress and rage. When you "bite your tongue," guess where the tension goes? Jaw Massage relieves chronic tension in the muscles of the jaw, resulting in feelings of calm and rootedness in the body as a whole.

1. Rub your hands vigorously to charge them and then, starting just below your earlobes, use your fingertips to massage the muscles of your jaw. Using small circular motions, work into and around the hinges of your jaw, and then into the muscles and bones of your lower jaw.
2. Breathe deeply as you make a thorough inspection across the territory of the jaw with your fingers.
3. Then, with your mouth closed, use your fingertips to massage your upper and lower gum line through the flesh of your upper and lower lips. Move your facial skin up and down and in small circles over the gums. When you massage your gums, it may feel both good and weird at the same time. Ignore the weirdness of the sensations, because this simple action is remarkably beneficial in a way that you wouldn't necessarily expect. You instantly improve circulation to the gum tissue and thus help reinvigorate them, and since they are

connected to kidney energy, you literally infuse your kidneys with new energy.

4. When you feel complete, take a few well-deserved Horse Breaths. Holding your arms away from your body shake your hands to fully discharge the stagnant chi.

Ear Love

Did you know that if you have trouble waking up in the morning, the best thing to do to bring your senses to life and help them greet the day is to tug and pull on your ears? All your organs have corresponding meridian points in your ears, so massaging and pulling on them stimulates the organs and sends positive energy signals, helping to bring them balance and harmony. The ears contain 120 points that correspond to other places in the body.

Caution: This is an area to massage with delicacy, even though you are using a firm and intentional touch, so move with care as you take a tour of your ears.

1. Rub your hands vigorously to charge them. Then cup your ears with your palms, firmly covering them, as if you don't want to hear what someone is saying.
2. Press your hands in against your ears firmly, holding for a breath. Then, as you exhale, release your hands, quickly moving them a few inches away from your head, with the palms facing your head. Bring your hands back to press on your ears and repeat this action twice more.
3. Now take your index fingers and thumbs and slide them behind the shell of your ears, as you bring the other three fingers (middle, ring, and pinky) in front of the ear and start to rub up and down quite firmly at a moderate pace as you breathe in and out. Rub up and down here ten times in total.

4. Anchor your index fingers in the central basin of your ears. Take hold of the thickest parts of your ears between your index fingers and thumbs and then use your thumbs to gently manipulate, twist, and pull your outer ears away from their centers. Start at the top crest of the ears and work your way down to your earlobes. Be creative as you do a full exploration of your ear—doing only what feels good. Breathe deeply and naturally.
5. After completing your massage, hold your arms away from your body and shake your hands. Also do a Horse Breath to release anything you've heard that now belongs in the past, to create space for new and beautiful, mellifluous sounds, speech, and music.

Wind-Palace Massage

The Wind-Palace Massage releases tension in the head, neck, and shoulders, key areas that can get very tight after bending our heads to read text messages and sitting in front of our computers.

1. Bring your fingertips to the occipital ridge at the base of your skull, where there are two distinct bony prominences. This is a place where many of your muscular attachments insert, so it can hold a lot of tension. As you breathe deeply, using your breath to move stagnant chi out of your body, start to make small circles inward, opening the energy of those spots.
2. Work your way now into the tissues surrounding the base of your skull, moving down the neck itself on either side of the cervical spine. Apply firm pressure, massaging your muscles in small circles.
3. As you are bringing life-giving chi to the back of your head and your neck and discovering all the tight and tender places that have been hiding there, take a Horse Breath to discharge stagnant chi, of which there is likely an abundance. It will feel good to be able to let go, as

you are liberating your muscles and sending new energy down your kidney meridian, which runs along the spine.

4. Perform the neck massage for several rounds of breath, using your intuition to know when the area feels complete before moving on and working your fingertips downward and outward, into the denser muscles of the shoulders.

Arm Clap and Brush

The Arm Clap and Brush opens and activates the lung and large intestine channels in the arms and relieves muscular tension and stagnation often caused by excessive typing on handheld devices.

Note: If you suffer from arthritis in your hands, carpal tunnel syndrome in your wrists, tennis elbow, or any shoulder ailments (for example, a rotator cuff injury), spend more time on the particular spot that is giving you trouble and focus your breath and energy there as well to increase the flow of chi to it and aid in healing.

1. Rub your hands vigorously to charge them. Then use your right hand to rub down the length of your left arm on the top, the deltoid side, from the shoulder to the back of the hand, as if you were polishing it like a piece of silver.
2. Flip your left hand over and work your way back up the inner arm to your chest. Start by brushing the *laogong* points in the palms of your hands.
3. Once you reach your shoulders, start the journey again, this time covering a greater expanse of the shoulder area, moving into your trapezius and upper back closer to the shoulder blades to the best of your ability to reach them. Send chi to that entire area of your body, breathing deeply the entire time and knowing that your breath is helping you unblock, stimulate, and harmonize the meridians in your arms and upper body. Repeat the brushing of the arm, up and down, twice.

4. Now form your right hand into a cupped shape, and start to firmly and rather vigorously "pat yourself on the back," so to speak, starting on the left side of your upper back. Continue, using a clapping action to thump on your left arm all the way down its length with the left palm facing down to the earth; once you reach the wrist, immediately flip the left hand over, so the palm faces up. Clap your own hand at least once here: this is a meeting of your two *laogong* points that will give an extra jolt of chi to both of your hands. After clapping, work your way back up on the inside of the arm.

Note: When you are clapping up and down your arm, it might sting a little, and that's a good thing. It means you are waking up the chi in your arms.

5. After clapping down and then up your left arm twice, brush your hand down the length of your left arm to move the chi that you have mobilized and unleashed off your skin and out of your energy field. Send the old chi into the earth to be recycled.
6. Switch to the other side, cupping your left hand and using it as the active hand to first clap down the length of your right arm and then up three times, and then brush it off.

Tiger-Claws Thymus Tap

The Tiger-Claws Thymus Tap clears the lungs, removing stagnation and activating new chi flow, and stimulates the thymus gland, which produces the T-cells in our blood that protect the body from infections, and are largely responsible for our immunity. As we age, the thymus gland shrinks. Tapping on it keeps it healthy, "fat," and able to perform its defensive duties for us, ensuring its—and our—longevity.

1. Inhale deeply and squeeze your perineum, your Root, making sure that your Bubbling Spring Points and Crown are open to receive chi.

Consciously bring all these energies together in your hands as you rub them together vigorously to charge them with the most potent healing chi possible.

2. Separate your hands to feel the buzz or pulse of the powerful chi you've just collected. Then unite the energy of your two hands by bringing them together and interlacing your fingers, holding your thumbs together side by side, facing your chest.
3. Tap your thumbs against your breast bone, making your first tap the strongest (like an accented syllable), followed by two lighter, shorter taps. Go at a waltz rhythm—TAP tap tap, TAP tap tap—because, yes, according to ancient Chinese texts, it just so happens that the thymus gland prefers the rhythm of the waltz to any other kind of dance rhythm, and so that is what it shall receive. As you tap, make sure you are breathing deeply and, most important, are focused on bringing the energy of love to your thymus gland, so that you are powerfully and silently focusing healing energy on it. Tell your thymus how much you appreciate all that it has done and continues to do for you in the area of immune defense and health.
4. Here comes one of my favorite parts of the love dance. After tapping your thymus for nine rounds of the waltz rhythm, very gently stroke the tips of your fingers down the center of your torso, running them down your central channel from your Upper Elixir Field to your solar plexus, bringing one hand over and on top of the other to replace it as it sweeps this area. This action should feel like petting a cat, and I imagine the sensation is one of the reasons why cats purr so loudly when they are stroked. This downward stroking will calm the area and seal in bounteous chi.
5. Holding your arms away from your body, shake your hands to release the stagnant chi you've liberated from your thymus gland.

True Mind Treasure

True Mind Treasure brings new awareness to your true mind and the emotions held there as it opens and activates the major energy pathways related to digestion and elimination, improving the overall function of those physical systems.

1. Rub your hands together vigorously to charge them.
2. Assume the Tiger Claws Open position with your hands. Use these open claws to tap on your belly, alternating hands, starting at your solar plexus (the tender spot just beneath your breast bone in your upper belly) and then moving to your left in a clockwise motion underneath your breasts and down the side of the belly until you reach just above your pubic bone, and then working up the right side of the belly, continuing back up to the solar plexus, breathing deeply as you make this circuit.
3. After a few complete passes, start to increase the perimeter of the circle. As you move down, actually tap on the surface of the pubic bone itself. Be prepared to feel pleasurable sensations! If you feel sensual feelings rising up inside you, let them fly free! Don't try to curtail or repress them. Rather than trying to "stem the tide," let the waves roll in, and breathe those lovely sensations right up into your brain, which in turn, will make your stomach feel even better. As you circle your stomach, make sure you keep breathing deeply and smoothly.
4. Take five passes, and when you're done, shake out your hands to release the stagnant chi you've liberated.

Riding the Roller Coaster

Riding the Roller Coaster opens and unblocks the central channel, sending signals that new chi can flow freely, enhancing emotional awareness, and improving digestion and assimilation.

1. Rub your hands vigorously to charge them. Then start tapping your solar plexus at a moderate pace, taking turns rather rapidly, alternating right and left hand. Use all your fingertips (but not your thumbs) to bring new energy to the stomach.
2. Breathe deeply and sense what you are feeling as you tap this area. Don't be surprised if you start to feel a kind of mild giddiness or anxiety, a feeling akin to riding a roller coaster on the downswing. The solar plexus is the seat of our emotions, and you may be tuning into feelings you've long been avoiding, as though you were revisiting the very events that may have initiated their pilgrimage here in the first place.
3. Continue tapping the upper section of your Middle Elixir Field for five breath cycles. As you inhale, silently think, "I am bringing new life-giving chi and love into my true mind." As you exhale, think, "I am letting go of what I no longer need."
4. After completing the five breath cycles, begin to pull chi down into your Lower Elixir Field using the tips of your fingers. Start to sweep your hands down over the solar plexus area you've just tapped, bringing one over and on top of the other to replace the other as it sweeps down your central channel to your Lower Elixir Field. This action should feel like petting an animal. As you stroke your body, send loving, healing energy to your true mind.
5. When you feel complete, shake your hands to remove stagnant chi, and do a few Horse Breaths.

Making Nice

Making Nice brings new, harmonious, loving chi to all the organs and the Lower Elixir Field. It calms anxiety, soothes indigestion, and improves elimination.

1. To soothe your true mind and bring even more healing energy into your Sea of Chi, rub your hands together to charge them. Focus on

keeping your Bubbling Spring Points, your Root, and your Crown open, so that you are actively channeling chi from earth and heaven into your hands. After charging your hands for several breaths, place your palms over your belly and send the bounteous chi you've harnessed directly into your organs.

2. Women should place left hand over right and men should place right hand over left. Circle your hands nine times over your stomach in a clockwise motion (start by moving your hands to your left and then down), pressing gently into it, as you breathe deeply and smoothly. Focus intently on bringing new chi into your organs to heal and soothe them, all the while becoming more and more aware of the sensations that arise for you as you "make nice" to your organs with these healing circles.
3. After completing nine circles clockwise, reverse direction and circle counterclockwise nine times. Moving counterclockwise (start by moving your hands to your right and then down) will detoxify your organs by reversing the flow of energy that they are accustomed to. The motion activates a variation on the healing response, causing them to release held toxins.
4. To finish, repeat one more round of nine circles in the original, clockwise direction. Then give your hands a good shake to release stagnant chi as you consciously let go of any negative thoughts and energy through your fingers, and do a Horse Breath.

Door-of-Life Love Tap

The kidneys are ruled by water and are responsible for cooling the body. Given that the body seeks balance, kidneys need their opposite, which is productive, focused fire. Keeping the kidneys warm, especially in cold weather, is important for nurturing their health and longevity. The kidney warming circles we'll do as part of the Door-of-Life Love Tap are just what the doctor ordered. They stimulate the smooth flow of chi in and around the kidneys and the adrenal glands, bringing nurturing life-force chi to the Door of Life. They soothe back pain and relieve stress.

1. Inhale deeply. Then, as you exhale, bend your knees and round your body forward in a large C shape, with your navel drawn up toward your spine.
2. Breathing deeply and smoothly through your nose, rub your hands together vigorously to charge them. Then place your palms on either side of your lower back, below your lowest ribs and above your sacrum, and infuse your kidneys and adrenal glands with new, life-giving chi.
3. As you continue to breathe naturally, with your head and neck relaxed, focus your eyes down at a slight diagonal in front of you at the floor, rooting your feet into the earth and consciously drawing chi up through your Bubbling Spring Points and Root.
4. Now make fists. Start to make small circles right over the kidneys, circling your fists inward toward the spine. Circle your fists on your lower back for five rounds of breath.
5. With alternating right and left fists, tap on your lower back using a gentle, but firm pressure. Be prepared to experience far greater sensation than you might have anticipated. Continue tapping those areas rather firmly, even if it feels counterintuitive. Of course, modify your love taps and make them gentler if your lower back feels exceedingly tender, but know that your own loving and intentional tapping can help disperse negative energy responsible for stagnation that led to what you now perceive as tenderness.
6. As you tap, inhale through your nose and exhale through slightly parted lips; exhale fear and inhale courage and confidence. Use your exhalation to release any discomfort you feel. Do a few Horse Breaths to help you release any feelings of surprise, stress, or frustration you may experience. Since you are giving love to the kidneys, you will likely be contacting fear, which is an emotion they govern. Know that

it's coming up in advance, so that you can move it out of the body and create space for new chi to flow.

7. Keep tapping your lower back for three breath cycles; then start to allow your tapping action to migrate higher and lower. If you encounter a tender spot, rather than moving away from it, linger on it compassionately and lovingly and breathe focused chi into the spot before moving on. In total, travel up and down your back at a moderate and mindful pace for nine breath cycles before immediately moving on to the next exercise.

Hindquarter Love Tap

The Hindquarter Love Tap activates the kidney and urinary bladder meridian and the lung and large intestine meridian as it releases held tension in the gluteal muscles of the buttocks, thus eliminating a potential source of lower-back pain.

1. Begin in the same inverted position as the last exercise. Still rounding forward in a large C shape and still in the flow of the Door-of-Life tapping sequence, begin not just to tap, but to hammer your glutes, covering the expanse of your entire buttocks. Increase the velocity of the impact of your fists against your body.
2. Breathe deeply and smoothly and focus now on making the tapping movements a substantive, vigorous action with each love "hammer" you do against your buttocks, and feel as though your fists are pounding against the flesh of your buttocks without apology. This should be a don't-hold-back, give-it-all-you've-got kind of thumping, because you are now working on denser tissues in the hindquarters, which appreciate a firmer, more intentional pressure with impact.
3. Be mindful and sensitive to your body, but think of this, as Mantak Chia used to say, as "beating yourself up in a good way, with love." We tend to beat ourselves up by berating ourselves with negative internal

diatribes. This is the opposite. This kind of tough love is the best, as ultimately it can even relieve back pain. Find the perfect pressure for your own body. Don't hold back or rear away (no pun intended) from intensity when it comes to your glutes.

4. Continue thumping on your buttocks for five rounds of breath. During the last few breath cycles, straighten your spine so that you are erect. This will change the way the thumping feels on your hindquarters: the flesh, now much softer and less extended, will move under your hands in a different way and respond to your touch slightly differently too. See which you prefer, as both are very beneficial.

Hip Love

The bones of the pelvis become more vulnerable as we age. Hip Love sends them a powerful energy signal to stay strong, as it liberates chronic holding patterns in the muscles surrounding the hip joints. It disperses stagnation in the liver and gallbladder meridians that run through the hips and relieves stress and frustration.

1. Standing tall, tilt your pelvis slightly forward and underneath you. Make fists with your hands and position your fists so that you can thump their pinky sides against your body.
2. In a pounding action that's similar to tenderizing meat with a mallet, with bent elbows, you will use your forearms and fists to strike firmly on the fleshy indentation at the side of your hip directly adjacent to your hip bone. Following the first several thumps you make to the sides of your hips, circle your forearms slightly forward and back to thump, establishing a smooth rhythm. Make these elliptical circles a total of nine times.
3. After nine smooth circles, skip the circling back motion and simply pound, firmly but gently, into the same spot at a more accelerated

pace. Be sure to continue to breathe deeply and smoothly throughout. Infusing the areas you are working with fresh oxygen can help you move stagnant chi out of your body and mind, so take generous Horse Breaths as needed.

Up and Down the Jing Channels

Up and Down the Jing Channels opens, activates, and harmonizes the leg channels that house the kidney and urinary bladder, liver and gallbladder, and stomach and spleen meridians, stimulating the *jing* (sexual essence, which is an essential longevity elixir) in the legs to rise.

1. Without pause, directly following the Hip Love exercise, inhale deeply and smoothly, consciously drawing energy up into your Sea of Chi from your Bubbling Spring Points and Root. As you exhale, start to thump down the outsides of your legs, using the pinky sides of your fists, going all the way down to your ankles with the same momentum you've built over the course of the past several minutes of love thumping—now reaching a crescendo.
2. Inhale again and start thumping on your inner ankles, this time turning your palms toward your inner legs before striking the flat part of your fingers between your knuckles against your legs. Travel up the inner line of the legs, coming all the way back up to the upper inner thigh and groin area.
3. Then, as you exhale, once again travel down the path on the outsides of your legs, waking up the leg channels as you go. Take another final pass up the insides of your legs while inhaling.
4. Immediately go down the outsides of the legs again, stopping and staying down at the bottom and exaggerating the rounding of your spine. This positions you perfectly to embark on the final sections of your legs that need to be thumped with love: your hamstrings and calves.

5. With your neck completely relaxed, head hanging heavy, and using slightly more force and impact with your fists than previously, start to thump on your hamstring muscles on the backs of your legs, alternating with your right and left fists.
6. When you are hammering at the hamstrings, I recommend that you use your fists with your palms facing the hamstrings, fingers snugly curled in against the palms and with the thumbs resting to the side of the index fingers, not across them. That creates a flatter surface to thump with.
7. After thumping on your hamstrings for several rounds of breath, without pausing move down to your calves and begin thumping them using the thumb sides of your fists. Your head should still be heavy, your neck relaxed, and your breathing conscious, fluid, and deep as you do so.
8. While still working on your calves, turn out your toes slightly and, switching to the pinky side of the fists, begin to pound into your inner calves, going up and down the lower legs. I recommend that while you are thumping, pounding, and hammering the legs, you take Horse Breaths whenever the spirit moves you and you feel you need a good release, a way to deal with all the surprising sensation you are experiencing as you travel up and down your legs, waking *jing* as you go.
9. Continue hammering for a few rounds of breath, and then rise up to an erect stance with your arms down by your sides for a breath.
10. Then, as the final step in this sequence, starting at the top of your legs, brush down all sides of your legs with both hands vigorously, as if you are brushing lint off a pair of black velvet pants. What you're actually doing is brushing off the residue of stagnant chi that you've just liberated from your leg channels.
11. Finally, hold your arms away from your body and give your hands a good shake. Do a final post-thumping Horse Breath as a reward for all the hard work and good loving you gave your legs and lower-body meridians in the last four exercises.

Blossoming Open

Blossoming Open mobilizes and lubricates the spine, expands the chest, and stretches the muscles of the neck and shoulders. In the process, it makes you feel tall, proud, confident, empowered, and sexy. It's one of the most powerful ways I know to invite joy and happiness into your heart.

1. Standing tall, inhale and join your hands in Tiger Claws Unite position in front of your chest.
2. Exhale, invert your wrists, and then extend your arms straight in front of you, palms facing away from you. Round your spine backward into a deep C shape in opposition. Bend your knees deeply, keeping them in line with your toes, while firmly rooting your heels into the ground.
3. Open your hands with your fingers spread wide out in front of you for a brief second and then transition, as you inhale, coming into an arching position with knees bent, and your head up, shoulders drawn down and back.
4. Place the heels of the hands into the spot where your torso and your legs meet with your elbows bent out wide to your sides, wrists flexed back, and fingers spread wide.
5. Without stopping, continue the motion of your deep knee bend, sliding your hands all the way down the length of your legs as you exhale and round your upper torso down toward the ground at the same time, letting your head hang down. Lightly clasp your ankles (or as close as you can get to them) with your hands.
6. Release the hold on your ankles and extend your hands down to the ground (or as close as you can get). Turn your hands so that their backs are touching. Spread your fingers wide and let your head dangle. As you inhale, skim the floor in front of you with your fingertips as a starting point for the next movement, which will be lifting your arms skyward. You will be inhaling as long as it takes you to rise to standing.

7. Beginning to inhale, extend your arms straight along the floor in front of you and start to rise up by straightening the legs and reaching your arms farther out in front of you, while lifting them up higher and higher in a continuous arc. Keeping your head down, allow your gaze to follow your fingertips until they reach eye level. At that point, continue lifting your arms in an arc up overhead in a kind of slow explosion, where you are opening your upper back and chest and coming into a moderate back bend with your uppermost torso. As you bend backward, open your heart center to receive chi from heaven. Imagine and feel the warming rays of the sun on your face and filling your heart with new, life-giving energy.
8. Slowly return to standing upright and lower your arms to your sides. As your arms are circling down, with the palms still facing down, at the last moment, turn your palms to face forward by your sides to begin again.
9. Repeat the above steps seven times.

Wing-Tip Flex

The Wing-Tip Flex should make you feel as though you are on a rooftop in the movie *House of Flying Daggers,* about to vanquish your first enemy. It releases held tension from digital technology overuse and repetitive actions by opening the meridians in the arms, wrists, and fingers.

1. Begin with your feet parallel and your legs together with your toes spread wide, with your arms by your side. The crown of your head should reach toward the sky.
2. Assume Sword Finger Position.
3. Now straighten your arms out in front of you at chest height, shoulder-width apart, with your index and middle fingers pointing straight up.
4. Then open your straight arms to the sides of your body, keeping them in line with your shoulders. Rotate your arms so your palms face the

floor and breathe in deeply as you bend your wrists so that your fingers point down toward the floor. Press the backs of your wrists away from the center of your body. Inhale and exhale in this position.

5. Inhale again as you flex your wrists and point your sword fingers up toward the sky, pressing the heels of your hands away from your body in opposite directions.
6. Focus on your breathing. You will start to feel what will likely be intense sensations in your arms and hands as you hold this final position. Breathe into these sensations, knowing that your breath will facilitate the smooth flow of chi to your hands through the meridians in your arms. As you breathe, continue to think of keeping the Bubbling Spring Points open in your feet and drawing chi from the earth up into your body and into your Lower Elixir Field.
7. Hold the position for eight complete cycles of breath, in and out.

Goddess Breaths

The empowering exercise Goddess Breaths reinforces inner confidence, self-esteem, and willpower. It opens and activates the navel center and solar plexus, clearing anger and doubt. As you perform this action, you should do it vigorously, with real conviction, as if you were Michelle Yeoh in *Crouching Tiger, Hidden Dragon* or Bruce Lee elbow-checking an enemy trying to sneak up on you from behind. Instead of thinking about an enemy, however, consider this a confidence-building exercise that represents the assertion of your power, because you are rooting your feet firmly into the earth when you are singing out your truth: *HA!*

1. Step your legs three feet apart, then turn your toes out, so that your legs are externally rotated, and bend your knees deeply, taking care to align your knees with your toes.
2. Inhale and reach your arms up to the sky in front of you with your

palms facing forward, away from you, and your fingers spread wide to collect heaven chi.

3. As you exhale, pull your arms down swiftly, forming fists with your hands at the sides of your hips, and make a *HA!* sound that comes from your solar plexus—your very core. Your elbows are bent and behind your body. The *HA!* sound is both an exhalation and a sound vibration, and it serves two purposes. First, it can help you move anger and frustration out of your body-mind. Second, it can be a primal declaration, a way of announcing yourself and taking your place in the world, as in, "I am woman (or man). Hear me roar!"
4. Repeat the actions of reaching your arms up and pulling them down to your hips several times. As you pull the arms down to your hips with bent elbows, root your feet even more firmly into the earth and feel the power in your legs and entire being. Start these repetitions slowly at first, like an engine that is warming up. Inhale and stretch your arms up to the sky, and exhale and pull your elbows back to your hips, securing them there suddenly and with great intention, almost ferocity, without going over the top.
5. Then, like an engine that has reached its stride, inhale as you lift the arms and exhale as you pull them down, and start to consciously direct the energy you feel building inside your own body. It is very likely that you will feel a tingling sensation moving up and down your spine. That, my friend, is chi!
6. Do twenty-one repetitions all together. On the last one, hold your deep knee bend with the elbows connected strongly to your torso and deepen the squat, feeling the burn in your muscles and the pride in your heart grow. Stay here for three complete breath cycles. Then rise, straightening your legs and lifting your arms up overhead with your palms facing in, bathing your Upper Elixir Field with the chi you've harvested for a few rounds of breath.
7. Then rotate the arms out, facing your palms away from your body, and with softly bent elbows slowly bring them in a half circle down

in front of you to spread the energy out into your aura, to strengthen it, and to help the new energy flowing through you emanate into surrounding space.

8. Finish by placing the palm of your right hand (if you're a woman) on your Sea of Chi and covering it with your left hand. (If you're a man, do the opposite: cover your left hand with your right.) Close your eyes and breathe chi into your body.

5

unleash and transform: kundalini yoga

I first discovered the magic of kundalini in the late 1990s, at a soundstage in Los Angeles, while I was working on the shoot for the world's first-ever Pilates video. Famed yoga teacher Gurmukh, Yogi Bhajan's primary female disciple and kundalini maven, was on the set next door, and through the walls our whole cast and crew could hear the cacophony of babies crying, mothers chatting, and directions being shouted across the room. We were ready to start filming, and just as our head of production left to ask next door for quiet on the set, a perfect stillness settled over the entire space—and not just Gurmukh's space, but everywhere. We were all hypnotized by the mellifluous sound of voices united in singing, "AUM."

Compelled by the pure sound, I rose from my seat and went to see with my own eyes how the miraculous change had happened. Thirty mothers sat cross-legged in a large circle with their new infants in their laps. Like a human incarnation of the Third-Eye Chakra, beaming out into space, right there at the center of the circle was Gurmukh, glowing in her white turban and dress. She smiled peacefully, eyes twinkling and luminous, looking at least twenty years younger than her then fifty-eight years. I stood in the doorway, transfixed, as she began the warm-up exercises. I watched this gathering of women moving in unison with eyes closed, gyrating to awaken their *kundalini shakti,* the primordial feminine energy, which she promised would activate their life force and deliver the power to manifest great health, creativity, and abundance.

Sign me up now! I thought. The exercises appeared to be so simple and accessible, but at the same time clearly very challenging. As I watched the women perform an exercise that made them look like birds ferociously flapping their wings, it struck me that they were assuming the "alpha role" with their bodies—not beating them into submission, but showing them that they were coming along for the ride no matter what and that it was something for their mutual benefit.

Now, this doesn't exactly sound like an endorsement, but it really looked as though they were doing battle on the mat, confronting themselves in order to be able to make it through the rigors of what she was asking them to do. Though the challenge was clearly daunting, they periodically broke into determined smiles, urged on by what had to be a strong belief in the payoff. It was compelling.

What won me over was Gurmukh's strong narration as the women pumped their arms up and down rapidly, many of them clearly looking as if they wanted to quit. "It's the mind that wants you to stop. Be true to your own power and move through the discomfort," she said as she cheered them on in her powerful singsong way. "Just three more now, and you'll feel a freedom and bliss unlike anything you've ever known, and you will know that you were the one who made it happen."

And it was true. I watched these new mothers go from sleepily rubbing their eyes to rising up like spring flowers, rosy cheeked and ready for anything. After each sequence they performed, they became brighter, and, strange though it may sound, they appeared to be moving *into* themselves. Energy was rising within their bodies and radiating outwardly, right before my very eyes. It was a remarkable transformation.

It wasn't until I did the first kundalini yoga practice of my own that I really understood what a triumph it was to complete even a single kundalini sequence. The magic is in movements that demand you go well beyond your comfort zone, successfully traversing what I like to think of as the "fire swamp" from the movie *The Princess Bride*. It's not just moving through the "discomfort zone," but surviving the signals your mind sends you beseeching you to abort your mission, as you're steadfastly working your way past pain into trusting the wisdom of your higher self. You have to move beyond what can feel like the "pain threshold" to claim the prize that waits for you, smiling, glowing, and rejoicing on the other side—your authentic self and your true radiance. This "breaking on through to the other side," I quickly figured out, was the serpent's secret. It was what held the power to vanquish the ego, which likes to deal in the currency of limitation, and introduced you to your higher mind, the place where kundalini devotees claim your infinite potential can be realized—where anything is possible.

Relating to the first three chakras, the seductive pull of ego, or the "lower mind," is a strong one, because it is concerned primarily with survival and getting needs met. When challenged or discomforted, it flips into a kind of primal fight-or-flight response, wanting to keep things at a status quo and return to the homeostasis it knows. Thoughts of doubt start to proliferate, telling you that you "can't make it through another minute." It drags you by the hair in order to get you back under its thumb, to return to the all-too-comfy passive couch of familiarity, running the show and returning you to the same negative loop of thoughts that yield the same unproductive results.

Mark Twain once said, "Never argue with a fool. Onlookers may not be able to tell the difference." When you try to argue with your lower mind, it reacts in much the same way that an anxiety attack can take you prisoner within seconds when you resist it. *All I have ever wanted,* I thought to myself, as I watched the women persevere through the trial by fire, *was to be free of the foibles and terrors of the lower mind and be able to soar above it.* This was my opportunity to do it.

Having suffered more than once in my life from severe anxiety, I was struck by the thought that this was an antidote if there was a next time—if I started to feel its creepy, relentless vine dance up my spine and into my throat. I have come to know in no uncertain terms that one must be able to recognize yin and yang in all things, to know how energies match one another. In this domain, where we are talking about cultivating the fire power to take on our own minds, we need something of equal strength and power.

The kundalini sequences I watched Gurmukh teaching demanded a sheer tenacity and determination, a pointed physicality, to make it past the anxiety and on through to the other side. Some of the moments seemed utterly impossible; the mothers were being asked to cross barriers that were utterly impassable—at least in their minds. The kundalini sequences are so challenging not because they require physical strength or ability, but because it takes something that powerful to move past the doubting mind of the ego to find liberation. In order to taste freedom, I had to make it through the gauntlet of the limited, objecting mind to land safely, truly safely, upon the shores of greater possibility—where I would discover my infinite self, my limitless potential.

It was this stoking of the inner fire that promised there was something better, beyond the familiar, beyond "good enough." And I wanted something better than the anti-anxiety drugs and antidepressants (as useful as they could be at times). It was this merging of body with will and love that could not only silence the doubting mind, but quell fear and separation (from rational thought and truth) and restore me to myself.

The Power to Weather the Storm

Though I may have first been introduced to kundalini in the late 1990s, I didn't really understand its power until I experienced a relentless string of anxiety attacks after a great personal loss in 2008. It was my mother who found articles on how going into the eye of the storm and inviting anxiety to pull up a chair and have some tea was the way to stop it in its tracks even before it had mounted its attack.

When I practiced this direct approach along with my kundalini, I felt as though I had won the lottery. I felt a kind of relief, safety, and peace of mind I had never known until then. I felt empowered. After experiencing its miraculous benefits, I knew that the next time I found myself on the edge of the fire swamp, I would have the right artillery to beat back those big, ugly fire rats before they could even start to think of nibbling at my heels.

Kundalini came to my rescue again just a few years ago when my healthy and powerful mother, who came from hardy eastern European Jewish stock, was diagnosed with multiple myeloma in late May 2013. Though she beat it and went into full remission months later, by January 2014 she had decided that she had suffered enough and stopped treatment. The cancer came back with a vengeance. By July 2014, she was moved to hospice and prepared for flight.

I was overcome with so much emotion, fear, and reckless anxiety that I didn't know what to do. I stood in my sister's living room, trying somehow to manage the agony of what was happening. I felt the rumblings of the inner tsunami building. Instead of being able to move past the shock to tears, which would have actually served as a release, I felt I was being dragged, bound and gagged, toward a precipice where a hungry pterodactyl waited, licking its lips and salivating. It had been years since I'd felt anxiety's vise grip, and I was frozen, incredulous that this slide into Hades could be happening to me again.

But this time was different. This time *I* was different. I was prepared.

I had my secret weapon. Exhausted, terrified, and shaking, I started my kundalini practice and with each *kriya* (exercise), I felt the thoughts of impending doom recede a bit more. The anxiety didn't just whimper and slink away; it shrieked like a banshee and ran out of the room at breakneck speed. And there I was—somehow standing tall, starting to believe that I might live to see another day.

Out of all the other practices I could have done, kundalini was what I chose in that moment, because I knew it was the only thing powerful enough to match the intensity and velocity of what was rising up inside me. Kundalini is what carried me through, changing my brain chemistry just minutes after I started the practice, so that I could return to myself. I broke through the shock and trauma to the heartbreak and sadness inside, so that I could finally cry and release my body from the enervating fight-or-flight response in overdrive. The kundalini practice helped me find the resilience that my anxiety claimed I lacked. With every breath, I knew on the deepest core level that I had inherited some of my mother's indomitable spirit and ability to be a survivor and that I was going to be okay.

When I went to visit my mother in hospice, I felt vulnerable, exposed in a way that made me feel enraged, but I didn't have the strength to express it. The doctors shared too much about how her body was deteriorating, being consumed by the myeloma, how one by one each of her functions was being overwhelmed. This magnificent light, my very own mother, was being swallowed up by the invaders in her body as the precious seconds ticked by.

To be completely present for her I had to call upon a new strength to strong-arm the hysterical tears and primal screams that wanted to erupt from me. I watched my mother, my soul mate, let her own tears flow after years of never wanting to cry. It was all I could do to contain myself. I had to let her know that it was all okay—it was okay that she had decided it was time, okay that she was finally crying. We would have had to say good-bye sooner or later, and although that day was here long before any of us could bear, we would all be okay. We loved her more than life itself. It was the hardest thing I have ever had to do in my life.

Aside from the stuff I am made of and what I have grown in the garden of my soul from every twist and turn and fall of the heart I have weathered, it was in large part the Unleash and Transform practice I did every day leading up to July 13—the last day that our eyes would ever meet—that gave me the courage I needed to be able to say good-bye to her and help her on her way when she finally flew away to start her next journey as pure spirit, waking energy in the beyond.

Snake Charming: Kundalini Rising

Now you should be starting to get a glimpse of the fact that all roads lead to Rome. In Unleash and Transform, we enter a new domain where our three elixir fields, our energy storage centers from qigong, become seven chakras, our meridians become *nadis* (energy pathways in the yogic tradition), and the three portals that seal the energy in your energy storage centers (your elixir fields) become the yogic equivalent, your three *bandhas,* or energy locks.

Here you will learn two empowering and energizing sequences, Charming the Snake and Kundalini Rising, that will distribute life-giving *prana* (energy) to every part of your body, almost instantly changing your mood and perhaps even lifting you to a place of natural euphoria.

Let me invite you now to your first dance with *kundalini shakti,* the energy of pure conscious awakening, the primordial divine feminine. Join me as we stoke the fire inside, coaxing the "coiled snake" to rise up out of her lair. *Kundalini shakti* is our sacred, sexual energy and one of our most precious endowments as human beings, holding the power to transform our lives. When you awaken it, you release the energy of bliss and tran-

The Chakra System

1. **Root Chakra** (*muladhara*):

   Location: Base of the spine in the tailbone area

   Emotional resonance: Security, safety, and grounding

   Color: Red

2. **Sacral Chakra** (*svadhishthana*):

   Location: Lower abdomen, about two inches below the navel and two inches in

   Emotional resonance: Creativity, joy, and enthusiasm

   Color: Orange

3. **Solar Plexus Chakra** (*manipura*):

   Location: Upper abdomen in the stomach area

   Emotional resonance: Personal power, expansiveness, and seeds of spirituality

   Color: Yellow

4. **Heart Chakra** (*anahata*):

   Location: Center of chest just above the heart

   Emotional resonance: Devotion, passion, and unconditional love for the self and others

   Color: Green

5. **Throat Chakra** (*vishuddha*):

   Location: Throat

   Emotional resonance: Independence, fluid thought, and clear, empowered communication

   Color: Blue

6. **Third-Eye Chakra** (*ajna*):

   Location: Forehead between the eyes

   Emotional resonance: Intuitive visioning and cosmic consciousness

   Color: Purple

7. **Crown Chakra** (*sahasrara*):

   Location: The very top of the head

   Emotional resonance: Pure crystalline consciousness, release of the body self, and connection to the divine

   Color: White

scendence, which makes you glow with a radiance far beyond what even great sex can achieve.

When you unleash your own *kundalini shakti,* there is nothing more empowering or fulfilling; you shine in an even bigger way, because you have made it happen for yourself. When you nurture your own life force, you come to intimately understand that your sexual energy *is* sacred, and you start to guard it like the precious jewel, the all-powerful secret, that it is, meant to be shared with only those who deserve it. This instills a new kind of self-love, respect, and appreciation for your own body, your *self,* and your soul. This realization alone wakes prodigious stores of energy inside and gives birth to much, much more.

Activating and unleashing *kundalini shakti* awakens your most primal, powerful, original sexual energy and your creative life-force energy. They are one and the same. You liberate your natural talents. You tap into your innate primal wisdom, your power to know, to act, to greet life with grace, resilience, confidence, and courage. *Shakti* means you are your own port in the storm, and you know how to drop down into deep calm, rest, and rejuvenation. *Shakti* is the discernment of what to keep and what to discard. It's the physical power to transform stagnation into vibrancy, to expel toxins and negativity from your body and your mind, and the mental and emotional wherewithal to let go of what no longer serves you. *Shakti* is the power to breathe deeply, to fully enjoy and appreciate the bounty of nature, to digest the nutrients your body needs, and integrate the experiences you live. *Shakti* is gratitude. *Shakti* *is* life.

Simply by moving through the kriyas that follow, we activate and balance our chakra and endocrine systems, raising our creative, sexual vibration and energy from the lower three chakras to the higher centers of refinement in our being, our upper three energy centers and our "higher mind," where earth meets with heaven and we manufacture the most potent elixir we know. The beauty of the practice here is in its innate simplicity. You only need to become acquainted with your chakras and the qualities and the parts of the mind, body, and spirit they correspond to in order to wake even more energy inside you to become the seasoned mystic of your own domain, charm kundalini upward, ever upward, where your own sexual energy becomes your fuel for life, your greatest tool for empowerment, and your own luminous energy.

the unleash and transform practice

TIME OF DAY: Morning

QUALITY: Yang

SUBTLE ENERGY: Opens and activates the chakra system.

BENEFITS: Mobilizes *kundalini shakti*, the primal life force, to heal and balance the endocrine system and organ function; fosters self-empowerment and healthy, balanced sexuality.

PROPS: Yoga mat, yoga blocks

The Practice:

Charming the Snake: Seated Practice

- Sufist Grind
- Heart Opener
- Child's Pose for the Crown
- Radiance Stretch
- Goddess Rolls
- Reaching Across Space and Time
- Active Cat
- Superhero
- Wings of Victory
- Taking Flight

Kundalini Rising: Standing Practice

- Archer
- Calling Destiny Home
- Shaking the Soul Tree
- Abdominal Pumping
- Corpse Pose (*Savasana*)

Before You Begin

The Kundalini Seat

For our kundalini practices (as well as our meditations in Chapter 10), you will learn a simple cross-legged variation called the Easy Pose and something called the Zazen Seat. There better be something "easy" in kundalini, because the practice itself is one of the most challenging and rewarding you will ever experience!

If for some reason you don't find either of the poses easy or accessible, you can always place blocks or bolsters directly underneath your knees to prop them up and relieve any undue tension or discomfort you may have been feeling without them. If neither of the seats is viable at all and doesn't suit you when you first begin the practice, you are welcome to sit in a chair.

Take note that although the positions may not be accessible to you when you first begin, after you dedicate yourself to practicing Awaken and Play for some time, it is highly probable that all the exercises in the kundalini practice will eventually become sequences you can do, and perhaps even one day without props. Keep in mind, as with all the practices, that they are *your* practices and, as such, intended to partner with you, facilitating your journey. They are not meant to discourage or intimidate you. Do whatever you need to do to modify them as your body indicates.

Easy Pose

1. Sitting tall, come into a good old-fashioned, conventional crossed-legged seat, as though you were sitting in front of a campfire.
2. With your spine tall and relaxed, bring your feet underneath your

knees, laying them on the outer edge, pinky side, of each foot, allowing your knees to fall out to the sides, with the hips comfortably positioned higher than the knees.

3. You can experiment to see which leg feels best stacked in front, and once you have found your best, most comfortable position, maintain it for a while and then you can and should alternate which leg is in front to balance the body.
4. You may find that you need a block or a cushion underneath you, so that you can sit more comfortably, because you want your hips to be higher than your knees and for the body to feel as comfortable and as easy as possible, as you don't want to be distracted by your seat even before you enter into the practice itself.

Zazen Seat

1. Sitting tall, draw your right foot in toward your groin and line the heel up with the midline of the body, laying your foot onto the pinky side, bringing it snug in as close as possible toward your Root. Lay the knee down to the side of your body, so that it opens out, falling naturally down to the floor.
2. Then draw the left foot in and repeat exactly what you did with your right foot, tucking it in, pinky side down to the floor, in front of the right foot, so that they are like fire logs stacked in front of one another, and again, lay the left knee down and out onto the floor.
3. As with the campfire seat, you may need a block or a cushion underneath you so that you can sit more comfortably and have your hips higher than your knees.

Kundalini Breathing

Breath of Fire

We will use the Breath of Fire for nearly every exercise in our kundalini practice. It awakens the body and enlivens the mind, clearing the sinuses and pathways to the lungs, warming the body, and creating a feeling of pure exhilaration and inner strength.

The Breath of Fire is one of the most powerful methods of breath control that we possess. It helps to release fear and relieve anxiety, appeases depression, and is a formidable opponent in helping to vanquish addiction. It reduces stress and alleviates pain. The very act of pumping the diaphragm and the abdominal center, as we know from qigong, keeps your Sea of Chi energy center awake and alive. Now with this added component of the breath charging it, your life force becomes even more powerful.

Because the pumping action has a direct effect on the navel center, where thousands of nerves meet and feelings register first, it cleanses negativity and balances the emotions. It regulates, harmonizes, and strengthens the nervous system and massages the internal organs, improving digestion and elimination. It increases lung capacity and enhances circulation, flushing impurities and deposits from the lungs, from the mucous lining and blood vessels themselves, cleansing the blood and aiding in detoxification. When practiced regularly, the Breath of Fire can actually produce such a relaxed, but conscious state in the mind that it mimics something called a global alpha rhythm in the brain, which usually occurs during quiet moments, while you're daydreaming or meditating.

And like your very own heartbeat, the Breath of Fire synchronizes your entire system to one rhythm, promoting greater internal harmony and health, generating a deeply beneficial internal heat that activates, opens, and balances the smooth flow of prana through the nadis, thereby dramatically increasing your energy.

Rapidly breathe a series of short, terse inhalations and vigorous, forceful exhalations, one breath quickly following the next, with a nanosecond of retention after each exhalation.

The most important thing to remember with the Breath of Fire is that you want to get into a hypnotic rhythm in which you let the breath "breathe you." And as challenging as it is at first, the Breath of Fire becomes another prime opportunity to practice effortless effort. When the physical component of the work starts to overwhelm your inner resolve and your lower mind tries to wrestle you to the ground, the breath will be your strongest ally.

Long Deep Breathing

The very foundation of all yogic breathing techniques is the two-part breath we use in Long Deep Breathing.

1. On the inhalation, breathing from bottom to top, fill and expand the belly, then the lower and middle rib cage, and then the upper chest.
2. On the exhalation, proceed in reverse, emptying first the upper chest and then the middle and lower rib cage, and then drawing the abdomen in to fully empty the breath from the belly.

Inhalation and exhalation are responsible for our life force itself and our very lives. With their own characters and qualities, they ask for different kinds of attention. Inhalation for example, was once synonymous with inspiration, reminding us that even in Western civilization the intimate links between breath and spirit were once acknowledged. During inhalation the chest expands and the lungs are filled with fresh air. But in the larger sense, inhalation signals the intake of vital energy, vital force, which makes possible the body's equilibrium and coherence, its activity and creativity.

The Kundalini Mantra

A mantra is a phrase repeated to aid in concentration. As you will come to know when you read the chapter on meditation, the mantra and your faithful breath are your guides. If the breath is your anchor, then the mantra is your compass. *Sat Nam* (literally, "true name"), which means "I am truth," "Truth is my name," or "I honor the truth within," is the central mantra most often used in kundalini yoga to connect with the divine; it reinforces personal power, true embodiment, and positive action, on the mat and off.

Applying the Locks: The Four *Bandhas*

Now that you're familiar with the different breathing techniques we will employ in our practice, it's time to safeguard the jewels. When you want to protect your valuables, your important documents, jewelry, mementos, what do you do? You lock them up. That is exactly what we are going to learn to do with our body's most precious possession by far: the breath. In kundalini yoga a lock is a muscular contraction or sealing of certain parts of the body for the purpose of retaining the breath. The three most common are the Root Lock, the Abdominal Lock, and the Throat Lock. When all three are applied at the same time, it is called the Great Lock. What's funny about learning the three locks in kundalini yoga is that previously we learned how to open our energy portals to receive heaven and earth chi, and here we are going to learn to seal them to further our energy cultivation abilities; we are simply traveling from China to India now and giving the energy "portals" different names, but the game is the same.

Root Lock

The first of our three locks, *mula bandha,* is the Root Lock. After the diaphragm descends into the abdominal cavity upon inhalation and the Root

Lock is applied by contracting the perineum and the urogenital webbing, the dense band of muscle between the genitals and the anus, the pelvic floor is raised and the breath you've just inhaled is compressed, or locked in, retained. The energy of the breath is sent deep into the abdominal cavity and held there. Internal pressure increases and, in combination with the other two locks, Abdominal and Throat, circulation increases and blood is exchanged optionally in the internal organs and surrounding tissues.

When you can root your own breath inside you, your energy gets locked inside where it can do its best work and strengthen you from the inside out, literally. When I apply the lock after inhalation, I can actually envision my breath becoming life-force "mist" inside me, a magic ether supercharged by my nurturing intention, circulating and nourishing everything it touches.

This later translates into "rooting to rise" in our actual yoga practice, when we root our feet into the earth to rise, to lift our bodies higher away from the earth. It is the rooting, the deepening into yin, into earth, that gives us the power to soar, to fly, to connect then to heaven, and it all starts with your own breath and how you consciously direct it. This is also what generates energy.

When you consciously commit to "guarding" your energy, as in becoming the guardian, the protector, of it, the one who savors the resource, it grows. Applying the first of the three locks, the Root Lock, is what establishes your innermost foundation and consecrates your commitment to the waking of your own energy.

Since I always learn the best through contrast, I believe you will too. We are first going to practice retaining the breath without applying the Root Lock and then see how different it feels when we do.

1. Sit in Easy Pose with your palms face down on your knees and inhale to three-quarters full. Hold your breath as long as you comfortably can, and while you do, tune into what this retention feels like. What is

the quality of the retention? Where is it exactly that you can sense the breath being held? Just before you feel as though you can't hold your breath any longer, exhale.

2. Inhale again, and now, just as you begin to hold the breath, coordinate your breathing and the contraction of your perineum and start to squeeze it at that very moment. Can you feel the difference? Can you feel how now the breath actually *is* locked inside? You can feel the "energy bathtub stopper" that you have applied. It's real. The Root Lock gives you a place to orient your senses, a "bottom," literally, a foundation, a floor from which the breath can then rise inside you. This is your first example of "rooting to rise."
3. As you squeeze your perineum, don't exert too much pressure; simply try your best to isolate the area and remember effortless effort, appreciating the subtle stimulation and lift that the contraction creates in your lower body, in your Root. Retain the breath as long as you comfortably can while squeezing, and then as you exhale gently release *mula bandha* and rest, taking in a few easy, natural breaths.

Abdominal Lock

The Abdominal Lock, *uddiyana bandha,* is also used to seal in the therapeutic compression, but this time it is located in the center of the abdominal cavity. When the Abdominal Lock is applied, the rectus abdominus, your central abdominal muscle does most of the work, helping you to draw your navel strongly toward your spine. And when you combine the Root Lock with the Abdominal Lock, not only does it encourage a healthy massage of the internal organs and glands, but it creates a powerful, propulsive force that pushes blood up into the chest cavity, just like a pump, temporarily relieving the heart of its normal workload.

Brief moments like these, of enhanced abdominal and urogenital contraction save your heart a substantial amount of work, because the locks create their own force that acts very much like your own heart. In fact, while you are maintaining your retention, you will become more sensitive and sympathetic to—more appreciative of—the beat of your own heart and its natural function, how hard it works all the time on your behalf. You will distinctly feel your heart slow down and beat in a more deliberate way. Imagine if you were to breathe this way even a few times a week how it would enhance the health and work life of your own sweet heart.

1. Sit in easy pose and bring your palms face down on your knees. Again, learning through contrast, inhale to three-quarters full, and hold your breath as long as you can and sense into what this feels like; then exhale and rest.

   Now inhale again, and this time imagine you are wearing a tight pair of jeans, and at the top of your inhalation, as you retain the breath, draw your navel strongly toward your spine, imagining that you are trying to pull your belly in and away from the waistband. Hold this contraction of your deep abdominal muscles for the duration of your breath retention.
2. As you are holding your breath with the Abdominal Lock applied, can you feel the difference, and now how when you draw your navel in with the lungs filled, you are in essence creating a greater internal pressure and sending the breath higher up into the chest cavity?
3. When you can no longer comfortably hold your breath, release both your breath and *uddiyana bandha* and return to a natural breath and rest.
4. It may strike you as funny if I were to tell you that applying the Abdominal Lock on its own, is actually harder on its own than when you apply it in concert with the Root Lock. It just makes more physical sense when both are applied, makes it easier to control the breath and energy you have retained and that is circulating inside you. Just wait until we get to *maha bandha,* where we apply all three locks together. This is the most powerful combination and exerts the greatest benefit on the body.

Throat Lock

The last of the three locks, the Throat Lock, *jalandhara bandha*, serves many functions. When you constrict the throat area, clamping down on the glottis at the back of the throat, blood is diverted and distributed to the lower body, facilitating more balanced circulation. The Throat Lock seals the breath down inside the lungs after you have inhaled so that it doesn't rise up, causing uncomfortable pressure in the throat, nostrils, and the eustachian tubes during compression. Finally, the action of dropping the chin slightly forward toward the chest creates a gentle traction for the spinal column, stretching the dura mater, the fascial sheath from the skull to the sacrum, stimulating all the muscles and nerves that run along the spine.

1. Before you begin, note that this one is harder to "find" than the other two, the Abdominal and Root Locks. In easy pose, with the hands face down on the knees, inhale through the nose to three-quarters full and contract the throat muscles by clamping down the glottis over the trachea, at the back of the throat.
2. At the top of your inhalation, with the Throat Lock applied, tuck the chin in slightly toward the chest, stretching the back of the neck, without sacrificing the length or integrity in your upper spine; don't allow the shoulders to roll forward at all. Your shoulders are relaxed and dropped down and back, open, your chest is expanded, and your neck is long and relaxed even as it's tilting forward.
3. Hold the breath here as long as you comfortably can, focusing on the breath and energy circulating, locked safely inside you.
4. When you are ready to exhale, raise the chin, leveling your gaze, so that your eyes are focused straight ahead, and let the air flow gently out of your nose. Then, return to your natural breathing and rest, taking stock, tuning into how you feel and sensing into the subtle energy flowing inside you as a result of your conscious breathing, your retention with the Throat Lock applied.

Great Lock

Now we will take everything we have just learned and apply *maha bandha,* the Great Lock, the mother of all bandhas. We will combine the three locks, activating and sealing the *mula, uddiyana,* and *jalandhara bandhas* to facilitate the flow of prana through the nadis and your central channel, the *sushumna nadi*. We will balance the left channel (*ida nadi*) and the right channel (*pingala nadi*), and this in turn will balance your overall subtle energy, emotion and logic, the left and right hemispheres of the brain, nourishing the energy in your kidneys and calming your mind to enhance mental focus in preparation for meditation.

We will apply Great Lock at certain strategic times throughout the kundalini practice. But for the most part, we will simply apply the Root Lock after most of the exercises.

Note: The Great Lock can be performed both with the arms down and hands on your knees, or with the arms sweeping up to the ceiling. We are going to learn the arms-up variation for our kundalini practice.

1. In the Easy Pose, as you inhale your breath to three-quarters full, sweep your arms up overhead and link your thumbs together, with your other fingers pointing straight up to the sky. Retain the breath, and as you do, squeeze the perineum, then draw the abdominal muscles in toward the spine and finally, drop the chin down toward the chest.
2. Deeply sense into the energy of your root, reaching down deep into the earth below, and your arms reaching up to connect to heaven energy. As you hold your breath, become even more attuned to the powerful oppositional energies vibrating inside you, as well as the circulation of *prana* throughout your body, delivering nourishment to every cell.
3. Retain your breath as long as you comfortably can, and then as you start to exhale, release the three locks, starting with the throat, lifting the chin

Kundalini Yoga

Sufist Grind

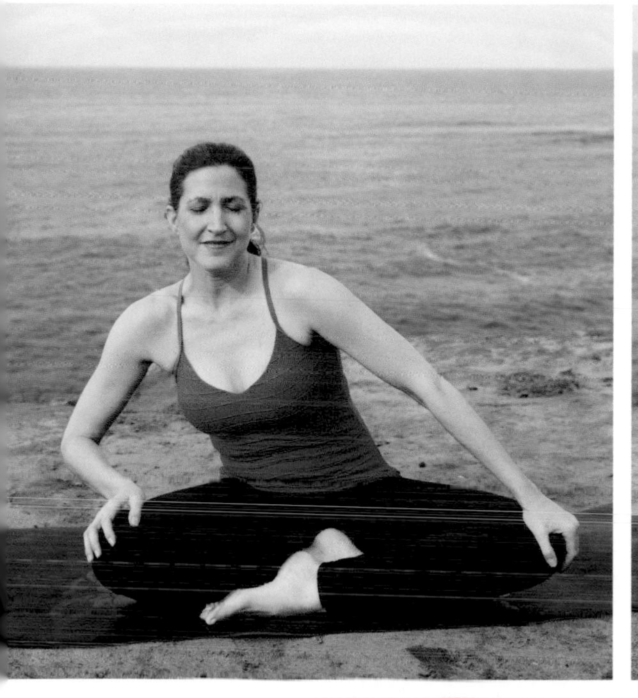

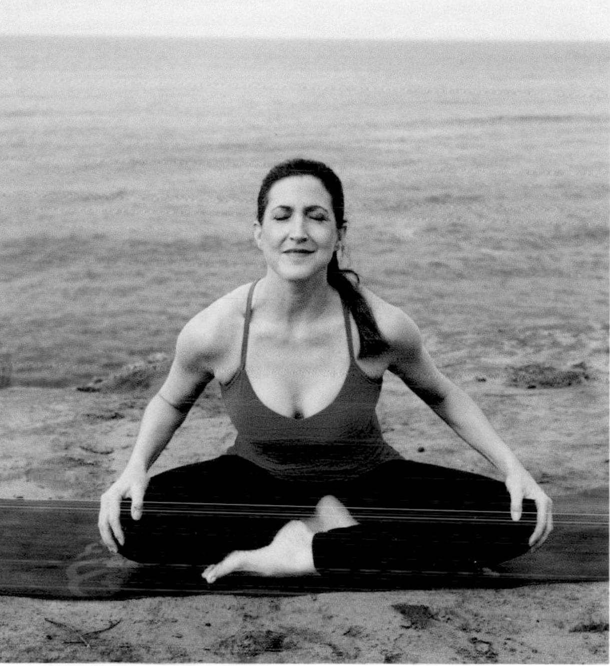

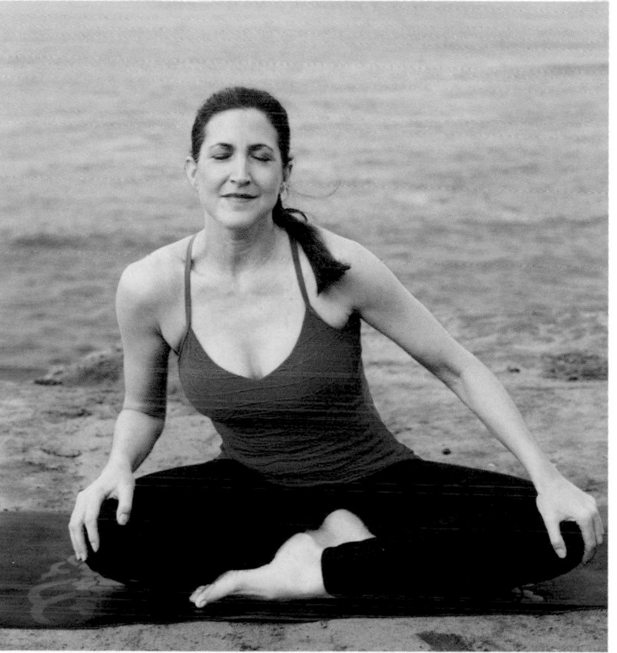

Heart Opener

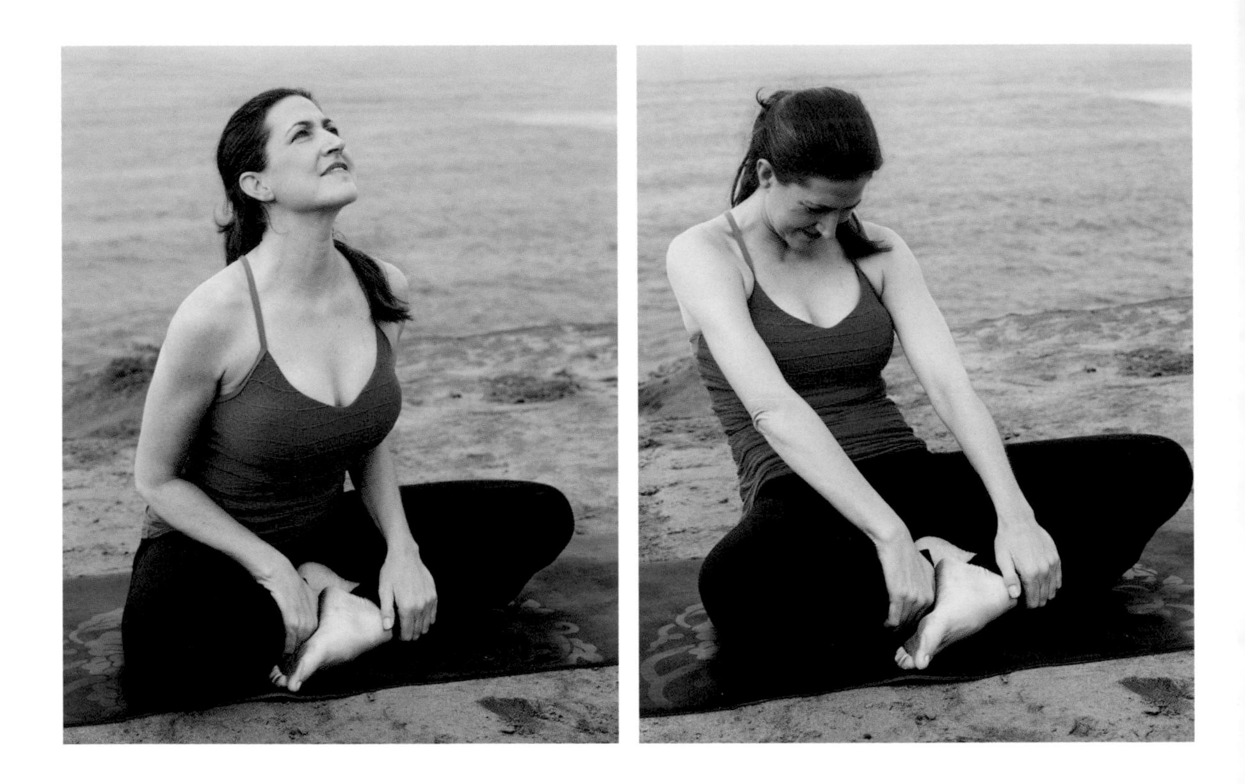

Child's Pose for the Crown

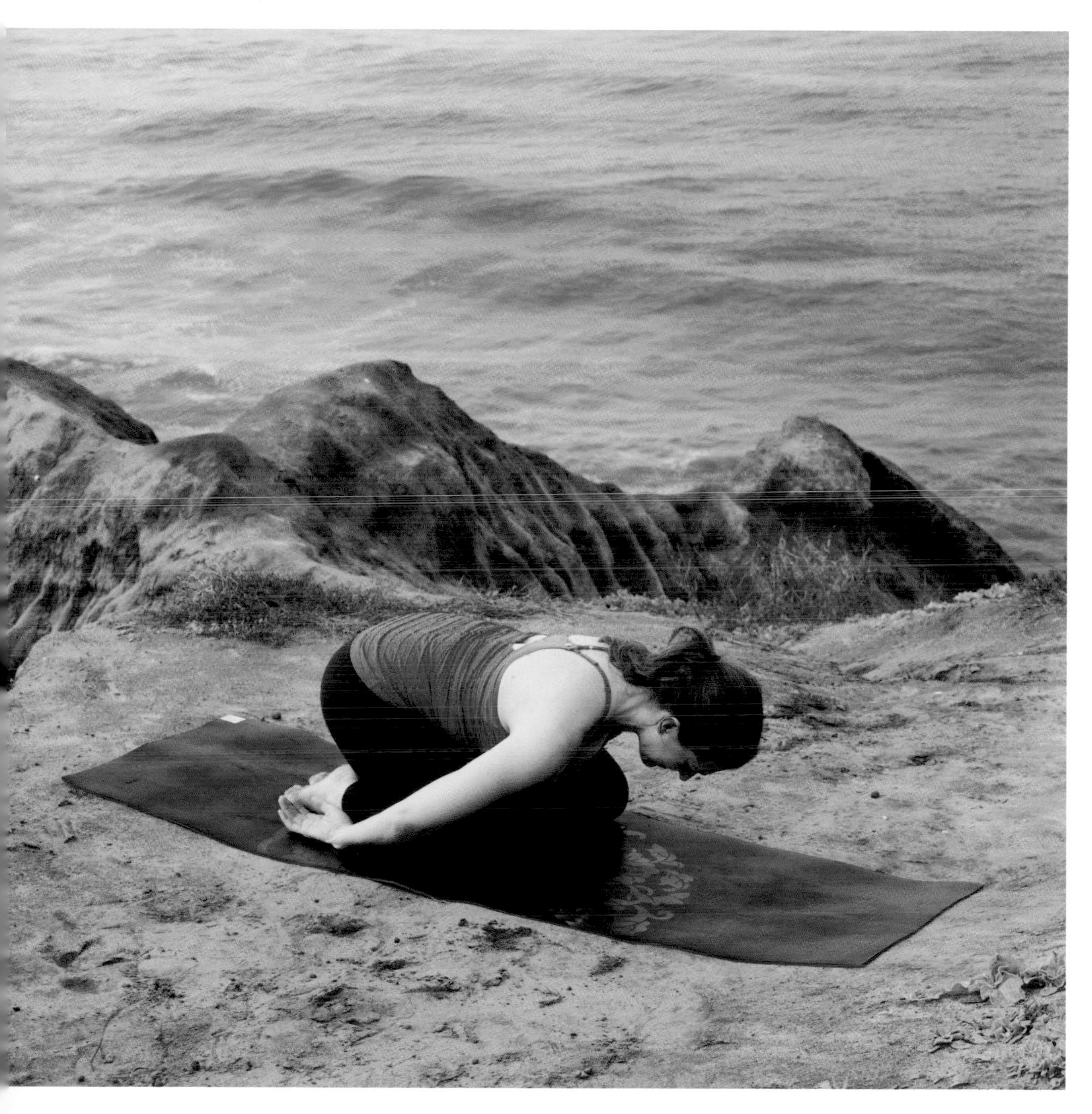

Radiance Stretch

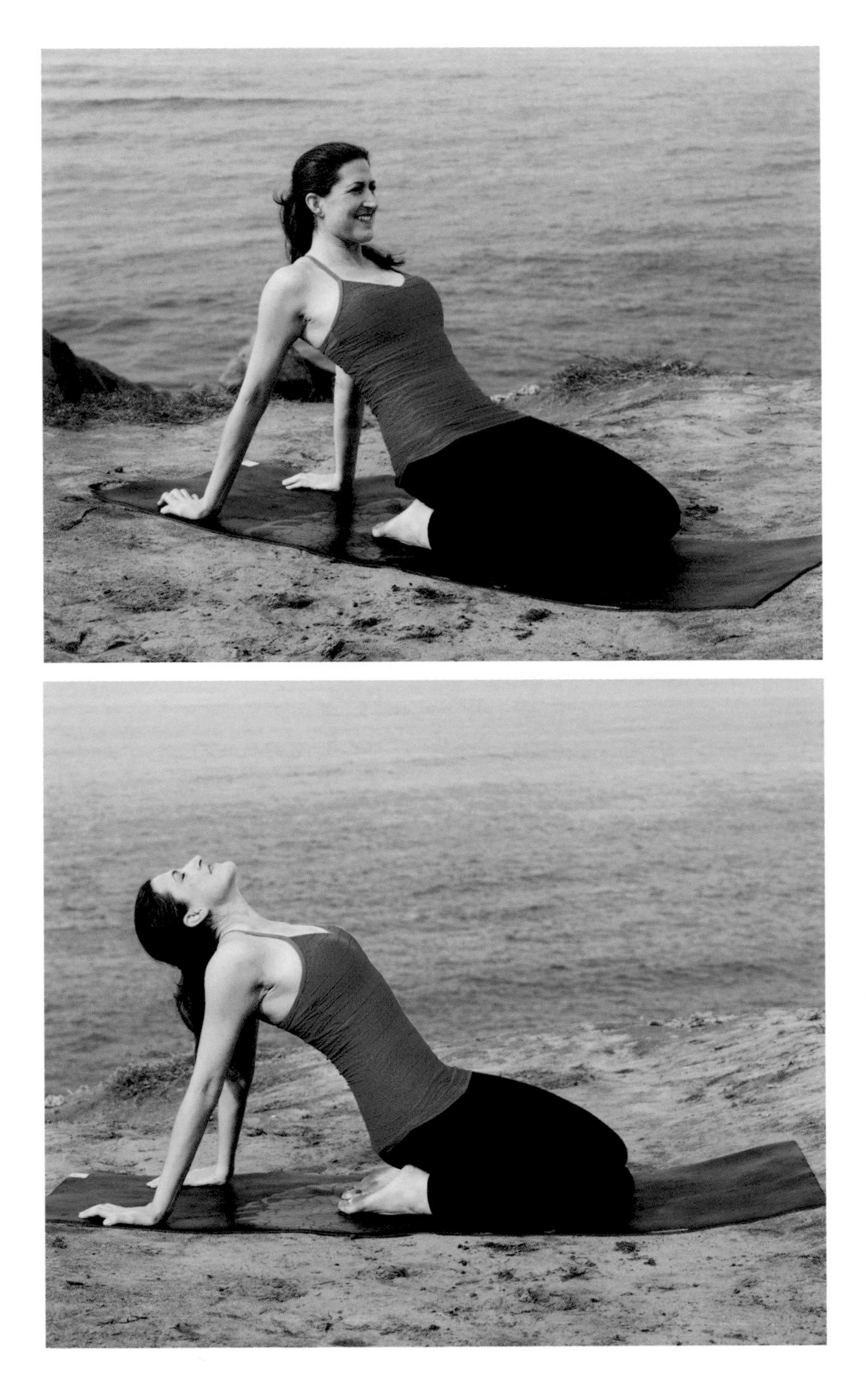

Goddess Rolls

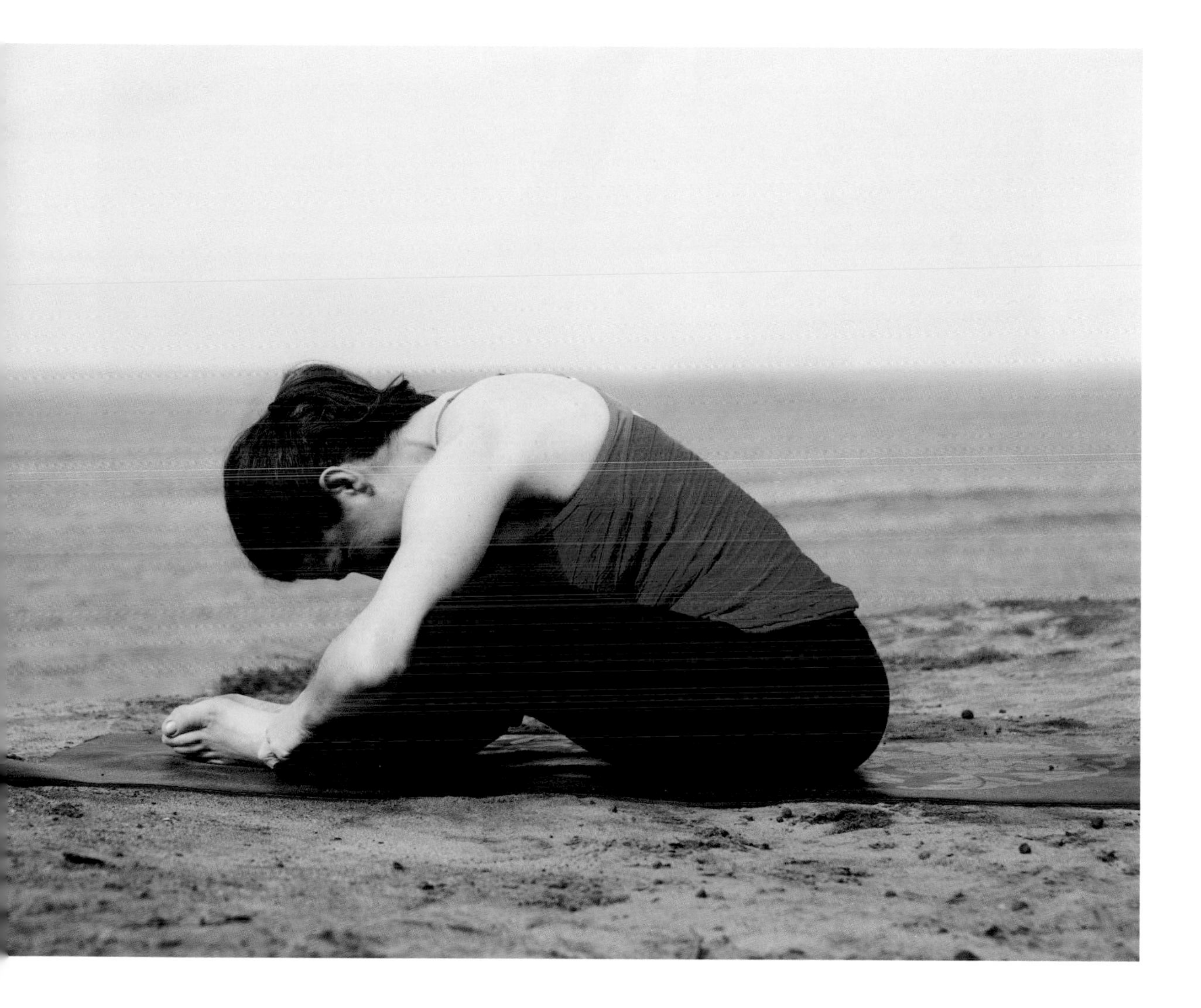

Reaching Across Space and Time

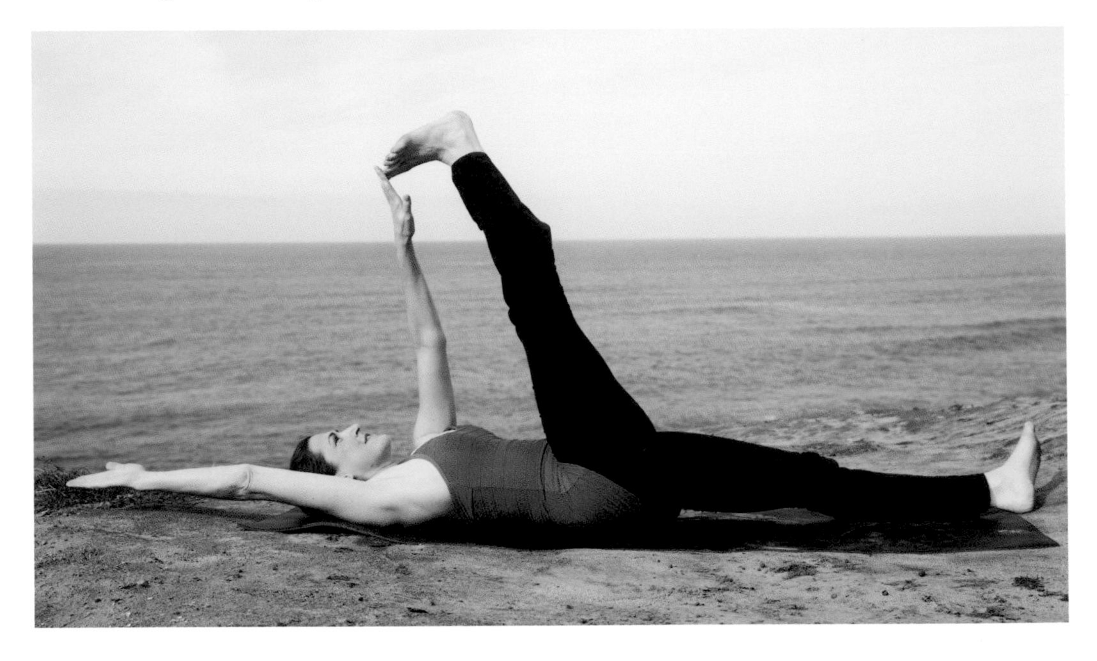

Superhero

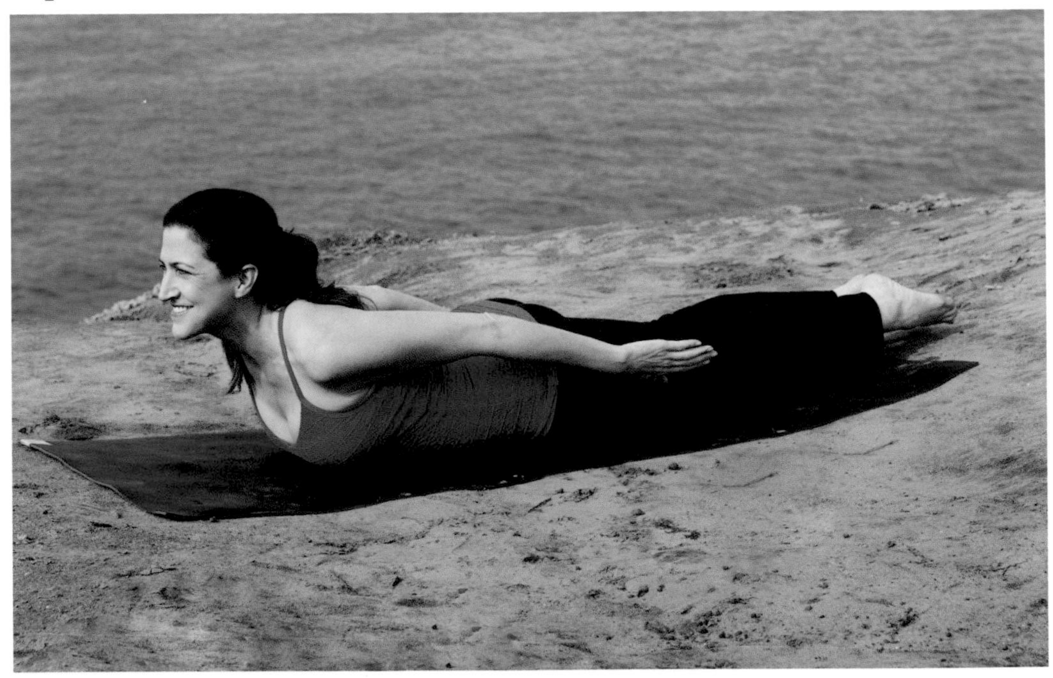

Active Cat

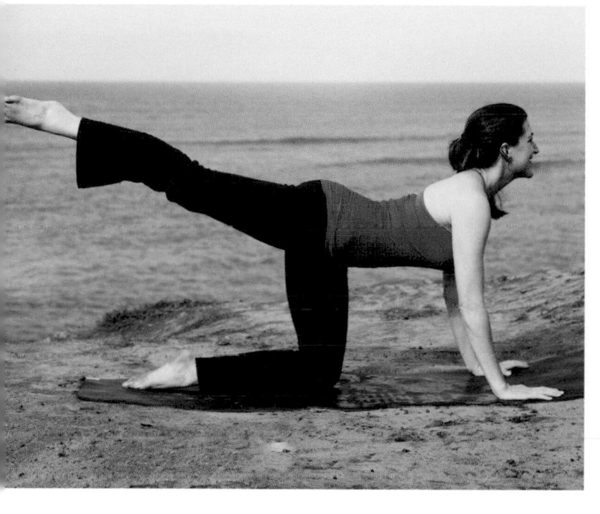

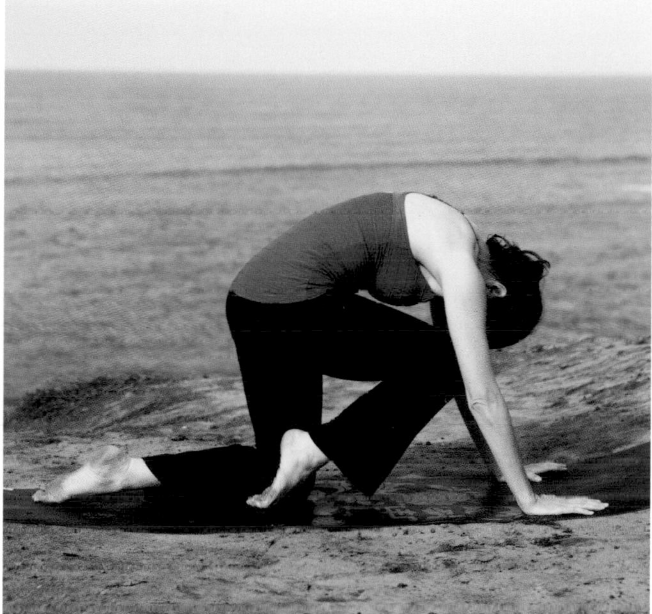

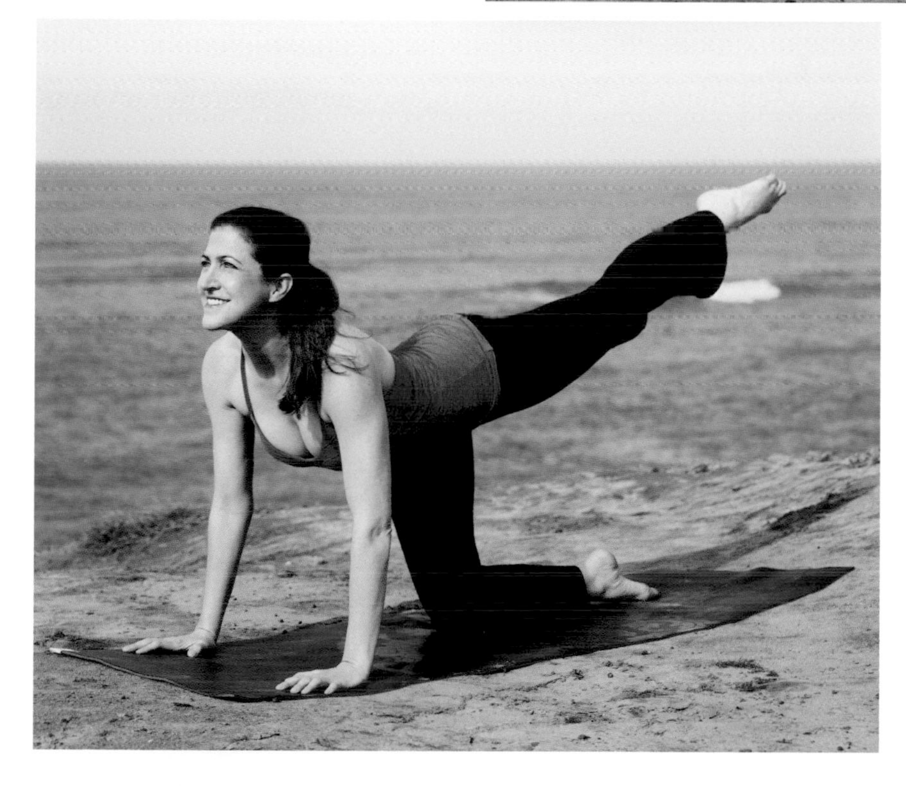

Wings of Victory

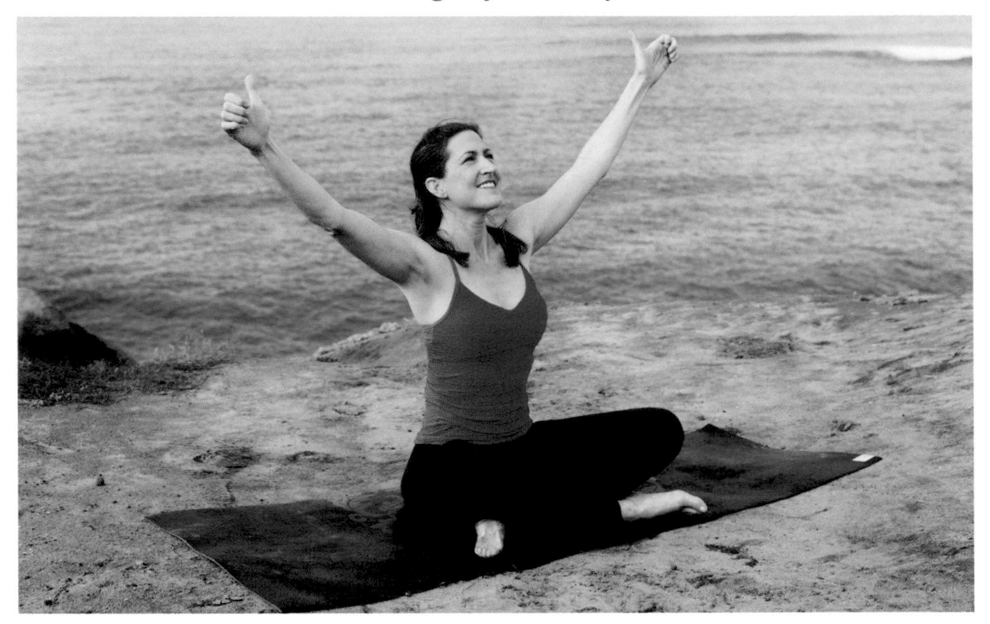

Taking Flight

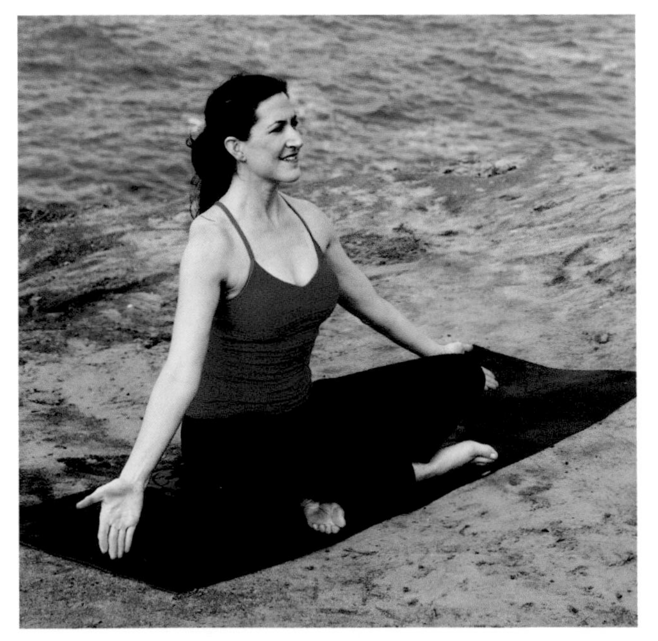

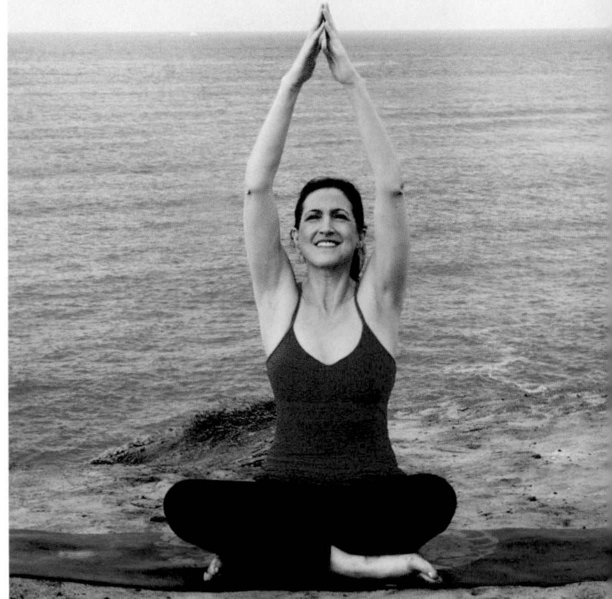

Calling Destiny Home

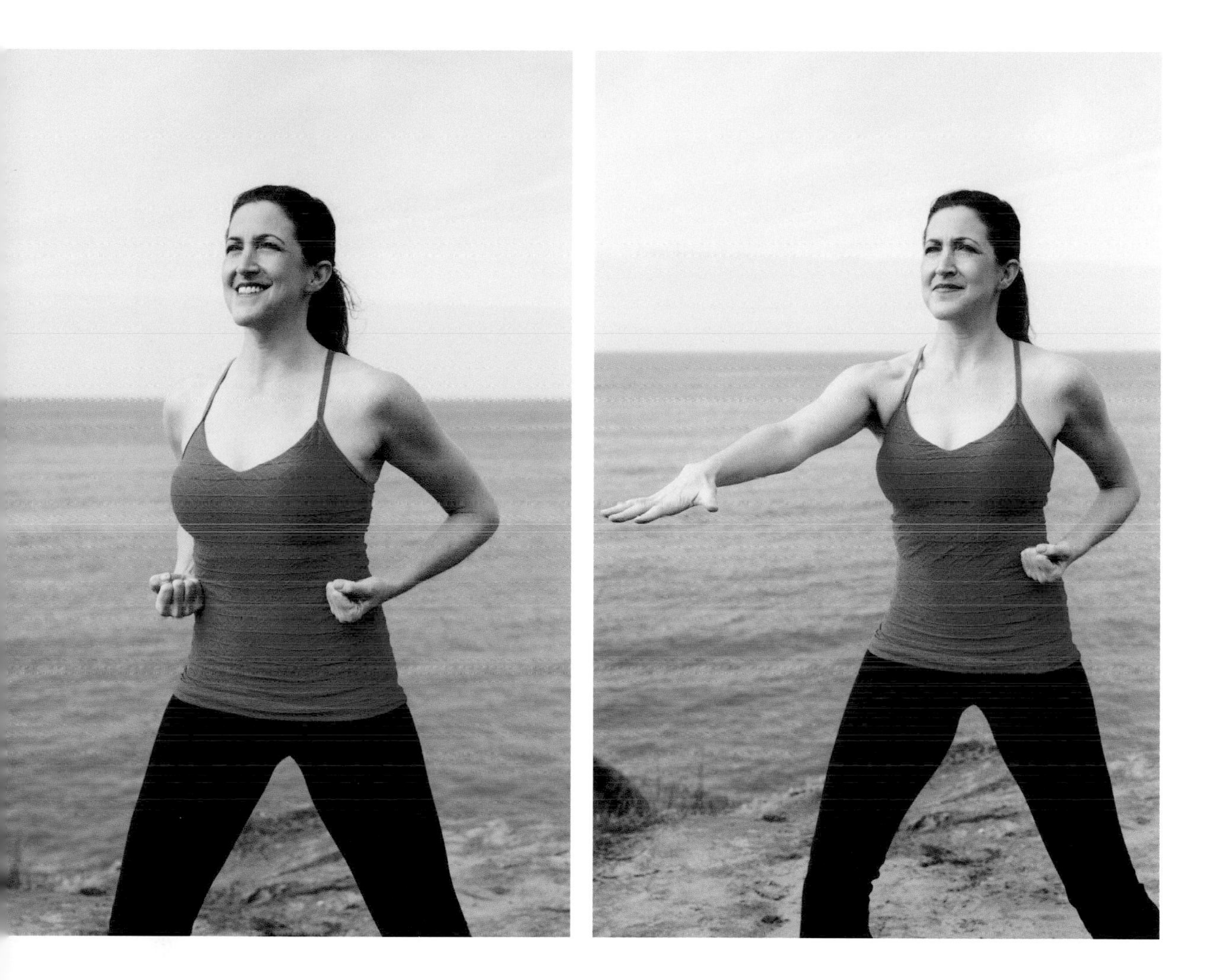

Abdominal Pumping

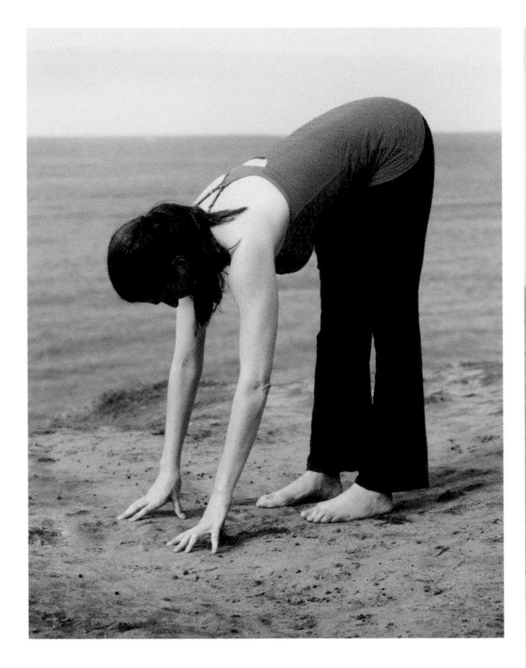

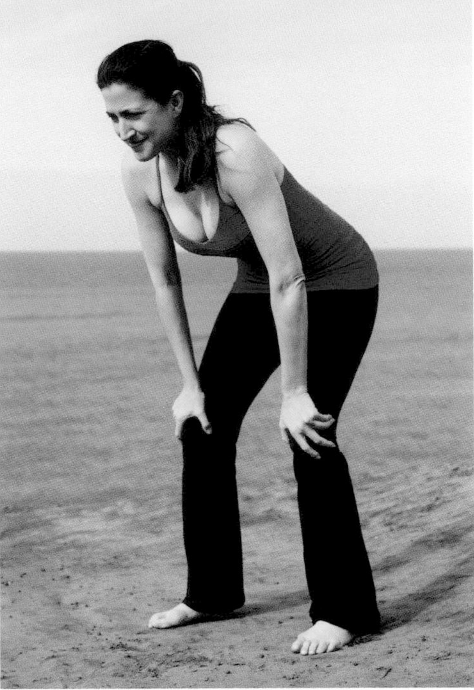

Shaking the Soul Tree

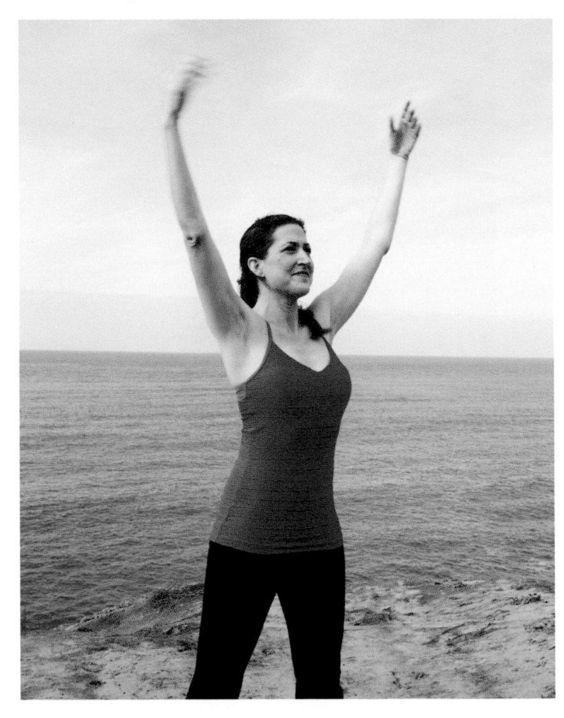

Corpse Pose

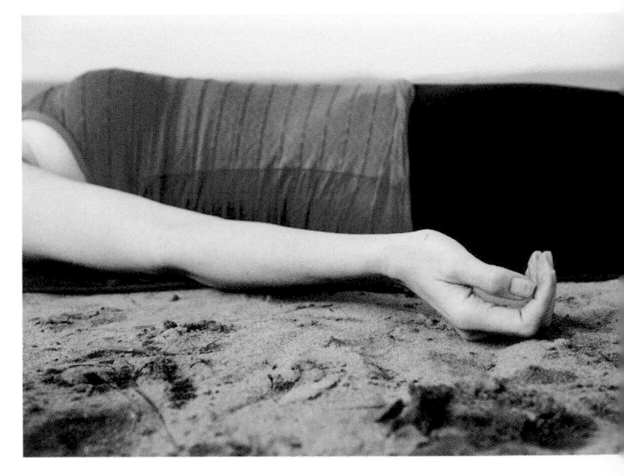

The Tibetan Rites

Spinning

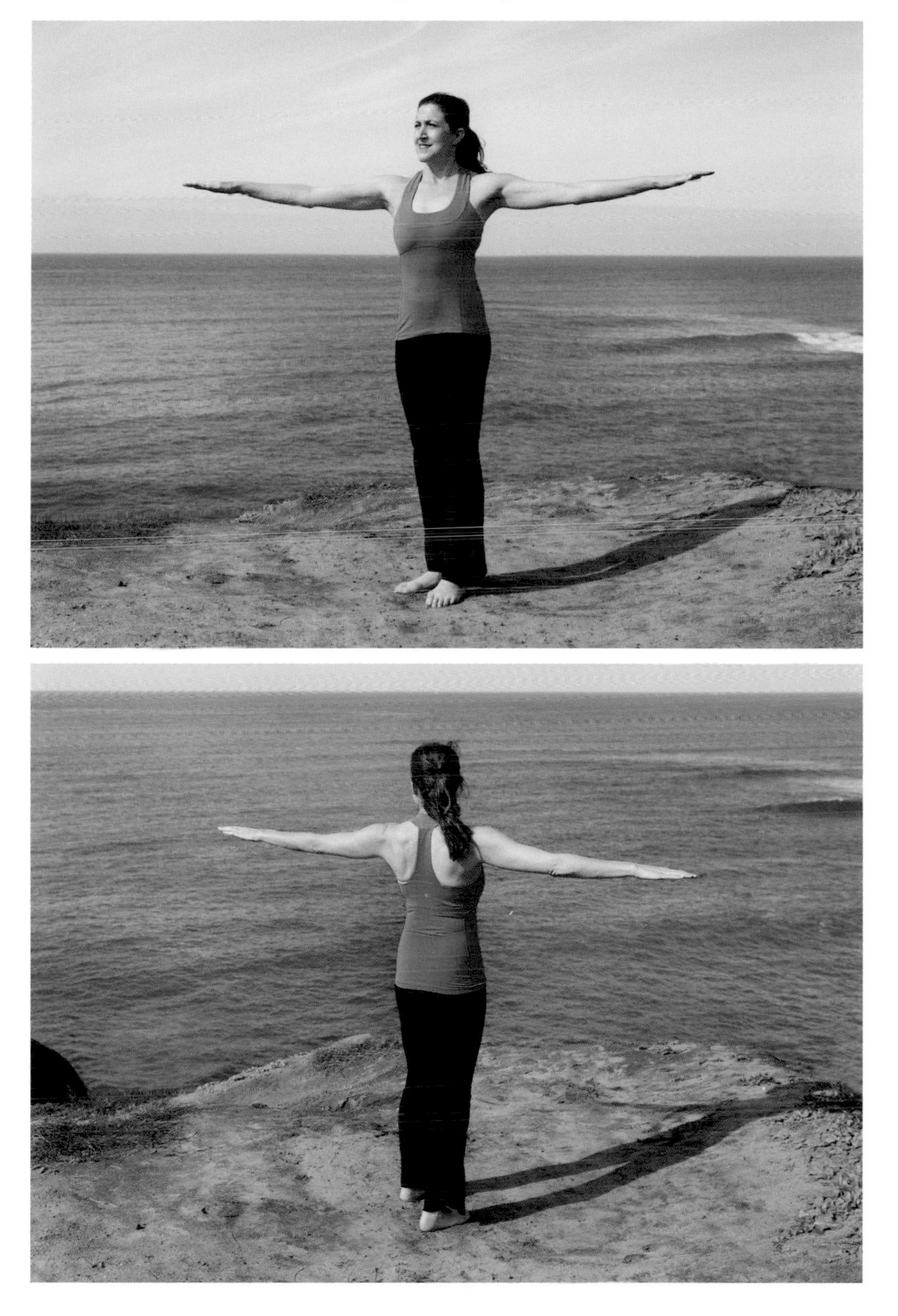

Leg Lift

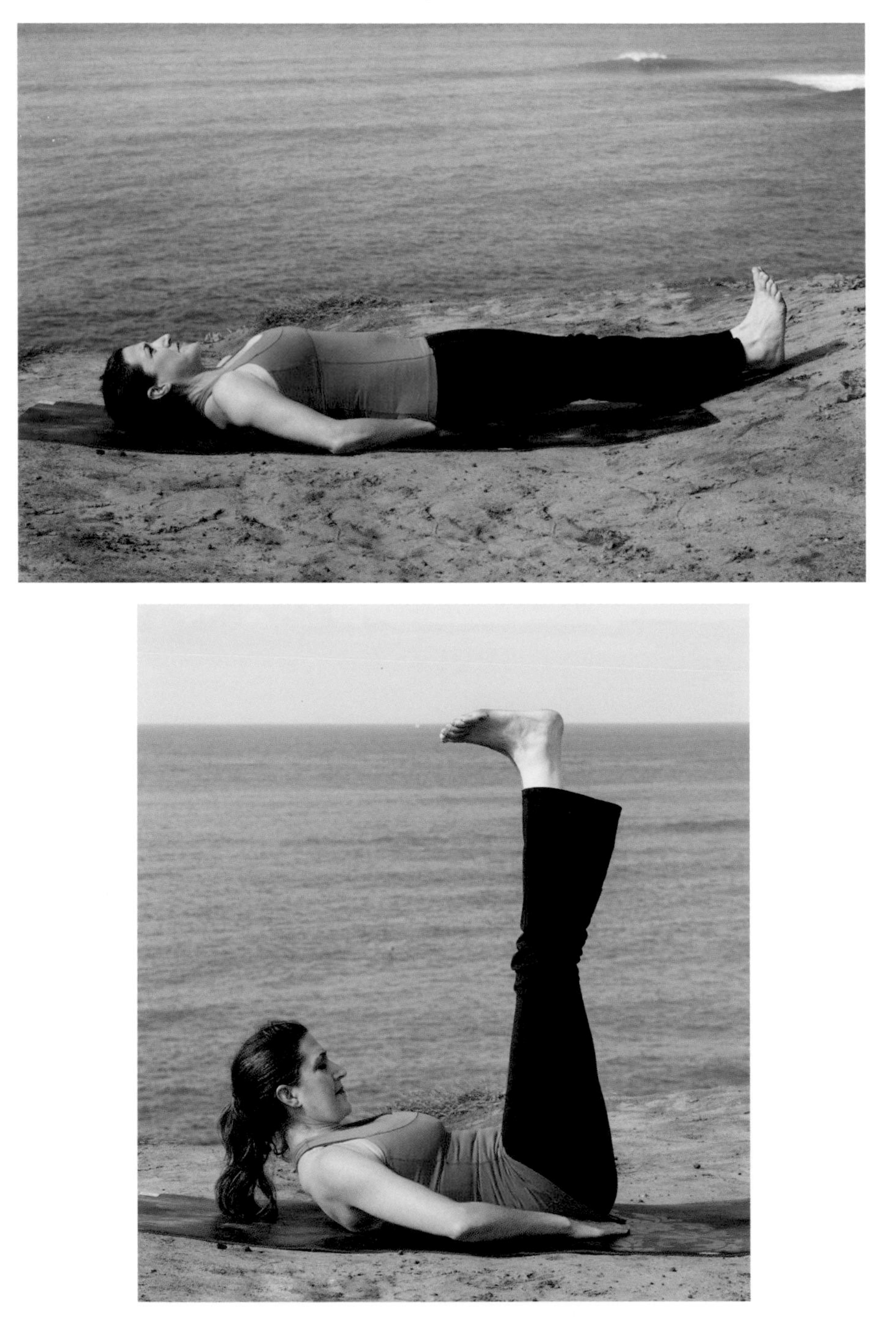

Camel

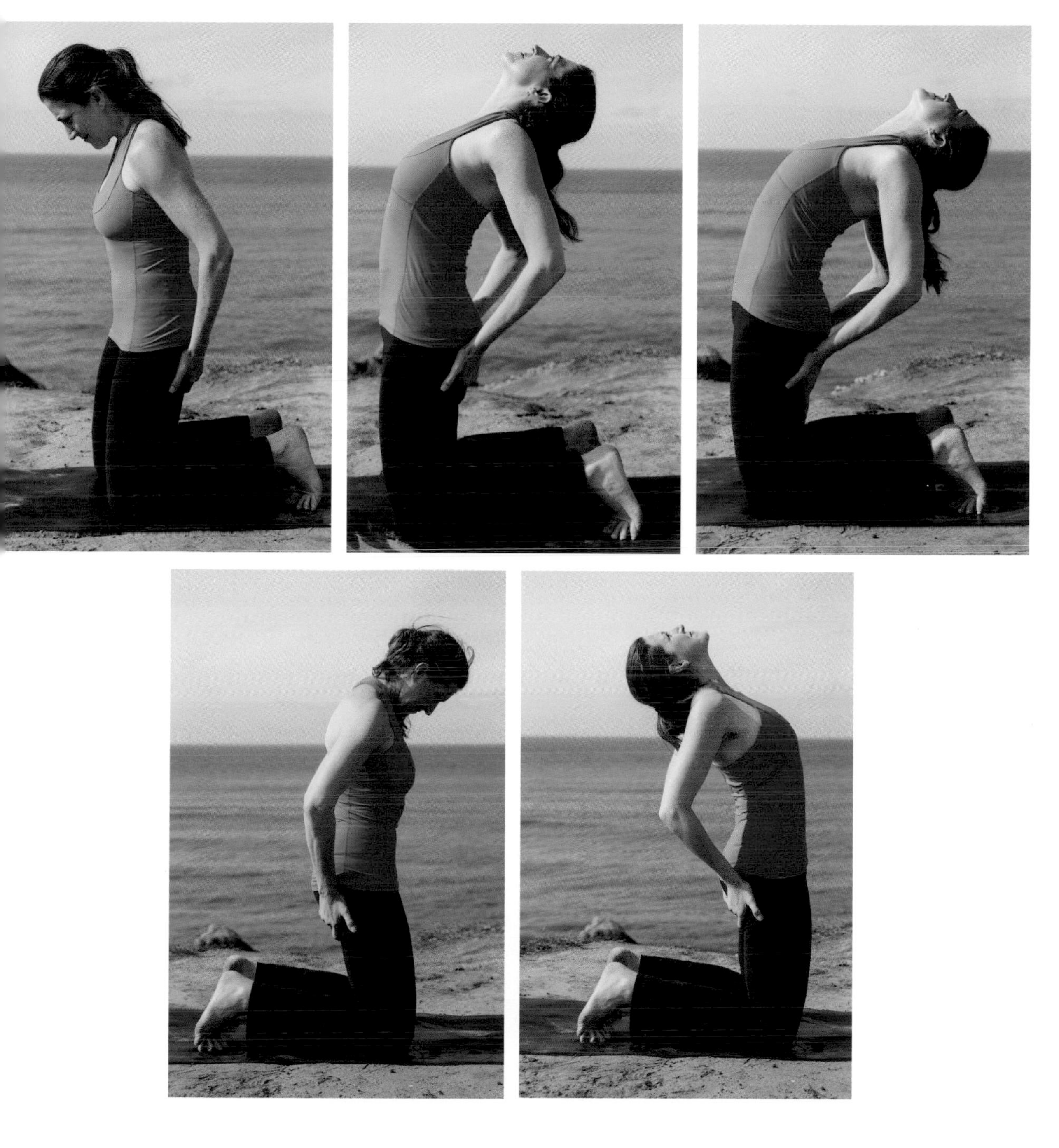

Tabletop Lever

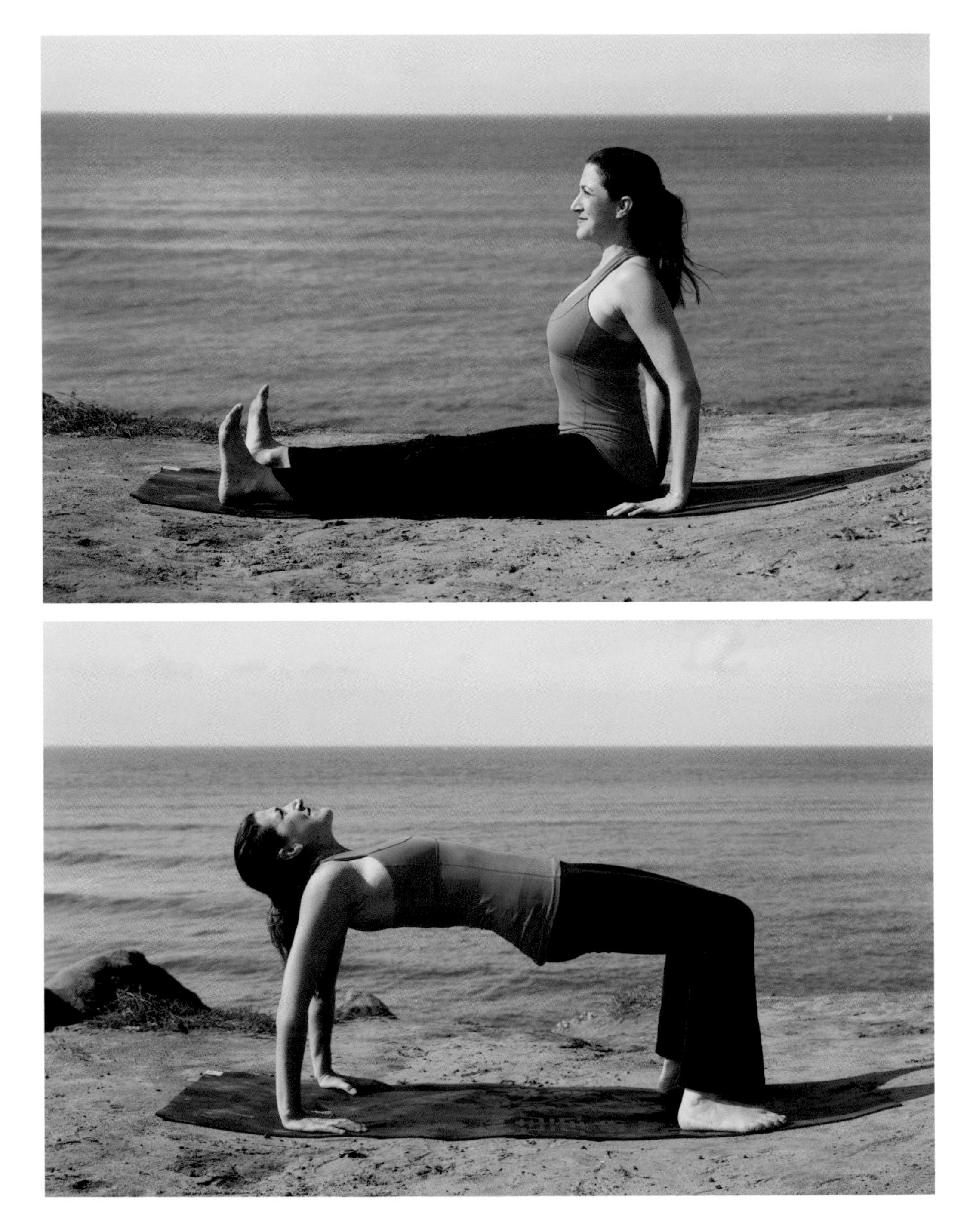

Up Dog, Down Dog

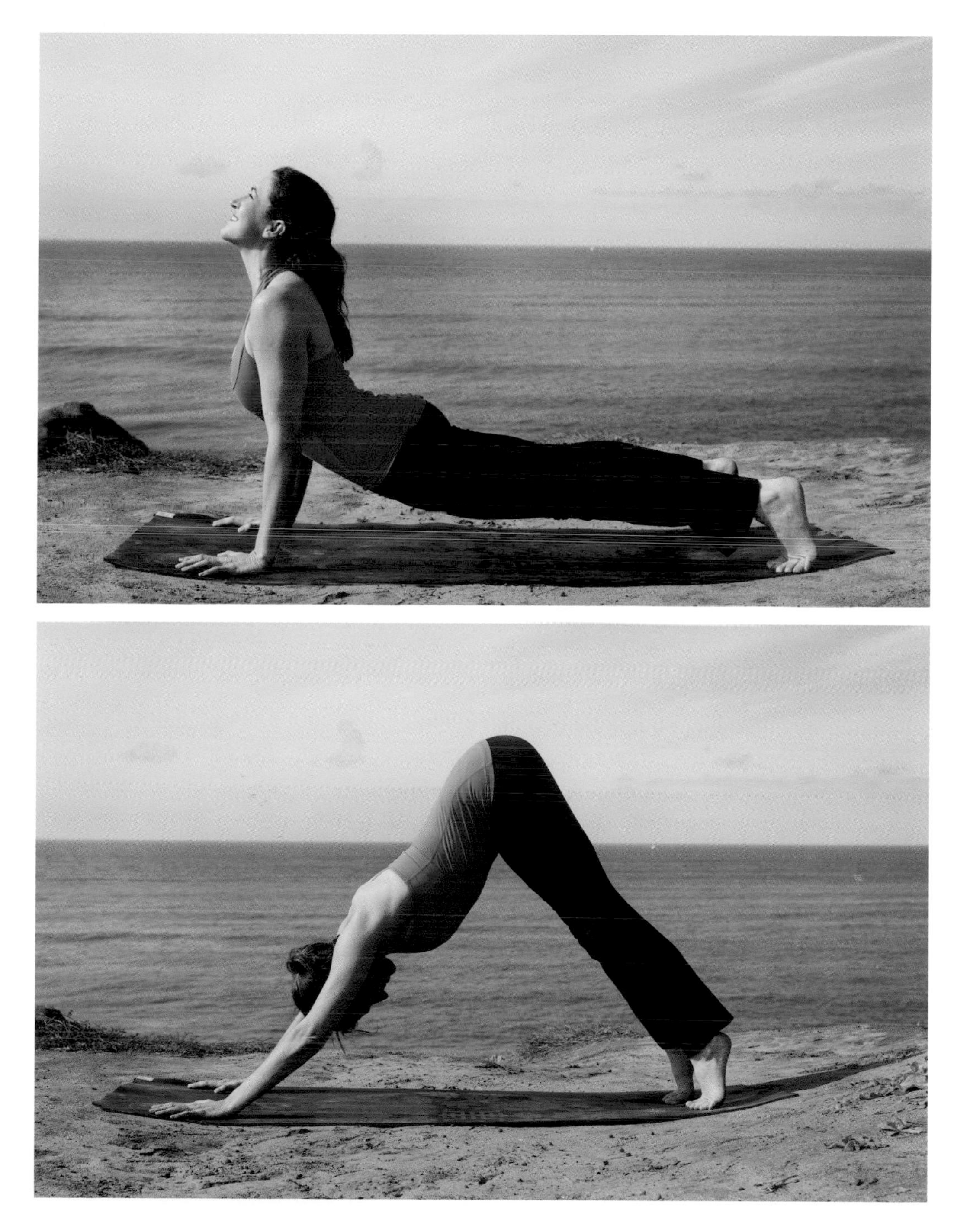

Abdominal Massage

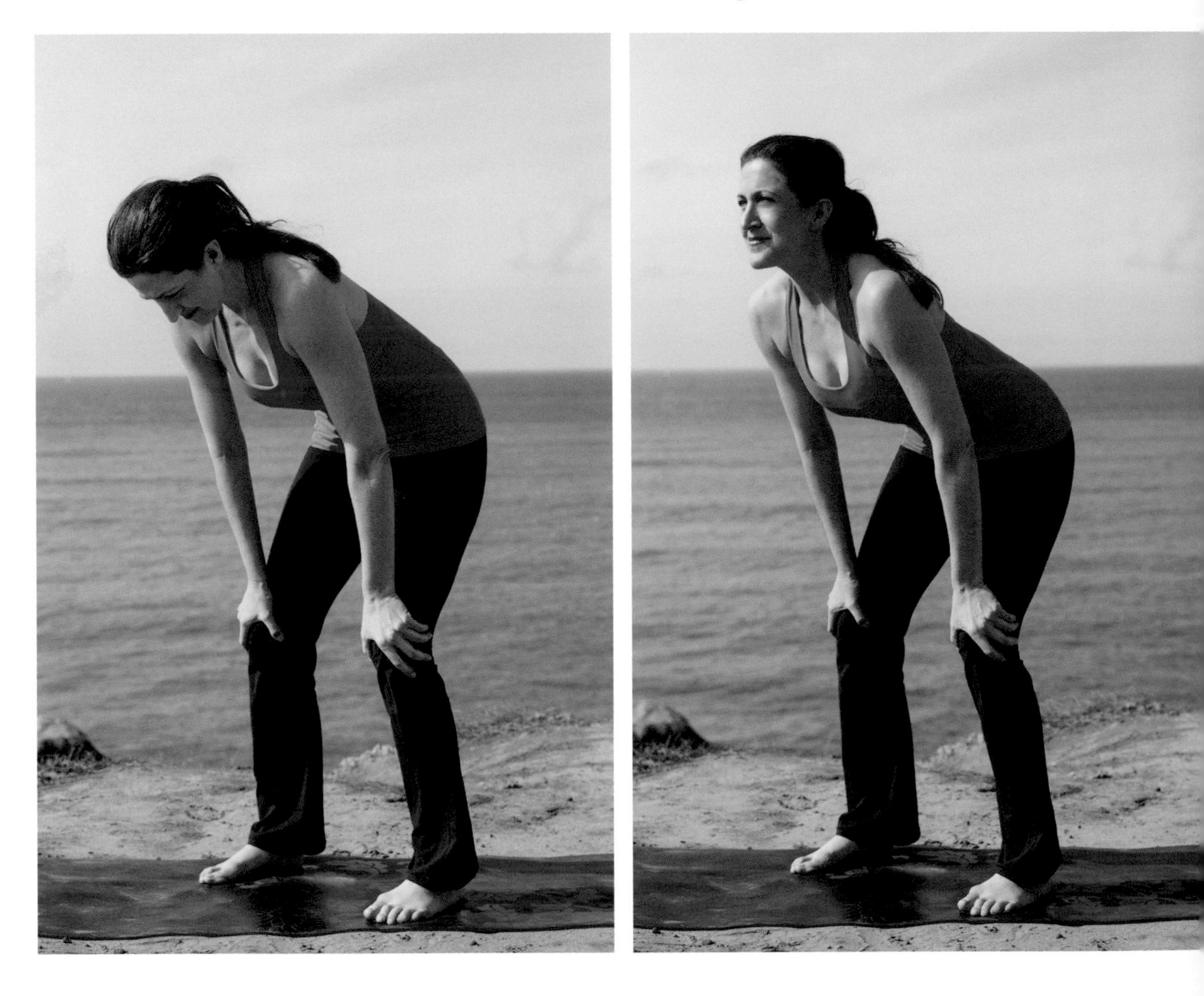

and leveling the gaze, release the belly and the root. Imagine that the air has suddenly become thick honey, as you press your arms down around you, slowly, with control, bringing your hands into *gyan mudra* where you will return to your natural breath and meditate for a few minutes.

Kundalini Hand Positions

Jupiter Hand (gyan mudra): Touch the tip of the index finger to the tip of the thumb, leaving the remaining three fingers straight but relaxed, and rest the wrist on the knees.

Root Mudra: Interlace your fingers and press the thumb tips firmly together.

Prayer Position (anjali mudra): Press your palms together, fingers pointing upward, in front of your chest.

Open-Heart Mudra: Press your pinky fingers and thumbs and heels of the hands against one another and open the other fingers like the thousand-petal lotus.

The Practice

Charming the Snake: Seated Practice

Sufist Grind

The Sufist Grind awakens the first and second chakras, lubricates the spine, nourishes and recharges the kidneys and adrenals, stimulates digestive "fire," necessary for good appetite and metabolic function, and massages and detoxifies internal organs. This exercise is so named because, thinking of your upper body as the pestle and your lower pelvis as the bowl, or mortar, you are "grinding" away at illusion. I prefer to call it a circle, because it feels smoother and silkier to me, like a snake's skin. As we are embarking on our warriors-of-love path in this practice, I would like to set the tone with the word "circle"; you are circling around your own globe, your own inner world, and starting the journey here in this new practice of kundalini.

1. Sit in Easy Pose or Zazen Seat, your spine tall and relaxed, and bring your hands to your knees with your palms facing down. Close your eyes and turn your inner focus up toward your third eye.
2. As you inhale, start to circle your upper torso to the right, in a clockwise motion, keeping your shoulders facing forward (you are not twisting) and your head level on top of the torso, allowing it to travel with your body.
3. As your body circles to the back, exhale and allow your spine to round naturally back before you inhale and arch the spine, extending the chest open as you come forward once again to start your next seamless circle. Your breathing should be smooth and deep as you round back and arch and extend forward. You will find that it instantly starts to calm and ground you.
4. Use your hands against your palms and your arms to leverage the body, facilitating its movement in opposition, and accentuate the opening arch of the spine as the chest moves forward and the rounding contraction of the spine as you circle back.
5. After you complete twenty-one circles clockwise, change the cross of the legs and repeat, this time moving counterclockwise twenty-one times.
6. After finishing the reverse, bring the hands into *gyan mudra* and meditate for a few breaths.

Heart Opener

The Heart Opener stimulates and opens the Root and Heart Chakras, makes the spine more fluid and flexible, and opens the heart to giving and receiving here and now in your life. Remember that your movement works in tandem with your breath, so slow at first is the way to go.

Note: If for any reason, as you are starting out, you experience cramping or "stitches" in your abdominal region, don't be alarmed. Just know that it's your body's way of telling you that you need to take it a little easier and work your way up to a faster pace, or that it's time to stop for a rest. You should resume when all is clear.

1. Sitting in Easy Pose, place your right hand on your right shin close to the ankle and your left hand on your left shin, and inhale deeply as you bend the elbows and pull the body up and forward, arching the spine, and opening the chest with the face up to the sky. I like to think of shining my heart open when I do this.
2. As you exhale, curl the spine forward, extending the arms straight, feeling the stretch between your shoulder blades. Gently drop your chin to your chest and feel a stretch in the neck. As you stretch the spine and open your chest, you open your heart, and you open your life.
3. Here is your first chance to practice your Breath of Fire with movement as well as your mantra, *Sat Nam*. Whenever you can incorporate it, inhale on *Sat* and exhale on *Nam*. As in our other practices, you are now going to learn another variation of subtle-body and outer-body multitasking. With both your breathing and the mantra, start out slowly and build to a hearty clip, a vigorous pace.
4. Ideally, you want to perform this exercise at a moderate to fast pace eventually, so start off slowly and work your way up to greater vigor.
5. Repeat this forward and back action up to one hundred and eight times.
6. Once you finish, bring your hands down to rest on your knees in *gyan mudra,* inhale deeply to three-quarters full, and retain the breath, applying your Root Lock by sealing the new energy inside and coax-

ing it up the spine. Hold your breath and your Root Lock as long as you comfortably can and then release, coming to meditate for a minute, connecting to the subtle flow of prana through your open heart and spine.

Child's Pose for the Crown

A powerful tune-up, the Child's Pose for the Crown activates and balances the master glands of the body, recharges the kidneys and adrenals, and stimulates the nerve plexuses along the spine as it stretches and soothes the lower back. It also awakens *ajna,* the sixth chakra, opening the window of our intuition and higher consciousness.

This exercise is naturally a little uncomfortable when you first attempt it, both because of the angle of your body and the action you are performing and because the breath exerts a kind of awkward pressure in your head and neck that you will need to focus your way through. It's an exercise that clearly lets you know just how effective it is from the minute you start doing it. Gradually, you will acclimate to the new sensations and even come to enjoy them. Whenever I do this exercise, almost more than in any of the others in the Waking Energy flow, I become immediately and keenly aware of how my glands are being massaged, activated, and "pumped" by the combination of the action of my breathing and my body position.

I appreciate the intelligence of this exercise, and I respect it for what it offers: the physics of the positioning and the way a very specific, beneficial pressure is exerted on all the muscles in the upper body and particularly the neck. It literally turns the body into a purifying engine for your subtle body, removing stagnation and opening the nadis for the smooth flow of prana. Here, more here than in most kriyas, you will be especially cognizant of how your body becomes an apparatus that assists you in your own energy cultivation.

This exercise helps you to burn through the noise of the mind, making your mind clear as it stimulates the master glands in what you will come to know in the chapter on the Inner Smile as your Crystal Palace. With bravery and determination, and with your eyes focused on the floor beneath you, think of this entire exercise as an homage to Mother Earth.

1. On your hands and knees, press your hips back so that you are sitting on your heels with big toes together and knees shoulder-width apart. Extend your arms in front of you and bend forward so your upper body is resting on your thighs. Allow your forehead to rest on the floor. Arms are stretched out in front of you, flat on the floor, palms down.
2. Inhale, and as you exhale, allow your entire body to release even more deeply into the floor as you draw the arms back behind you and allow them to rest on the floor at your sides with the palms face up to the ceiling.
3. Lift your head and your upper back about six inches off the floor so that your head and spine are exactly in line with one another, and with your gaze down toward the floor, begin the Breath of Fire. For your first attempt at this exercise, just focus on getting comfortable with your Breath of Fire, since it's the first time that you will be attempting an accurate example of greater intensity with the rhythm and power of the breathing. Forgo trying to incorporate *Sat Nam* into your breathing, as this is a more challenging exercise; as you become more practiced, I welcome you to add *Sat Nam* as a layer.
4. Continue to lengthen the crown long away from the tail, keeping the spine energized, with your mind focused entirely on the steady rhythm of your breathing. Continue your Breath of Fire for up to three minutes.
5. After completing your Breath of Fire in the Child's Pose, lower your head to the floor and rest for three full, complete breaths.
6. Then rise up on your knees. As you inhale, filling the lungs to three-quarters full, practice retention by applying the Root Lock and bring your hands into *gyan mudra*. Hold your breath as long as you

can without straining and then release the breath and meditate for a minute or two.

Radiance Stretch

The Radiance Stretch is a simple sequence that brings a glow to your face and a sparkle to your eye. A powerful liver detoxifier (complexion and vision are both related to the liver), it stretches the quadriceps and the spine, particularly the muscles of the shoulders and neck, opens the heart, and increases your lung capacity. It vigorously awakens the third chakra, *manipura,* as it conditions the first and second chakras as well.

> *Note:* At no point should you feel any pain in the knees; if you do, it's a sign to back off and choose a variation that feels better. Trust your instincts.

1. On your hands and knees, draw your knees together, and do your best to keep them in that position for the duration of the exercise. Lean back, bringing your arms behind you with your fingertips actively touching the floor (like a cat that's landed from a jump). Open your chest and lift your chin slightly. You will feel a significant stretch in your thighs and hip flexors, the front of your hips, and this is a good thing.
2. For this exercise, which is a variation of the Hero's Pose, you have three positioning choices, depending on what suits your body the best.

    Variation 1: You can stay here, in this more upright position.

    Variation 2: If you feel more open, you can bend your elbows behind you, increasing the range of motion of the exercise, and stretch more deeply into your thighs.

    Variation 3: If you feel ready for a back bend, you can release completely onto your back, coming into full Hero's Pose, with your arms overhead, folded at the elbows, framing your head, with your head and your back resting comfortably into the floor.

3. Once you choose your preferred position, establish a focused gaze on a point in front of you, begin the Breath of Fire, and continue for up to three minutes. If you can, once you establish a healthy rhythm in your breathing, layer *Sat Nam* into your breathing, inhaling *Sat* and exhaling *Nam*.
4. After you complete your three minutes, rise up carefully, sitting on the heels (or coming into Easy Pose), inhale, and retain the breath, squeezing your perineum in the Root Lock as you bring your hands into Root Mudra. Right away you will feel on some indescribable, subtle level a clear connection between the awareness of your perineum and sexual organs and the exact energy that your hands in this special configuration are rendering. Like the resonance of a bell, I promise you will feel the vibratory, relational connection of your Root and your actual hands. Root Mudra makes you feel a deep and instant connection to the earth.
5. Release the hands onto the knees, palms face down, and meditate on your beautiful liver for a minute, letting go of anger and ushering in love and empathy for yourself.

Goddess Rolls

Goddess Rolls is an instant energizer! If you have time to do only one exercise in the morning to feel awake and alive, this is the one to do. It activates the area below your navel center that houses your life force, massages the spine, the kidneys, and adrenals, and opens the hips, turning stored tensions into creative inspiration and balancing the first and second chakras.

1. Sitting tall, bend your knees wide out to the side in a butterfly shape and draw your feet in, approximately six inches away from your groin, holding onto your lower shins at the ankles, and bring the soles of the feet to touch (the fronts of the feet will separate slightly as you move).

2. Round the spine forward over your legs and feet, and as you inhale, like a child on the playground, rock all the way back onto your spine, just up to the top of the shoulder blades and before you come up onto the neck; as you exhale, rock forward with some jolly momentum and allow your head to naturally fall as close to your feet as possible.
3. Inhale as you rock back and exhale as you round forward, pressing your elbows into the inner line of the legs to gently push the backs of the knees down into the floor in the butterfly position, progressively stretching the groin muscles open more and more each time you rock and roll.
4. Eventually, you will become so open, free, and flexible that your head will touch in between the soles of your feet, coming to nestle there for a second or two as your body rounds forward.
5. Repeat twenty-one times. After your last repetition, come into Easy Pose and bring your hands into *gyan mudra* with your eyes turned up to gaze at your third eye, and meditate for a few breaths.

Reaching Across Space and Time

Nothing builds your courage, will, and determination like Reaching Across Space and Time. When you stretch your arms away from your legs with the energy and intention that this exercise calls for, you truly feel as though you are reaching across space and time. It strengthens the abdominals, increases flexibility in your hamstring-gluteal connection, and stimulates and balances your third chakra, clearing anger and ushering in self-love that arises from a job well done, the kind of self-fulfillment that is born from deep commitment.

1. Lying on your back, lengthen your legs straight out along the floor with your feet firmly flexed, hip-width apart, and stretch your arms high overhead with your fingertips reaching as far away from your feet as possible. Reach farther than you ever have, and apply the

principle of opposition, in which the energy of your fingertips is as far away from that of your feet as possible.

2. Lower your navel toward your spine to activate your abdominals and make sure that your ribs are drawing together, so that your spine is safely anchored to the mat beneath you rather than arching up off the floor. You should feel a slight space between you and your mat, which means you are encouraging the natural curve of your spine against the floor without pushing or straining to get it down to the floor.
3. Inhale as you flex the left foot and, using your deepest abdominals, lift the left leg up, bringing the toes of your left foot up to touch your right palm, which should meet it at around a ninety-degree angle above your chest. As you exhale, lower both the left leg and the right arm back down into their starting positions. Because this exercise is especially challenging on a few different levels, you will want to rely on your compass, your mantra, so from the very start, inhale *Sat* as the leg comes up to touch your hand and exhale *Nam* as the leg and opposite arm descends.
4. Then immediately, without pausing, repeat the entire sequence using the right leg and the left arm, inhaling to lift the right toes up to touch the palm of the left hand. It is as though you are aiming your toes like an arrow at the bull's-eye, the target of your opposite hand, and it should feel satisfying each time you are able to spatially perceive with exactitude the "sweet spot" of your own palm. This sensation is similar to the satisfaction you would feel while playing tennis or baseball, when the ball connects to the sweet spot on your racket or bat. It takes practice to hit your toes into the middle of your opposite palm, but when you do, there is no mistaking the solidity and the integrity of the connection. Don't get frustrated or angry if you miss the bull's-eye, because the point here is to *clear* anger. Do your best, and over time, with practice, your coordination and spatial awareness will improve, resulting in a feeling of great satisfaction and pride.
5. After you complete about five sets, alternating sides, I guarantee, you

will want to stop. Don't! Keep going, and challenge the voices in your mind that say, "No" and "I can't." Call upon Kali, the goddess of destruction and transformation, now and remember it isn't perfection we're after. It's the bravery you bring to your yoga practice that makes all the difference. Think of how incredibly powerful you are becoming, clearing anger, committing to yourself and a higher purpose. Keep going! You will be so proud of yourself and enjoy an unparalleled satisfaction that will build on itself, strengthening your resolve for when you need to call upon it next.

6. Ultimately you will want to work your way up to doing this for up to seven minutes, but try three minutes to start. After completing your three minutes, hug your knees into your chest and rock side to side to massage your spine. Then send your legs up to the ceiling and give them a vigorous "shake" before hugging them back into your chest and finally releasing them back down long on the floor beneath you, where you will bounce them out and then come to stillness for a breath or two. Then come into the Child's Pose and rest for a few breaths.

Active Cat

The Active Cat is a combination of the commonly named Cat Pose and Cow Pose. It opens the heart, releases neck and shoulder tension, makes the spine more fluid and flexible, provides a gentle massage to the internal organs, and activates the first and second chakras, which stimulates the kidneys and adrenals.

1. Come onto your hands and knees in Tabletop position with your back aligned straight and parallel to the floor, hands lined up directly underneath your shoulders, fingers spread wide apart, and arms strong and straight, toes tucked under and heels lined up with your lower legs.
2. As you inhale, arch the spine down toward the floor, releasing the

pelvis, roll the shoulders back and down away from the ears, and look up, coming into cow pose.

3. As you exhale, release the toes and relax them flat down into the floor as you press the hands more strongly into the earth, creating opposition with which to arch the spine and pelvis upward, coming into cat pose.
4. Repeat the cow-to-cat movement, inhaling as you come into cow and exhaling as you move into cat for a total of eight times and then pause, returning to neutral, Tabletop position.
5. Now inhale and extend the right leg straight out behind you and up as high as you can go, while keeping the arms strong and straight and the neck long as you focus your gaze up.
6. As you exhale, bend the knee and draw it in toward your forehead as you lower the head down to curl the spine into cat pose, coming as close to the right knee as possible.
7. Inhale, extend the spine and the leg behind you, and look up as you speak *Sat* silently inside. Exhale, rounding the spine underneath you to make forehead and knee meet as you silently speak, *Nam*. Start slowly and then build like a steam locomotive up to a moderate to vigorous pace, tuning into your body's wisdom to inform you as to which pace suits you best today. Repeat the Active Cat, the action of extending and contracting with control and ease, inhaling and stretching out with *Sat* and exhaling and tucking under with *Nam,* for a total of one minute. Then switch to the left side and again, starting slowly to acclimate to what the left side of the body feels like and needs, building your way up to real vigor for another minute.
8. After completing the second side, come to rest in the Child's Pose for a few breaths. Rise up to sit on your heels or come into Easy Pose and meditate for a breath or two. Bring your hands into Root Mudra and, as you practice your Long Deep Breathing here in meditation, tune into the abundant new subtle energy moving through you.

Superhero

The Superhero powerfully strengthens the muscles of the back, upper arms, hamstrings, and glutes as it stretches the chest, improves digestion, and reduces stress. It stimulates the lymphatic system, flushing toxins from fatty tissues like the breasts, making it a potent preventive agent; recharges the kidneys and adrenals; balances the third, fourth, and fifth chakras, opening the heart; and enhances confidence to help you express your creativity and speak your truth.

There are two distinct parts to this exercise. Get ready to feel like Superman flying through space and time.

1. *Round 1:* Lie on your stomach with your hands forming a pillow under your forehead, legs outstretched behind you, with the tops of your feet flat against the floor.
2. Lengthen your neck so that you can bring your chin onto the floor where it will rest as you bring your arms behind you, with your palms facing up to the ceiling.
3. Inhale *Sat* as you lift the arms up behind, strong and straight, as high as you can, and as you exhale *Nam* with control, bring them back to the starting position. Repeat this action twenty-six times, and when it gets challenging and your triceps start to burn, use this feeling as an incentive to keep going—you are releasing toxins and burning them away with your powerful inner fire and intention.
4. After you finish your twenty-six repetitions, rest with your head down on your hands and rock your hips gently from side to side.
5. *Round 2:* Bring your arms back behind you, interlace your fingers, and stretch your arms up off your back as you squeeze the inner thighs together and lift the legs as high up off the floor as you can.
6. If possible, press your palms together as you lift and lengthen the arms off and away from your back. With your gaze directly forward and your shoulders rolled back, start the Breath of Fire.

Variation: If it's not possible for you to keep your palms pressed together here, simply link your thumbs together with the other fingers extended long away from you, or keep your arms long down by your sides and off the floor a few inches.

7. Know that the Breath of Fire can be a little awkward in this prone position and may take some getting used to, but it is incredibly beneficial to the internal organs, particularly the digestive system. Stay the course, and *Sat Nam, Sat Nam, Sat Nam, Sat Nam* your way through it, knowing you are nourishing your primary energy batteries, opening your heart, and building inner confidence as you do—real incentives to keep going strong.
8. Continue the Breath of Fire at a moderate pace for up to three minutes. Once you have finished, release your hands, but keep the arms outstretched long behind you and the legs strong and straight; lift your arms, legs, and upper body as high up off the floor as you can with one last deep, full inhalation. As you exhale, release everything into the floor and rest with your hands underneath your forehead once again, bathing in the glow of sweet success and a job well done.
9. Press back into the Child's Pose and rest for a few breaths before rising up through the spine, where you will sit back on your heels and bring your hands into *gyan mudra,* with your gaze turned up and in toward your third eye, simply meditating for a few breaths on your beautiful, open heart and powerful body.

Wings of Victory

Oh, how I love Wings of Victory! This exercise will put you through your paces, but it is amazing, incredibly uplifting, and fulfilling. It instills a feeling of real power and inner confidence, restoring your belief in yourself. It stimulates your lymphatic system and strengthens your heart, specifically the venous return. (One of the reasons that musical conductors are so long-lived is that they are constantly moving their arms above their hearts, aiding in the blood flow back into the heart; this exercise simulates that very action, resulting in untold benefits.)

It activates and strengthens *anahata,* the Heart Chakra, helping to release anger and disappointment and usher in love and forgiveness. This kriya and the next one, Taking Flight, both work with the sacred geometry of the heart. The sixty-degree angle at which we hold our arms is a direct conduit for moving heart energy, for opening the heart up to receive nurturing, healing universal love, and to then give back to the world—again, love in abundance.

Whenever I do this exercise, I think of one of my favorite birds, my beloved albatross, which spends most of its life "on the wing" using a technique called "dynamic soaring." As they fly, albatrosses angle their wings into the wind in order to gain height and move into the "boundary field," a smoother current that exists above the frictional layer of headwind that would ordinarily slow them down. This current enables them to stay in the air, sometimes traveling as far as ten thousand miles without flapping their wings, before landing to refuel. They move like true tai chi adepts, flying with the flow, literally extracting energy from that field to buoy them and carry them aloft, a true real-life model of effortless effort. And you thought kundalini was hard!

1. Sitting in Easy Pose, raise your arms up overhead into a large V shape, a forty-five-degree angle, and fold the tips of the fingers, just the first knuckles, in toward the palms with your thumbs pointing straight up to the ceiling.
2. Focus your gaze on a point in front of you. I suggest using creative visualization here, perhaps a cherished goal you want to pursue in your life or a person important to you. When the going gets tough, you'll want to have this image readily available to help vanquish negative thoughts and the desire to quit. (Trust me, you may want to quit—but you won't!)
3. With your arms outstretched, separate your thumbs from your other

fingers and feel as though your thumbs are conduits for heavenly energy to beam down into your body, not only through your Crown Chakra, but literally through your thumbs.

4. Start the Breath of Fire, inhaling *Sat* and exhaling *Nam*. Now that you are becoming more practiced with the Breath of Fire, see if you can actually jump right in and establish a more vigorous pace from the onset of the exercise.
5. As you pump your diaphragm in and out, stoking your inner fire, stretch your arms out even more expansively, spreading those big, beautiful wings, the biggest wings you've ever seen, out into space. As you think of rooting even deeper into the earth, rise! Like the albatross, feel your boundlessness, feel your infinite power, feel your radiance rising up through your body!
6. Continue inhaling and exhaling powerfully for up to three minutes, feeling your heart opening and *kundalini shakti* rising inside you to do her nurturing, energizing work.
7. After completing your three minutes (you can work up to as much as seven or eight minutes in this exercise), sweep your arms overhead, linking your thumbs together and stretching your other fingers straight up to the ceiling as you apply *maha bandha*, the three locks done simultaneously, holding your breath as long as you can.
8. When you are ready to exhale, release the locks and let your arms float down with your fingertips extended, the backs of the hands coming down to touch the floor where we will not pause, but go directly into Taking Flight.

Taking Flight

The sacred geometry of the Heart Chakra comes alive in Taking Flight, a graceful and demanding kriya that connects the upper chakras to the lower three, strengthening the will and summoning your deepest commitment, as it tones and strengthens the arms and shoulders, muscles of the back, and sides of the waist.

1. In keeping with our aviary theme, we will now take flight. Coming directly from Wings of Victory, with your arms outstretched down to your sides and fingertips grazing the floor, as you inhale, raise your arms up and around you, bringing your fingertips to touch overhead, and immediately exhale and bring the arms back down to barely touch the floor.
2. Inhale and raise the arms strong and straight up overhead as you speak *Sat* and exhale as you sweep them back down with *Nam.* Start rather slowly and deliberately, fully feeling into the power of your long wings, working your way gradually, over the course of ten or so repetitions, up to a very vigorous pace, inhaling up, exhaling down, like a bird who is ready for takeoff, flapping its wings to make real speed for the ascent.
3. When your arms start to get tired, which they most assuredly will, think of how strong you are, how limitless, how your mind wants you to believe otherwise, but fly past it and ask it to come along with you—take flight into your greatness!
4. Continue strongly lifting the arms up and down for three full minutes (or fifty-two times), saying *Sat Nam, Sat Nam, Sat Nam, Sat Nam.* Know that when the going gets tough in your life, this very exercise and what you are cultivating here and now will help you to call up the vitality and grace you need to meet adversity and rise above it.
5. Now, end on a high note. On your final upswing, just as we did with Wings of Victory, link your thumbs together and stretch your other fingers straight up to the ceiling as you apply *maha bandha,* holding your breath as long as you can.
6. When you're ready, exhale, bringing your hands into Prayer Position overhead and then draw your prayer down, pressing the flat of your thumbs in front of your third eye, where you'll rest for a few breaths

meditating on your accomplishment, your dedication to yourself, your power, your infinite nature, and your great flight.

Kundalini Rising: Standing Practice

Archer

The Archer activates the first, second, and third chakras, opens the hips, stretches and strengthens the muscles of the legs, ankles, calves, feet, chest, shoulders, and back as it builds inner fortitude and courage to stand your ground and heed destiny's call. It also strengthens the nerves to such a degree that our bodies can fight off anything, creating a powerfully "divine" energy shield, amplifying the radiance into a grand protective aura that guards against negative energy.

1. Stand tall, with your feet deeply rooted into the earth at the front of your mat in Mountain Pose: feet together, big toes touching in parallel alignment, legs together, arms at your sides, upper body stacked on top and aligned with your navel, which is drawn in toward your spine, and your tailbone long, drawing down and back.
2. Step back with your left foot, placing it at least three feet behind you and slightly turning the left toes outward to form a sixty-five-degree angle to your right foot, which is now pointing straight ahead. Keep your left heel active and stretching back.
3. With both legs strong and straight in their alignment, bend the front knee in line with the big toe, squaring your hips to face the front of the mat, and as you do raise the arms up in front of the chest with your hands facing one another, three inches apart and your fingers outstretched.
4. Gazing at your destiny, you are going to pretend that you are drawing your arrow back in your archer's bow. Slowly and surely, relax the shoulders back and down. Come into a thumbs-up position with both

hands (hands in fists, thumbs pointing straight up). Keep your right arm extended, feeling a strong and vibrant connection to the heart, with the chest opening wide. Then bend the left elbow parallel to the ground and bring the hand back in line with the left shoulder. You are pulling the string of your bow back and drawing your arrow back into "let fly" position, literally forming your left hand in such a way that you feel the arrow in it. You will likely feel a stretch in your chest and left armpit.

5. Lift your upper chest proud and tall as you brighten the thumbs-up position with your right hand, energizing the fingers, lifting your gaze slightly higher than the horizon line, deepening the front right knee bend, and straightening the left leg even more strongly, rooting it into the earth.
6. Focus on a point in front of you, and with your feet deeply rooted into the earth let your upper body soar and call to it as you begin the Breath of Fire at a moderate to vigorous pace. As you breathe, keep gazing at your beautiful destiny, why you came here, why you came to earth. Think of the gifts you were meant to share. Merge with those gifts. Merge with your destiny, with the will of the divine.
7. Start your *Sat Nam* mantra right away and continue breathing powerfully for three minutes. Once you finish, inhale deeply and retain the breath as you apply the Root Lock. Suspend and retain the breath and open the heart, and when you can't hold your breath any longer, deepen your front knee bend and literally let your arrow fly—releasing the fingers of the front hand into bright, long, straight, extensions of your inner commitment and what you wish to manifest out in the world. Send your arrow to hit its mark!
8. Then, using your inner leg strength and abdominals, step your left foot forward to join your right foot in Mountain Pose. Let your arms hang down by your sides, and just breathe and feel. Close your eyes and just absorb the benefits of the Archer and the Breath of Fire. Feel yourself deeply grounded to the very core of the earth and bask in

your own radiance. It is palpable. Feel that love in your heart, feel it swimming and dancing around.

9. Now repeat on the opposite side, stepping the right foot back and moving through the entire sequence, performing the Breath of Fire for three minutes, then retaining the breath with the Root Lock, and letting your arrow fly when it's time. When you finish, come into Mountain Pose once again, stand in your greatness, and feel your deepest desires manifesting as you stand in your power.

Calling Destiny Home

You will pull your destiny toward you in Calling Destiny Home as you root your feet firmly into the earth and open your heart to usher love into your body and your life. This exercise instills a powerful sense of self-confidence, manifesting your wishes with every reach and pull you perform; it balances the first, second, and third chakras as it tones and strengthens the arms, shoulders, and abdominals.

1. Standing tall with feet slightly wider than hip-width apart, bring your hands into natural fists with your thumbs clamping down on the index and middle fingers; rest your fists at the sides of your waist and lift your gaze just above the horizon line, so that you grow even taller and feel proud and capable even before you start.
2. Keep your left hand in a fist and, as you inhale, reach your right hand out in front of you with your palm facing down and fingers spread wide apart as if you're casting a magic spell on the space in front of you.
3. Then right away, without so much as a pause, exhale and pull the right hand back into a fist at your side, and a nanosecond later send the left hand out in the same way to perform the same action as you inhale, *Sat.*
4. Exhale, *Nam,* and pull the left hand back in as you inhale again and send the right hand out, continuing in this way for up to three minutes, moving with real power and verve, like a true engine of self-love

at a moderate pace increasing to a vigorous one. Get your hips and upper torso involved, letting them naturally follow and emphasize the movement of your arm as it extends out in front of you and you pull your destiny in, drawing into your being, into your life, exactly what you wish for, what you want to manifest.

5. As you cast your nets out with each reach of the hand, manifesting your magic, envision each thing, person, or situation you want to usher into your life and pull it toward you with absolute belief in yourself, faith, and utter conviction, making each reach and pull very deliberate, filled with love for yourself and gratitude for this chance to speak with the universe in this special way.
6. After you have completed three minutes, on a great big inhalation extend both arms out in front of you, this time with the palms facing up and the chest open, the eyes lifted to the sky, opening your heart and celebrating this powerful loving homage to yourself and your deepest desires. As you exhale, slowly draw both arms back, bringing your hands into Prayer Position in front of your heart.

Shaking the Soul Tree

Shaking the Soul Tree resets the entire nervous system and strengthens the arms, shoulders, and abdominals. It washes your psyche and system clean of sadness and heartache and replaces them with clear vision, deep insight, wisdom, and prodigious inner strength and calm. This kriya will give you nerves of steel, so that you can rise to any occasion.

This is another exercise where you might want to abandon ship about thirty seconds in. Do not quit! The rewards are limitless. Not only are you strengthening your will, commitment, and determination, but you are burning through old, heavy, hardwired emotional programming as well as newly acquired stresses and upsets. This exercise has the power to help heal broken hearts and devastating disappointments. Keep going, and when you are finished, I assure you, you will feel a thousand pounds lighter in body, mind, and spirit.

1. Standing tall with feet slightly wider than hip-width apart, bring your arms up above your head to form a narrow V shape.
2. Keeping the arms strong and straight, but the wrists and hands soft, with the palms facing one another, start to flap the hands vigorously in the air in a back-and-forth motion, so that they look like the highest branches of a tree being whipped around by ferocious storm winds.
3. Rather than performing the Breath of Fire here, you will do Long Deep Breathing and concentrate on shaking the arms to keep the hands in constant, deliberate motion.
4. Keep shaking your soul tree for three minutes or even longer if you are so inclined, and when you have completed your time, bring your hands into Prayer Position overhead and draw the hands down in front of your heart center and then in front of the midline of the body. Open your hands, drop them down by your sides, and then reach them around back.
5. Interlace your fingers, trying to keep the palms pressing together if you can, and as you pull the hands down and back toward your heels and the floor, open your heart to the sky and breathe deeply, feeling the stretch of your chest, shoulders, and arms, all the muscles you have just worked so intensely for the past several minutes.
6. After a few breaths, release your arms down by your sides and turn your palms to face front, which will naturally open your chest and encourage optimal posture. Stand relaxed and tall, basking in your own energy and radiance.

Abdominal Pumping

Abdominal Pumping activates the abdominal center and the Solar Plexus Chakra (*manipura*) to receive powerful life force, stimulating the thousands of nerve plexuses and nadis that emanate from this center. It prepares your entire breathing apparatus for the work ahead, enhances lung capacity, loosens and relaxes the diaphragm, flushes the internal organs, infusing them with highly oxygenated blood and moving stagnant blood and toxins out, boosts overall circulation, and stimulates and strengthens digestion.

1. Stand tall with feet slightly wider than hip-width apart and lean forward, placing your hands on top of your thighs so that you can fully support the weight of your upper torso, or if you're more open and flexible, bring your hands down to press into the floor with palms flat.
2. Inhale deeply and draw in as much air as you possibly can without overexerting yourself, and then exhale immediately and powerfully, completely emptying the lungs.
3. Once the lungs are fully emptied, strongly contract the abdominal wall in and up toward the spine and hold it up and in for as long as you comfortably can.
4. Then rise to an erect position, breathe naturally for two breaths, and then repeat, coming into a forward bend with your hands on top of your knees, inhaling deeply and then fully emptying the lungs.
5. With the lungs completely empty, powerfully contract the abdominal wall once again. This time, start to pump the abdominals in and out, like a bellows stoking a fire, for as many repetitions as you can (optimally thirteen) until you feel the need to take your next breath.
6. When need to inhale once again, breathe in as you rise to stand, and then take two smooth, deep natural breaths.
7. Repeat the sequence one more time, then return to standing, and take two deep breaths before moving on to the next exercise.

*Corpse Pose (**Savasana**)*

Because the kundalini practices are heavily yang in nature, it is important to end with a yin pose to restore balance. Please follow the instructions for the Corpse Pose given at the end of Chapter 8.

After the Corpse Pose, make your way into a seat, with your hands in Prayer Position in front of your heart. I'd like to invite you to chant my favorite part of completing a kundalini practice. Say the following blessing:

May I live in great health, happiness, and wholeness.
May I come to know my sat nam, my truth, my true identity,
and find a peace within myself that illumines my life.
May the longtime sun shine upon me,
all love surround me,
and the pure light within me guide my way on.

Onward and Ever Upward!

Now that you have performed Unleash and Transform, some of the most challenging sequences and paces you have ever put your body through for its greater good, you have been officially initiated into kundalini. When you read the words "onward and ever upward," you now know exactly what they mean, because you have lived the feeling they inspire. It has risen up inside you like irrepressible laughter, like the ocean's swell, like the celebration of reaching the summit after an arduous climb, like the thrill of falling in love.

You have called upon an inner resolve, that tenacity and determination, that celebration of life that you were born with—your own power, health, peace, joy, and bliss! You have stoked the fire within and developed some powerful tools that not only brought you closer to yourself, but also helped you to pull back the curtain on a brave new world. You are now starting to understand just how strong and unlimited your potential is, that nothing can stand between you and your destiny. No disease, no discomfort, no one's ego, including your own, can have power over you. You are learning how to cultivate your most exquisite gifts to share here on earth.

As your inner radiance rises and permeates your being, you are able to trust that because of the energy you are cultivating, you alone have the power to draw to you what you need and want in life. Your own true beauty is found in the balance and flow, arising from the perfect marriage of strong nerves and healthy glands that produces the elixir of resilience and gratitude.

Now more than ever, you have started to wake your own energy and be true to yourself—to your eternal self. You have gotten your first taste of the mystical kundalini's magic spell. You now know how to access the power to great health, creativity, and abundance, inspiring you to reach your highest potential in every area of your life.

6

your own fountain of youth: the tibetan rites

About twelve years ago, on retreat in a remote village in Costa Rica, I was awakened before six o'clock one morning by a loud whirring outside my window. To my surprise, when I pulled the curtain back, I saw a tall, handsome, shirtless man, spinning like a whirling dervish with palm fronds in each hand, smiling and singing to himself. Without a moment's hesitation, I got out of bed and walked outside onto my porch to get a closer look.

It was clear that I was observing a private ritual. The devotee, completely dedicated to his work, was in his own world. After what seemed like an eternity, he stopped spinning, tossed the palm fronds on the ground, placed his hands on his hips, puffed his chest out, and took very deep breaths. He then lay on the ground, lifting his legs effortlessly up to a right angle with his head up. He sliced the air like a knife with his legs, lifting and lowering his head in tandem with the movements, not missing a beat. Mesmerized, I started counting, four, five, six times, all the way to twenty-one!

Leaping up with such ease that he appeared to levitate, the handsome stranger stood with his hands on his hips and took two deep power breaths, then dropped to his knees to begin the yogic Camel Pose. Placing his hands on the backs of his legs and arching his back, he inhaled and expanded his chest as if he had no bones, dropping his head back as he pressed his hips forward. In the same rhythmic motion he had established in the previous exercise, he inhaled as he arched back and exhaled as he brought his head forward, softening his chest—again, going all the way to that mysterious number: twenty-one. He inhaled again deeply, and then without a moment's hesitation he began another exercise.

Now it was Tabletop Pose, but instead of simply holding the pose, he literally swung his body back into Staff Pose, then right back up into Tabletop, in a powerful, unbroken rhythm. With each repetition of the movement, his skin seemed to glow brighter. I am sure he felt me watching him, but he stayed in his ritualistic bubble, transcending time and space.

When he moved into Downward-Facing Dog, rather than simply holding it, he flowed right into Upward-Facing Dog, and then down again, his face and upper torso gliding effortlessly down toward the earth as if he were a dolphin diving into water. Then he started a pumping, pulsing rhythm with his movements that seemed to create a kind of invisible energy shield repelling everything away from his orbit. He made the rest of the world disappear. His movements appeared so effortless. He was laughing at gravity.

After twenty-one repetitions of the Down-Dog and Up-Dog combination, he moved more slowly and deliberately. Standing still, he took a deep breath and exhaled like a lion. Then with his hands on his slightly bent knees, he contracted his abdominal area with such force that he carved a kind of canyon out of his own midsection. Suddenly, all I could see was his rectus abdominus (the central abdominal muscle) flaring out like a cobra, as if it were undulating inside his belly. Seamlessly, he moved the snake in and out and side to side—the kind of abdominal rippling a belly dancer might perform.

I recognized the esoteric breathing and abdominal massage to be the same that only special sects of yogis perform. I had seen it demonstrated at an ashram in upstate New York many years earlier. Now, as then, I was in awe.

After repeating this abdominal ritual three times, he rose to an erect stance, took three power breaths, and brought his hands into Prayer Position, with his palms pressed in front of his heart and his eyes closed. A full five minutes passed as I waited, breathless.

He opened his eyes and smiled. I will never forget what he said afterward—not to me, but to the panoramic world around him—the mountains, the trees, flowers, and birds: "*Pura vida!*" (Life is good!). Then, before I could even grasp that it was happening, he had broken the "fourth wall" of his sacred ritual. He looked right at me with an even bigger smile and said, "Come, I will teach you."

Right there on the grounds of a gorgeous Costa Rican outpost, in my best sleepwear, with this handsome superhero as my very own private instructor, I became privy to a thousand-year-old secret ritual.

I swear to you that when I stood where he had been spinning and pumping and breathing, I felt an incredible rush of energy shoot through my body. I must have gasped aloud, because he laughed gently and said, "*Si, cara* (Yes, my dear) . . . just ride it." In an elegant, dulcet-toned English accent, he softly said, "Close your eyes and breathe it in."

In that moment, my perception of time changed. I must have lingered there for ten minutes before he gently interrupted me with his hand on my shoulder. I wanted to continue swimming in that sweet vortex of liquid velvet—the enveloping energy spiraling up into my body from the earth below.

With a knowing smile, my charming, radiant new friend told me to stretch my arms out at shoulder height with my palms facing down to the earth and spin clockwise, "the direction of time," so that I could "surrender my ego to the universe." I loved the idea that by spinning I could relinquish my ego and my judging mind and travel into a realm of real substance.

"Where are my palm fronds?" I asked coyly.

He chuckled and told me that he had added them to the original movement that his father had taught him as a child, so that he could feel as if he was flying. When I said I wanted the full effect, he retrieved them, and with the anointed palm fronds in hand, off I went, my arms outstretched. One revolution, two, three, and by the fourth I was incredibly dizzy. Somehow I managed to say, "I think I need to stop!" With that, he gently held my shoulders and told me to rotate counterclockwise once and breathe deeply so that the dizziness would subside.

"How long did it take you to be able to spin twenty-one times?"

He laughed, flashing a perfect smile, his eyes sparkling, and said that if I practiced every day, adding a revolution every few days, I would reach twenty-one before long. He explained that this would mean that my "vestibular apparatus"—my balance, spatial awareness, and stability—had become strong and vital.

And that's exactly what I did. I got back on the horse, palm fronds in hand, and started to spin again. This time, I made it to five repetitions before I started to get dizzy. I then placed my hands on my hips and took the three superhero "power breaths" I saw my friend take earlier. Once I took that second breath, with my hands on my hips, my feet firmly planted in the earth, I started to believe that maybe I could be a superhero too.

Then, following his meticulous cues, I got down on the ground and performed an exercise that looked like a "leg chop." My years of Pilates served me well in using my core strength and being able to maneuver my legs up and down, but I could feel that something else was going on entirely—something deeper was being opened and released inside my own body. It felt like a new kind of strength and vitality bubbling up from a deep well inside me. My entire body was coming alive in a way that was foreign, but not completely unfamiliar. It was exciting!

Each exercise took on an entirely new dynamic and texture, different from anything I'd ever done, ushering me into what felt like an altered dimension. I had to surmise that it was because of the breathing, the incredible focus, and the rhythm—that powerful, unbroken, steady, forward-moving rhythm that was implicit in each exercise he instructed me to do. It swept over my body like a wave, until I suddenly felt as though I was part of everything around me.

The sun had only just started to rise and I am decidedly *not* a morning person, yet I felt as if I were ready for anything. After my final power breath, I looked at my new mentor and said, "I've never felt this awake and, may I say, powerful at six forty-five in the morning!"

To which he replied, "We were meant to rise with the sun and align with its rhythms. It gives us natural power and energy. If we sleep through the dawn, we miss it—we miss this precious opportunity. When you add these secrets to what you already have here in nature, you have something very, very precious. I am very glad that I could share this ancient secret with you. Promise yourself to do it every day, and you will have a long, happy life."

I nodded. But then remembering the yogic abdominal undulations he had performed earlier, I asked why he hadn't shown them to me.

"The Sixth Rite is one that you must build up to. It requires great concentration and focus. When you are able to channel your procreative energy into your higher mind, you will start to develop a spiritual consciousness of the divine, of higher realms. You must be ready. Once you have practiced the five rites for many moons, you will know when the time is right."

As casually as he had performed the movements, he handed me a yellowed, tattered book containing the rites that had clearly been his for a long, long time. I felt so honored, as if I were receiving an ancient artifact, and wondered if I had earned the right to receive such a valuable gift. Smiling knowingly, as if were reading my mind, he opened his arms and gave me one of the all-time best hugs of my life. Embraced against his powerful, vibrant body, I could feel the energy of his being literally bouncing off his skin and into mine, as if it were beaming out all the way to the sun and back and, together, we were somehow creating a rarefied circuit, a channel. I couldn't remember a time when I felt so energized and alive!

Feeling almost out of body, I heard my voice come barreling out of nowhere, "How old are you anyway?" I braced myself, embarrassed for blurting out such a thing to a man of such generosity, quiet grace, and dignity—but he had nary a gray hair on his head and looked not a day over thirty-five.

"I am sixty-six years young, my dear," he smiled.

That was all I needed to know. Whatever he was doing, I wanted to do it.

Little did I know that he had shared the famed Tibetan Rites, also known as the Rites of Rejuvenation. Because I was privileged to learn these secrets from a master, I will now teach you yet another way to wake up the kundalini energy inside you and taste the sweet waters that flow from your very own fountain of youth.

The Tale of the Tibetan Rites

Legend has it that an ancient sect of Tibetan monks discovered the secret to eternal youth and passed it on generation after generation for thousands of years. Cut off from the outside world by the vast, largely uninhabited Himalayas, this treasure remained shrouded from the rest of the world. Until the end of their days, these monks retained their youthful vigor. By practicing the Rites of Rejuvenation daily, they learned energy cultivation and refinement. They understood that by dedicating themselves to a daily rejuvenating ritual, they would strengthen and balance their outer body as well as their inner emotional lives and connection to spirit.

Reversing the aging process wasn't their chief goal, although it was a natural consequence and welcome bonus. By dedicating themselves to their bodies, they made them into extraordinary vessels for balance and health—the perfect vehicles with which to reach higher levels of consciousness and evolution while on earth. For these Tibetan monks, the Rites of Rejuvenation were a profound link to realms that enhanced their development as spiritual beings. By cultivating greater awareness of their internal energies and how to harmonize and harness them, they became closer to their body's capabilities and more masterful in influencing how they functioned. So refined and sophisticated was their practice, legend has it that they were able to leave their bodies at will, while in prayer, and transcend the earthly realm entirely.

This attunement allowed them to use them to use their bodies as vehicles to attain enlightenment. In the process, it became clear to them that they did not have to grow old and infirm. If they embraced a life of action, wisdom, and devotion, anything was possible. For generations, they dedicated themselves to raising the consciousness of the planet.

In the late 1930s, retired British naval officer Peter Kelder met a decorated British military colonel named Colonel Bradford (a pseudonym) in southern California. Kelder was a man in his sixties, stooped and using a cane. He shared his discontent that he had deteriorated and that he was determined to restore himself to his former military glory. Also tired and feeling older than his years, Bradford had decided to travel to India in search of a remote sect of Tibetan clerics who had allegedly discovered the secret to eternal youth. Bradford shared his plans to find them and bring the teachings back with Kelder, whose curiosity was piqued.

Years passed, and Bradford reappeared on Kelder's doorstep miraculously looking like a virile, younger version of himself. Bradford told Kelder he had learned the rites he'd been seeking from a sect of lamas living at a monastery in the Himalayas. He had seen no old people there, only wise old souls in young vital bodies. Due to the extraordinary power of this ritual, he swore, many of the monks lived well to one hundred and beyond.

Thrilled with the transformation the rites had produced in his own body, Bradford documented them in detail and eagerly taught the rites to Kelder. A few years later, enthused about the work and its results, Kelder started writing his own books about them. First, he published *The Eye of Revelation* (1936), then *The Original Five Tibetan Rites of Rejuvenation* (1939), and finally *The Ancient Secret of the Fountain of Youth* (1985). In the last book, he described fully, for the first time, the philosophy behind the rites, which he called *youthing*. The Rites of Rejuvenation were now introduced to the Western world.

The Tibetan monks were "plugging into the source," harnessing universal energy for their benefit and for humankind as a whole. Sharing these rites with you here is my way of continuing the tradition.

"Spinning Wheels" of Energy

The chakras are individual vortexes of energy, or "spinning wheels," and their speed and fluidity are the keys to vibrant health. When all the chakras are spinning at an optimal rate, they remove stagnant prana and distribute pure prana throughout the body, resulting in total rejuvenation. When the chakras dance together, they flow like a fountain that perpetually renews itself.

The body naturally seeks homeostasis. The momentum of health and healing that takes place when you engage in the Tibetan Rites is akin to keeping plates spinning in a magic act. Once the chakras are set in perfect motion, they require very little effort to sustain, because, like the whirling dervishes of Rumi's Persia, they prefer motion over stillness.

Once the chakra system learns how to function at its optimal speed, it lays down its own new and improved way of being, establishing something akin to muscle memory, so that little is required to maintain it. The new energy that the rites introduce to the subtle body, the very thing that initiates the change and brings the chakras into balance, is what also maintains it long after you finish performing the movements. Each time you perform them, this muscle memory builds, resulting in greater stamina, flexibility, and power in your life—the body just keeps getting stronger and stronger.

Because of our sedentary lifestyle, the spinning of our chakras tends to slow down. A slow-moving, underactive chakra system causes the corresponding organs and parts of the body to stagnate and deteriorate. When we have to cope with the stresses of life, the chakras can respond by speeding up too much, leading to a condition of excess, causing nervousness, anxiety, and exhaustion. Neither state is desirable.

If this cycle continues, the chakras continue to function "in the dark," without conscious awareness on the part of the human they belong to, and the pranic energy is blocked, often leading to accelerated aging.

The Tibetan Rites normalize, then optimize, the speed of our spinning chakras. By spinning at the same rate as one another, they work in harmony and lead to a heightened state of awareness and empowerment. The result is vibrant, superhero-like vitality!

As the speed of any particular chakra is increased, the life force of that particular chakra becomes stronger and more directed, moving from your center outward to your extremities, and the kundalini energy stored at the base of the spine is urged to travel up the spine. The Tibetan Rites are similar to our Unleash and Transform practice, but here you can access and distribute *kundalini shakti* in a shorter amount of time.

Not only can the series produce an internal wellspring of health and vitality, but it will also shape your outer body beautifully. You won't believe how incredibly toned and sculpted the series can make you look—and if you're dedicated to a consistent practice, it can happen in seemingly no time at all.

Turning Back the Hands of Time

Judging by how my dashing mentor looked that memorable morning in Costa Rica, it's true that you can turn back the hands of time. Because each of the rites engages every muscle of the body, it produces a beautiful musculature that includes longer, leaner arms and legs and a well-defined abdominal core—not to mention the grace that comes from coordinating whole-body movements with breathing.

The seven chakras influence not only how well and how long we live, but every aspect of who we are and how we experience life. Just as a massage can soothe an aching muscle or the right nutrient can stimulate a gland to function well, practicing the Tibetan Rites balances and stimulates the chakras and encourages them to function at peak efficiency. When the Tibetan Rites are practiced regularly, they actually work so effectively to bring harmony and balance to the endocrine system that, in essence, the aging process is slowed, defied, and in some cases reversed. The stimulation and opening of the chakras in turn activate all the glands of the endocrine system, which is responsible for the body's hormonal and metabolic functioning as well as its aging process.

The Tibetan Rites positively affect the overall functioning of all body systems. With a newfound vitality, you will boost your metabolism, find the optimal weight for your body, and experience increased physical strength and flexibility, total-body toning, relief from joint and back pain, reduced stress, restful sleep, improved memory, mental focus, heightened creativity, better eyesight, hair growth, enhanced energy, youthful vigor, rejuvenation of organ systems, and reinvigorated sexuality. All of this, in turn, balances the mind and emotions.

Even though I know you may want to explore the "reinvigorated sexuality" benefit, I suspect that what's really calling your name is finding your optimal weight—or adjusting your weight "set point." Because the rites regulate hormone production, they improve metabolic function. This means better assimilation of nutrients, better sleep, and increased energy. As a result, you lose weight. You look better, look younger, feel younger, and act younger—because you *are* younger!

In the process, your weight set point is lowered, perhaps even lower than it was in your youth, allowing your body to naturally release any extra weight you've been carrying around. This happens not only because your body's subtle systems are stimulated, opened, and balanced, but because of the vigorous pace at which you perform the rites, with every muscle participating in the challenge. Add to that the deep breathing you engage in while performing the rites, which circulates essential life energy throughout the body, helping it rid itself of toxins and burn stored fat cells.

Once you start to reveal the body that lies beneath that extra weight through consistent practice, you will automatically start to feel rewarded for your efforts. You will feel more confident and empowered. In fact, your first and second chakras are also stimulated, which are specifically responsible for feelings of security, creativity, and sexual expression. As you feel more sensual, you may very well be moved to share your new confidence with another, and *voila!* There is your reinvigorated sexuality.

With the chakras spinning optimally, your energy will actually extend beyond your physical body, creating a kind of shield of protective energy around you like an "orb" of guardian prana. This orb, which extends out at least five feet in every direction around the body, is the *etheric body*. It interacts harmoniously with the environment and can also literally protect us from people who are less aware or who are engaging in malevolent behaviors.

The Tibetan monks believed that we draw in energy without being aware of what we are taking in. All kinds of emotional energies enter our etheric body in this way. Psychically, we can attract negative emotions belonging to other people that relate to the emotions we ourselves are carrying. Fear or anger inside us can act as a magnet to pull in similar energies from other people. When we bring focused attention to our own chakras and move the stagnant, negative energy out, we then automatically activate our protective shield and keep others' negative energies at bay.

When we consciously activate the protective orb, it provides us with an overall "glow," a youthful health and vitality that shines from the inside out. You become your own sun. The Tibetan Rites are mortals' answer to a mere taste of the enlightened masters' decades-long training on the mountaintop. What they can accomplish in ten minutes to improve your overall health and energy has greater immediate impact than almost anything else you can do in life.

The Tibetan Rites

The body doesn't require complicated maneuvers to function well. It just wants to move, and when you add conscious breath and intention into the mix, you have a winning combination—an unbeatable combination. The Tibetan Rites were the prized health and longevity secret for Tibetan monks for generations. You may think they are mysterious and complex, but they're actually remarkably simple to learn. The Tibetan Rites require nothing more than your focus and a small investment of your time to reap prodigious rewards. The entire routine can be completed in less than ten minutes, but it helps you achieve more than most regimens can do in hours.

It's very important to do The Tibetan Rites exactly as they are presented, without altering the form or sequence, so that you too can experience the phenomenal benefits. Each of the exercises is performed up to twenty-one times, because the ancient Tibetans believed twenty-one to be a perfect, mystical number. It represents the seven core chakras multiplied by the three realms of body, mind, and spirit.

This incredible little jewel of a series does it all. It shapes and tones the entire body; enhances flexibility, grace, and poise; empowers; builds confidence and inner resolve; and literally stimulates the entire chakra system for total body balancing, strengthening, and awakening. It is age-defying, revitalizing, and super immune boosting.

your own fountain of youth practice

TIME OF DAY: Morning or evening

QUALITY: Yang

SUBTLE ENERGY: Balances and harmonizes the chakra system.

BENEFITS: Dramatically increases overall energy; encourages weight loss; enhances physical strength, flexibility, and stamina; instills peace of mind; restores youthful vigor, reawakens sexuality, and boosts libido.

PROP: Mat

The Practice:

Spinning
Leg Lift
Camel
Tabletop Lever
Up Dog, Down Dog
Abdominal Massage

Before You Begin

On your Tibetan adventure, all I ask is that you be kind and patient with yourself, that you listen to your body and respect its limits when you attempt the exercises here. Some of them can be challenging and could test your resolve. Please note that because the Tibetan Rites are so powerful, you may experience some detoxing effects at first—anything from dizziness to nausea, lethargy, or achy muscles. These symptoms are often signs that your body is actually responding favorably to the practice and is trying to rid itself of stagnation and toxin buildup. The solution for these symptoms (though you may not experience them at all) is to be patient, drink lots of water, and rest when needed.

Soon, with consistent practice, your body will adjust and stabilize and you will start to feel wonderful. If you start gently, you will be inspired by the results of your efforts and amply rewarded. You will see and feel almost immediate results: increased energy, strength, and stamina and a sense of true overall well-being. Here are some additional things to remember before you begin:

- For your first attempt at the Tibetan Rites and only if you are relatively healthy and fit, do each exercise three times. Then gradually start to add a repetition each time you perform the rites, working your way up to seven repetitions, then fourteen, and ultimately twenty-one.
- If you are inactive, overweight, or have health problems, begin by doing one of the first three exercises each day. As with all the other practices in this book, do only what you feel comfortable doing. This may mean only one of each exercise for the first week. That's okay! Remember, Tibet . . . I mean, *Rome* wasn't built in a day! Build up to two of each exercise the second week, three of each exercise the third week, and continue in this way until you've reached at least seven repetitions. You may increase the number of repetitions you do daily or perform the exercises at a faster pace as long as your body feels good when you do them.
- Twenty-one is the maximum number of repetitions of each exercise you should ever do. If you want to enhance your program, do the whole ritual at a faster pace, but not more than twenty-one of each exercise each day. More than twenty-one repetitions of an exercise in a day could adversely affect your chakras, creating imbalances in your body.
- None of the rites should be so intense that it makes you feel exhausted. For example, you should be able to speak comfortably after performing any of the rites. If you can't or feel as though you are

"losing your breath," it means that you should slow down. When performing the exercises, the main emphasis should be on your breath and fluency of movement rather than on speed and number of repetitions. If you're overly concerned with the latter, that's your ego talking, and the whole point of performing these, really, is to renounce it! Remember that when you are tempted to push yourself unsafely past your limits.

Tibetan Breathing

An important part of the Tibetan Rites is a conscious synchronization of breathing while performing the movements. Before beginning the exercises, practice the following basic four-part breathing technique.

Four-Part Breath

1. Inhale deeply through the nose.
2. Hold the breath as long as possible in comfortably filled lungs. Do not overfill.
3. Exhale completely through the nose.
4. With empty lungs, hold the breath out as long as you can.

After finishing each rite, come into the Superhero Power Breath Stance before moving on to the next rite.

Superhero Power Breath Stance

1. Make your way onto all fours, tucking your toes under and pressing your hands into the ground, raising your hips to the sky, straightening the legs as much as possible, and pressing the chest toward the

thighs to come into Downward-Facing Dog Pose, forming an inverted V shape with your body.

2. Walk your feet up to meet your hands and roll up sequentially through the spine to a tall stance with your feet hip-width apart and hands on your hips.
3. Take three full, deep breaths, inhaling through your nose and exhaling through your mouth with your lips pursed in the shape of an O to release tension in the face, specifically the jaw.

The Practice

Rite One: Spinning

Children naturally spin while they play. Since Waking Energy is about reclaiming your original self, here is your chance to remind your body of something it already knows how to do. Become a child again. Without thinking too hard about it or giving in to preconceived notions about how it might make you feel, prepare to be surprised—it could be fun! That's why children do it! So why not seek it out, the way a venturing child would?

Spinning stimulates the body's total energy system, waking up all the chakras. It gently accelerates the overall flow of your life force. By bringing the vortices to an optimal speed, spinning has a calming effect on the mind and the emotional body. When we spin clockwise, the Tibetan monks say that negative residues are flung out of the body. The bridge between the left and right hemispheres of the brain is strengthened and balance improves.

This exercise strengthens the vestibular apparatus—the balancing mechanism in the inner ear. With regular practice, your initial dizziness will stop. The spin will become easy and fluid, even at very fast speeds. This is the same motion practiced by Sufi whirling dervishes, who twirl at rapid speeds for long periods of time to achieve a state of prayerful transcendence.

1. Stand erect with your arms outstretched horizontal to the floor and your palms facing down. Without moving from your place, slowly start to spin in a clockwise direction, rotating around that one spot on the floor, breathing naturally, and working your way into spinning as fast as you can without losing control.
2. It is important to keep your eyes focused on a point at your starting place, or "spot," in the front of the room for as long as you can, until your head turns naturally to follow the rest of your body as you spin. Then turn your head around quickly and find your spot with your eyes as soon as you can, leaving your gaze there while your body rotates until you have to turn your head again. Spotting will enable you to preserve your equilibrium as you spin and diminishes the dizziness that occurs as a natural consequence of the spinning action.
3. Continue to spin until you start to feel dizzy. Once this happens, stop. Feel free to rest, to sit or to lie down until the dizziness subsides and resolves entirely. When you first attempt this exercise, you may not be able to spin more than a few times without getting dizzy. As your chakras attune and your inner balance mechanisms get stronger, you will be able to spin up to twenty-one times without getting dizzy at all.

Rite Two: Leg Lift

The second rite connects you more deeply to your emotional life and the seat of your "true mind." Physically, the Leg Lift tones and strengthens the deep abdominal and "corset" muscles of your trunk as well as your glutes and muscles of your back. It also serves to increase flexibility in your hamstrings and lower back. By raising your head to the chest, you create an extra stimulus to the Solar Plexus Chakra (*manipura*) as you stimulate and open the *sushumna nadi,* your central channel, distributing that new, life-giving prana throughout your entire subtle body.

1. Use a thick mat to support your spine, and lie down on your back with your legs outstretched along the floor. Extend your arms down by your sides with your palms pressing flat into the floor and your fingers close together.
2. Inhale as you raise your head off the floor, gently tucking your chin into your chest with your eyes focused on your navel.
3. As you lift your head, first draw your knees to your chest, and then extend your legs straight up to the ceiling with your feet fully flexed. (If possible, let your legs extend over your upper body, slightly behind your head, but do not bend your knees.)
4. Exhale as you slowly lower your head and your legs down to the floor simultaneously, with your eyes focusing up at the ceiling and your feet flexed. Protect your lower back by drawing your navel to your spine and activating your abdominal muscles.
5. As you inhale, press the backs of your arms into the floor, lift your head back to the upright position, with your eyes focusing on your navel. At the same time, strongly lift your legs back up to the starting angle, with your abdominals deeply engaged and your feet flexed up to the ceiling.

Tip: As you repeat the movements, develop a rhythmic, moderate pace, inhaling as you lift your head and legs, exhaling as you lower them. Use the inhalation as a force to lift your head and legs back up, as if they were literally slicing through the air with strength and energy, like a piston.

Rite Three: Camel

Rite Three opens your solar plexus and heart centers. The Camel is a classic back bend, but performed in combination with a forward upper-body contraction in a strong, fluid fashion. We begin life by drawing energy in through the umbilical area. This rite provides an opening and extension, a powerful lifting and opening of the entire trunk, which is the opposite of a defensive, contractive stance. By performing this motion, you raise new, conscious, positive energy from the first, second, and third chakras to the fourth, the Heart Chakra (*anahata*), where all four chakras become unified and vibrate together in a heightened and tranquil awareness.

1. Kneel on the floor with your knees under your hips and your toes tucked under in a stretched position. Keep your body erect.
2. Place your hands on the backs of your legs just under your buttocks.
3. Inhale to prepare. As you exhale, tilt your head and neck forward, tucking your chin against your chest.
4. Then gently move your head and neck backward as far as possible. At the same time, arch your spine backward on the inhalation, allowing your eyes to follow your trajectory back.
5. Exhale as you lift your head and upper back to return to the original position.

Tip: Establish a rhythmic breathing pattern. Breathe in deeply as you arch your spine. Breathe out as you return to an erect position. If possible, keep your eyes closed while performing this rite to eliminate distractions and keep your focus inward.

Rite Four: Tabletop Lever

Rite Four stimulates the second chakra, the Sacral Chakra (*svadthisthana*), the home of our sexuality and creativity, where emotions are exchanged between other chakras as well as interpersonally. The Tabletop Lever activates the nadis and the energies to and from your groin and down your legs, stimulating and augmenting your sexual and kidney prana reserves. It also connects your second chakra to your Heart Chakra, raising your sexual awareness to a higher, more conscious level, leading it to embrace the loving aspects of your heart and all that it holds. Physically, this rite strengthens and tones your legs, glutes, and abdominals as well as the major muscles of your upper body and back.

1. Sit on the floor with your spine tall and your legs extended straight out in front of you about twelve inches apart.
2. Flex your feet and place your palms flat on floor next to your hips with your fingers pointed toward your feet. As you press your palms into the mat, straighten your arms and press them more firmly against the floor to grow taller and lift into perfect posture.
3. Inhale deeply, then exhale, while dropping your chin to your chest and gently tucking it forward against your chest.
4. Bend your knees, and place your feet flat on the floor, still keeping your legs hip-width apart.
5. Press your hands into the floor by your sides, inhaling and tilting your head backward as far as it will go. Engage your buttocks and abdominals fully to lift your hips into a position parallel to the floor, as you push up into a Tabletop Pose with your arms straight behind you. Your face should be looking skyward.
6. Be sure to breathe in as you raise your body into the Tabletop position and hold your breath as you engage all your muscles while in the "up" position. Breathe out completely as you come down.
7. Once you have established a stable position with your feet, inhale and lift yourself up into your hips-raised position. The trunk of your body should be in a straight line with your hips and upper legs, horizontal to the floor. Let your head fall back gently, with your eyes focused upward, keeping your head in line with your spine.
8. Exhale and push even more firmly away from the floor with your arms. This will create more height in your upper body, so that as you come down into your original starting position from Tabletop, you'll be able to lift your body high enough to glide down, seamlessly slid-

ing your bottom back and through your arms before you immediately begin your next repetition in a steady, unbroken rhythm.

Tips: After the second repetition, the action should become quite vigorous, building momentum like a steam engine. Exhale as your body swings strongly back into the seated preparation position. With each repetition, focus on rooting your feet even more solidly before lifting your hips up to a position perfectly parallel to the floor. Do your best not to let your feet slide. Ideally, your feet should stay in the same place through this whole exercise, and because the movement is accomplished by pivoting at your shoulders, your arms should not bend.

Rite Five: Up Dog, Down Dog

Note: If you have tight shoulders, you will need to gradually work into being able to fully tilt your hips upward. Honor your body's limits here, and know that with practice you'll be able to move into greater range before you know it.

Because your body is moving in concert with the energy rising up your spine, propelling *kundalini shakti* up along the central channel, the fifth rite, brings an immediate and positive change to your subtle body. Up Dog, Down Dog is the most powerful rite for unifying and optimally setting the speed of the chakras, which in turn then stimulates and opens the organs they are connected to. The alternation in it makes you feel extra strong and invigorated—as the Tibetan lamas say, "Brings a happy glow to your face."

On a physical level, it's a total-body strengthener and significantly increases the power of your abdominals as they control and stabilize your arms and legs. It increases overall stamina and enhances grace, spatial awareness, and balance.

1. Begin on all fours with your toes flexed under, and your weight evenly distributed between your knees, your palms, and the balls of your feet. Make sure the hands are directly under the shoulders and spread your fingers wide into the ground as you firm your arms.
2. Inhale and press into your heels, straightening your legs as much as you can, lifting your buttocks skyward. Maintain a flat back and lower your head, so that your body comes into Downward-Facing Dog Pose, forming the shape of an inverted V.
3. Exhale and, keeping your arms perpendicular to the floor and drawing your navel to your spine, press your hips toward the floor until your legs are strong and straight behind you. You'll transition through a Plank position (parallel to the ground) and press the hips down so that they're grazing the floor, deeply arching your spine, and rolling your shoulders back so that your chest is open, as you come into the Upward-Facing Dog Pose.
4. Continue now by swinging your body back up into Down Dog again, as you exhale and push the earth away with your arms strong and straight, and right away again glide your body down with graceful control into Up Dog.
5. This is a bit of a brainteaser, but you'll inhale whenever you're on your way *up* into Down Dog and exhale on your way *down* into Up Dog.

Tips: Throughout this rite, your hands, arms, legs and feet should be kept so energized that not only are they straight, but they actually make you feel as though you are pushing the floor or ground away (by employing the principle of opposition, which you'll officially learn in Pilates). Follow the deep breathing pattern used in the previous rites, but on this one in particular, really exploit the up and down pumping action of the body, breathing in very deeply as you raise your body, and breathing out fully as you lower it, expelling the air to cleanse your lungs and move stagnant prana out of your body.

Rite Six: Abdominal Massage

The Tibetans say that this special sixth rite will turn you into a superbeing. For the Abdominal Massage to be truly effective, the monks say that you must practice celibacy, primarily because you preserve your life force more effectively by not "giving away your power." For instance, when men ejaculate, they give away their power because their primary source of energy is in their sexual essence, and by abstaining they retain it.

However, if you have read Chapter 5 and feel comfortable with your level of proficiency with the Unleash and Transform practice, you've earned the right to try this one. Not only does this massage detoxify the internal organs; it stimulates *kundalini shakti* and concentrates it in the third, the Solar Plexus Chakra, in an extra powerful way, making it available for more potent and immediate distribution throughout your entire subtle body.

1. Stand comfortably and exhale as you bend forward from your waist, placing your hands on your knees.
2. Expel the last bit of air from your lungs and without taking in new breath, return to an erect position.
3. Place your hands on your hips, with your fingers to the front, and press as hard as you can while sucking in your abdomen. This will raise your shoulders and chest.
4. Holding in your abdomen, squeeze your perineum to emphasize the upward thrust.
5. Hold this position. With your eyes closed, bring your internal focus to the third eye, the point between your eyebrows, so that all the energy from your lower chakras will be encouraged to rise up to the higher energy centers with your conscious attention as the driver.
6. Repeat three times. Lie down on your back in a fully relaxed position and rest for a few minutes afterwards.

Tip: When you must take a breath during the sixth rite, breathe in through your nose and then exhale through your mouth as you drop your arms down to your sides to relax. Take in several normal breaths through your nose and mouth before beginning again.

As you practice the Tibetan Rites, you will actually feel the silent pulse of perfect rhythm that connects us to all of life, energy, and nature. You will feel like a child again, spinning color wheels of energy in harmony with one another and with your breathing, awakening the circulating, flowing energy body within you. You will experience yourself as a vibrant microcosm of the universe, at one with the universe and forever young.

7

empower and flow: pilates

Now it's time for me to introduce to you one of my oldest and truest friends, Pilates, a vibrantly energizing, dynamic yang exercise series that connects you to the center of your fire power like no other. Pilates brings energy cultivation to new heights with the added dimension of an invigorating, muscular reinforcement of the core of the body. You are now ready to meet your muscular core, which works so beautifully in tandem with your subtle energy body.

Pilates serves as a kind of keystone to Waking Energy. A keystone is the balancing element in the structure of an arch; it creates strength in the arch by receiving the equal pressure of the stones to its right and left. In our Waking Energy arch, Pilates stands in the middle, supporting yang forces on one side and yin forces on the other. As a keystone, it is a perfect meeting point between these two types of subtle energy, inviting you to apply all the knowledge of subtle energy you've acquired thus far.

The Empower and Flow series will supplement your present abilities by introducing you to a realm of power you've not yet explored: pure yang. The series is designed to balance the musculature of your body. Like kundalini yoga, as Pilates raises the heat in your body, it purifies and enlivens your entire system. From the Hundred onward, you won't stop until you've completed your last Seal and are clapping for more, feeling fully alive, awake, empowered, and ready for anything.

Pilates is ingeniously designed to meet you exactly where you are, never giving you more than you can handle, but always challenging you in such a way that you surpass your preconceived notions of your capabilities. It imbues you with a sense of purpose by dangling a carrot of promise before you, landing it in your hands just long enough to whet your appetite, and then tempting you to climb higher.

When you embark on the Empower and Flow practice, you'll discover that the way it combines subtle body awareness with powerful core strength will both make demands on you and reward you. Because of what it asks of you physically and mentally, Pilates rewards you with the strength to take on more. The combination is winning—unbeatable, really—because it gives you the energy to *want* to do more. What makes Pilates unique among exercise programs is that the workout itself perpetually surprises you. With regard to building strength and physical capability, you'll find that it's unmatched by the mind-body modalities you may have tried elsewhere, because the way it combines subtle energy awareness with strength demands literally sculpts the beautiful physical body that you can see. Like kundalini, it continually raises the bar, asking more of you physically and mentally, inspiring you to deliver, creating a kind of new extraordinary belief in your own potential.

Catching Fire

A childhood spent in ballet studios finally paid off during the summer of my thirteenth year. Not only was I accepted into the prestigious

School of American Ballet, where talented young dancers are groomed to one day join the New York City Ballet (NYCB), but I also signed up for a conditioning class using an approach then called "Contrology." The class was taught by the late Eve Gentry, one of Joseph Pilates's protégées who was a guest teacher that year for NYCB's summer dance intensive.

I remember the first day I stood at the door with fourteen other young ballerinas, our hair obediently pulled back into little chignons, eyes wide, mouths closed in expectant, dutiful silence, barely breathing. Our teacher, Eve, seemed to float into the room: a slender, elegant woman with a twinkle in her eye, the embodiment of effortless grace.

She told us that we were there to strengthen our bodies—our *center* or *core muscles*—so we could become better dancers and prevent injury. She told us that the class we were about to do had been invented by her mentor, Joseph Pilates, a friend of Mr. Balanchine. Designed to use the body as an integrated whole, this exercise system would help us increase our competitive edge. She said it would enhance our overall performance and have us jumping and turning like Mikhail Baryshnikov in no time. At the mention of Baryshnikov, I was sold.

I dutifully followed Eve's instructions. I stood at the head of my mat and crossed my arms in front of my chest as she directed us to do. I lifted the crown of my head upward so that my reflection in the mirror across from me made me appear taller than I ever thought I could be. I used my *powerhouse,* the belt of muscles extending from the buttocks up and around through the abdomen into the upper torso, to lower myself gracefully to the floor.

I was told to lie down, lift my legs up to the ceiling, and then lower them down to an angle where my back was held flat against the mat only by the strength in my abdominal muscles. At the same time I was to pump my arms up and down at a rapid pace by the sides of my body for ten ten-count breaths. "Pumping" felt like flapping to me, because it was so foreign and difficult for my gangly young body to do. I was cued to keep my upper body lifted and my eyes on my navel while my legs were extended. It felt nearly impossible.

By arm flap number twenty-five, I was in agony. I didn't think I'd make it to fifty, let alone one hundred. I felt my abdominals burn for the first time: they were on fire! I could barely breathe, never mind keep my legs up or smile, as Eve mercilessly commanded we do. "Keep those arms pumping. Get the blood moving. Keep the oxygen flowing. Inhale, two, three, four, five. Exhale, two, three, four, five!" I thought I was going to die.

After I finished the workout, I called my mother to complain bitterly about the strange exercise class I'd just taken in which I had lain on my back and flapped my arms up and down a hundred times, after which I got severely punished for the next forty-plus minutes by having to perform gymnastic movements that made my stomach ache in ways I'd never known it could. Instead of indulging my complaints, she told me she was sure that the class would prove to be very useful and important to me and that I should attend as many of the "strange exercise" sessions as I could. She had a good feeling about them.

Later that same day, I wandered into an empty rehearsal studio to practice some phrases from the morning's repertory class. I moved into the final bars of the most challenging choreography and prepared to do the ever elusive triple pirouette that marked the end of the phrase—a flourish I'd been hungering to master. Every attempt I'd made before had ended in frustration and a double pirouette—or at the most in a sloppy, overexerted double and a half. I prepared once again for the triple. I took a deep plié. Then my arms moved into port de bras, encircling my newfound center, and in what was soon to become an unforgettable slice of time my head turned and my body followed effortlessly for one, two, then three turns! Gliding gracefully, I finished in fourth position. I had done it!

With that, I understood for the first time what effortless effort meant, and (no pun intended) there would be no turning back. Considering the results of working my core, the next conditioning class just couldn't come soon enough.

That summer, even when I encountered exercises that were harder than I imagined they would be, I persevered, just as my mother had told me I should. Because of the nature of the work and how balanced and symmetrical every movement was, I couldn't rely on my old ways: I couldn't just mimic a movement by watching it and then repeating it, as we did in dance. I couldn't "cheat," counting on my stronger "workhorse" muscles to compensate for my weaker ones. In order to successfully execute *any* movement, my weaker side had to participate as well. I had to think, to really concentrate, and I had to do it quickly—dialoguing with my body within a span of seconds and asking it to comply and partner with me. For the first time, employing the muscles I "found" in Pilates, I used my body as an integrated whole.

As if overnight (and that's the magic of the work, how quickly it reeducates you), I developed an entirely new interior awareness. I'd been introduced to another aspect of the mind–body connection: how my precise and focused, fully conscious efforts affected my body and how immediately it responded. Pilates pulled me in. I couldn't get enough. Even with my innocent, thirteen-year-old scope of understanding, the mental focus and discipline it required was mysteriously compelling. I was awestruck. The Pilates method fascinated me and captured my imagination.

Old Tricks No More

It wasn't until I returned to my regular dance schedule in the fall that I was able to fully appreciate the benefits I had reaped. Instead of feeling depleted after a full day of classes, I felt inspired, invigorated, and enlivened. My stamina had increased, as had my focus and drive.

Pilates made me feel omnipotent. So much so, in fact, that in all my inflated teenage, self-aggrandizing glory I stopped doing it consistently for a while—just because I thought I didn't need it anymore. I thought there was nothing I couldn't do.

Amazing as it was, the "work" of Pilates seemed to work for me even after I took a break from it. In my mind it had managed some miraculous rearranging of my cellular biology and had remade me into a better, stronger version of myself; I was a mortal turned superhero. My range of motion and overall physical capability for a young woman my age exceeded the norm, and I shamelessly exploited the extra edge that Pilates gave me in the same way that bodybuilders use steroids. It never occurred to me that my body would betray me.

Drago's: The Magical Beehive

After pushing myself past my limits and sustaining the first of my near career-ending injuries (the famous hip injury in London), Pilates took on even greater meaning. After miraculously recovering in such a short time, I knew I had to continue my Pilates journey when I returned home to the States—and the only place for me to go was to 50 West 57th Street in Manhattan.

The first time I walked into Drago's Gymnasium, I was humbled. There stood Romana Kryzanowska, another protégé of Joseph Pilates. I felt as though I'd entered something like an epic European cathedral, perhaps Notre Dame, which commanded only silence and awe. Drago's was unlike anything I'd ever seen. It was like a magical beehive, a busy body shop of physical and mental conditioning. One room, approximately fifteen hundred square feet in size, was designated for the Pilates apparatuses, Joseph Pilates's genius inventions, large-scale mousetrap-like machines rigged with springs for isometric resistance. Romana held court in this Pilates haven.

As I scanned my surroundings, I saw clusters of clients paired with Pilates apprentices deeply engrossed in their movement plans. All were on apparatuses and following different regimens to suit the needs of their bodies on that particular day. From just a glance, I knew I had to do whatever it took to get an entrance pass to become a part of this underground society.

Keep in mind that this was the early 1990s, long before anyone in the mainstream knew what Pilates was. Only the New York elite practiced it; only celebrities, musicians, and members of old, established, affluent New York families were exclusively privy to the gifts of this private club. On any given day, as an apprentice, you could have right there on your Pilates machine, ready for a session, Gloria Vanderbilt, Jill Clayburgh, or Mr. Glick, the first-chair violinist of the New York Philharmonic. Mr. Glick, who then was easily seventy-five, showed off inversions that would shame a twenty-five-year-old.

At Drago's, I was invited to participate in a tradition steeped in discipline, hard work, and sweat designed to keep a well-oiled human machine operating at peak efficiency. In so many ways, it was more challenging than dance, and I was continually surprised by my body's untapped abilities. To understand this is to understand Pilates at its essence, its very raison d'etre—building self-belief through the core, your seat of will and determination. After every single workout I ever did, after moving beyond my own self-doubt and rising to the challenge of performing what I was asked to do, my incredulity was replaced by an enormous endorphin rush—my prize for having worked so hard in such an integrated, focused way. After every workout I felt fulfilled, powerful, proud, and never more alive!

Pilates carries the *music of movement,* as I like to say. The earliest discoveries I made with Romana at Drago's about the singularly dynamic combination of fun and challenge, acknowledgement of the self and of the human body in all its glory and capability, are being passed along to you directly through me just as they were given to Romana by Joc Pilates himself. *Integrity. Dedication. Determination.* When I think of the Pilates sessions I grew up on, what they required of me and how they made me feel, those three words come to mind. I live them to this day and am thrilled to share them with you.

the empower and flow practice

TIME OF DAY: Morning

QUALITY: Yang

SUBTLE ENERGY: Activates all energy pathways and the lymphatic system.

BENEFITS: Defies the aging process, balances the endocrine system, supercharges the immune system, improves flexibility, and sculpts and tones the muscles

PROP: Pilates mat

The Practice:

Hundred
Rollup
Rolling Like a Ball
Single-Leg Pull
Spine Stretch Forward
Open-Leg Rocker
Saw
Single-Leg Kick
Pendulum
Classic Teaser
Swimming
Seal

Before You Begin

The *principle of opposition* is the principle at work when you create an equal and opposing isometric resistance to a movement. It's a self-imposed resistance that involves using muscles with intention and stretching them to their utmost in diametrically opposite directions. It's a highly effective way of lengthening and strengthening. When you use intention as you're executing a movement, the muscles of that part of the body develop as a testament to that intention. All your muscles reflect your effort and intention when you create oppositional resistance.

The Practice

Hundred

The Hundred powerfully increases cardiovascular activity, getting the heart pumping and lungs working, and stimulates the lymphatic system as it strengthens and tones the abdominals and muscles of the arms and legs. It enhances coordination and builds stamina.

1. Lying on your back, draw your knees into your chest and stretch your arms along the mat down by your sides. Inhale deeply. Then, as you exhale, curl your head, neck, and upper shoulders off the mat just high enough so that the tips of your shoulder blades are still connected to the mat. As you do, raise your arms a few inches off the floor, reaching your fingertips as far away from your body as possible.
2. Right away, extend your legs straight up to the ceiling, rooting your tailbone into the mat. Squeeze your heels together as you externally rotate your legs, bringing your toes slightly apart.
3. Then lower and lengthen the legs down as far as you can with control, just to the point where your abdominals are engaged and your lower back is securely rooted into the floor—no farther (your point of control, where your back is connected fully to the floor and your abs are engaged), and start to pump your arms vigorously up and down as if you are slapping the surface of water. In time with the arm movements, use this breathing pattern: inhale, one, two, three, four, five; exhale, one, two, three, four, five. Breathe in through your nose and out through your mouth. Because of the rapid arm movements, the breathing in this exercise has an effect somewhat similar to that of the Breath of Fire. When you become more skilled, breathe in and out through your nose only. Do not allow your abdominal muscles to pump in and out with the breath. Maintain your navel-to-spine connection.

4. Pump the arms with real intention and purpose. Each time you inhale, think about bringing new life into your heart, lungs, and cells. Each time you exhale, think about expelling stale, stagnant air and drawing the navel to the spine that much deeper.
5. After completing ten ten-count breaths, curl your upper back just a little bit higher, drawing the abdominals in the most deeply yet, expelling the last thread of breath in the process and stretching your fingertips and toes to their utmost lengths. Then draw your knees back into your chest, hugging them in as you release your head, neck, and shoulders back down into the mat.
6. Repeat for a total of ten sets of ten breaths.

Transition: After hugging your knees into your chest at the end of the exercise, do not linger. Move on immediately. With control, using your powerhouse, lower your legs to the mat, and raise your arms overhead and backward, until they come to a position six inches off the floor behind you.

Rollup

The Rollup assists in spinal articulation, making the spine more fluid and flexible as it strengthens and tones the abdominals and stretches the hamstrings. The trick to experiencing the most accurate and optimal expression of this exercise is to impose your own isometric resistance on it by employing the principle of opposition.

1. Lying on your back, stretch your arms long overhead about six inches off the floor, and lengthen your legs down away from your torso.
2. Draw your ribs together and anchor your back to the mat to the best of your ability, so that there is little space between your back and the mat. Your abdominals should already be fully engaged in order to maintain this starting position.
3. Make sure the legs are fully extended and the feet are flexed, with big

toes touching, as you squeeze the inner thighs together. Drive your heels into the floor to activate the backs of your legs, particularly the hamstrings.

4. Inhale with your arms in the overhead position. Then, as you exhale, lift your arms and circle them forward over your chest, peeling your upper torso off the floor as you reach your fingertips forward. Curl your body forward, coming into a deep C shape. Keep going until you are stretched over your straight legs. Your arms will be extended straight out in front of you at shoulder height, parallel to your legs. Your eyes should gaze down at your belly button.
5. As you curl forward into the stretch and deepen the navel-to-spine connection, maintain the feet in the flexed position. Keep your knees as straight as you possibly can and your feet squeezing together. As you round the body forward and stretch your arms and feet away from you, feel as if someone is hugging you around the waist and trying to pull you backward while you fight to reach forward and stretch through your fingertips. In this manner, you'll feel your core muscles activated in the deepest way and achieve the greatest range of motion and stretch in your spine and hamstrings.
6. Repeat five to seven times.

Rolling Like a Ball

Rolling Like a Ball massages the spine and related supporting muscles, bringing improved circulation to the nerve plexuses that insert themselves in and around the spine. It also strengthens the abdominals—and sparks laughter, giving you a bonus endorphin and serotonin charge that lifts your spirits instantly.

1. Sitting just behind your tailbone, round your spine, and pull your knees to your chest, wrapping your arms around your knees. Lift your feet away from the floor and balance on your buttocks with your toes

pointed down toward the floor, making yourself as compact as possible and assuming a shape that resembles a small ball. Keep your knees shoulder-width apart, your navel drawn deeply toward your spine, and your head tilted downward, eyes gazing at your navel.

2. Do your best to squeeze your heels as closely to your buttocks as possible, bringing your heels together with your toes slightly apart and pointed down to the floor.
3. As you prepare to roll back, draw your shoulders down away from your ears. Also press your knees into your elbows and your arms against your knees to create your own isometric resistance. Again, make sure that your head is down and your eyes are focused on your belly button.
4. Inhale, then rock back, going only as high as the base of your neck and no farther. Always take care not to rock onto the cervical vertebrae (which can be delicate). Then, using your powerhouse and your outgoing breath as the engine, immediately rock back up on the exhalation—again coming to arrive at the point of balance. Hold here for three short counts before rocking backward again.
5. Repeat five to seven times.

Single-Leg Pull

The Single-Leg Pull builds the core and massages the internal organs even as it lengthens and tones the muscles of the legs, shoulders, and arms.

1. Lying on your back, with your head lifted and eyes on your navel center, hug your right knee into your chest, clasping the right ankle with the right hand and the right knee with the left hand, and extend your left leg along the floor.
2. Double-pulse the right knee, squeezing it deeper in toward the chest, as you breathe in twice in tandem with the movement of the knee. The

rhythm is inhale-inhale. Extend your elbows wide out to the sides of the body, pressing into your lattisimus dorsi muscles on your upper back under the shoulders, so that the shoulders move down and away from your ears. Extend your left leg out and away from your body, reaching through your toes as far as you can.

3. Switch sides and hand positions, drawing the left knee into the chest and clasping the left ankle with the left hand and the left knee with the right hand. (Learning this first transition and the next few may take some patience and concentration, as you must coordinate your hands with the switching of the legs.) Then double-pulse again. The rhythm is exhale-exhale. Use short, perfunctory, staccato breathing as you hug the left knee in toward your chest, making sure that your breath is working in tandem with the movement.
4. Keep your head held high and in the same position you started with, looking at your navel throughout the exercise. Continue in this way, hugging one knee tightly into the chest while reaching the opposite leg away and breathing in and then out in the two-beat rhythm—employing the principle of opposition.
5. Repeat for a total of six sets (right and left make one set).

Spine Stretch Forward

The Spine Stretch Forward uses the principle of opposition to increase flexibility in the spine and hamstrings and build postural muscles and awareness.

1. Sitting up as tall as you can, extend your legs straight out in front of you, spreading them slightly wider than hip-width apart and flexing the feet strongly. Bring your arms behind you, tenting the fingertips into the floor to roll your shoulders open, down, and back, coming into perfect posture.
2. Maintaining the posture you've established, lift your arms out in

front of you, holding them at shoulder height, shoulder-width apart, with your fingers energized and reaching forward.

3. Inhale and squeeze the buttocks underneath you, getting a boost and growing even taller, reaching up to the ceiling through the crown of your head. As you exhale, maintain your arms at shoulder height and curl your body forward over the legs into a deep, but lifted C shape, imagining that you are curling up and over a beach ball and lifting your abdominals so as not to let your stomach touch it.
4. Inhale as you rise back up to sitting, articulating through the spine, rolling up bone by bone, making sure that your head is the last thing to lift, until you return to the starting position, further refining and perfecting your posture. Squeeze your glutes to get an extra boost and lift your gaze so that you are looking slightly above the horizon line, which will help you to lift your entire body higher.
5. As you exhale, draw your navel deeply to your spine and curl forward again, reaching your arms strongly toward the wall in front of you. As you round into the C curve this time, stretching your spine and keeping your legs strong and straight, feet flexed, try to bring your head as close to the floor as possible, deepening the stretch.
6. Repeat five to seven times.

Open-Leg Rocker

The Open-Leg Rocker strengthens the abdominals, stretches the hamstrings, massages the spine, improves balance and coordination, and inspires a playful determination.

1. Balancing on your buttocks just behind your tailbone, with your pelvis curled under, lift your legs straight up in front of you, shoulder-width apart, and clasp your ankles. Keep your arms strong and straight. You'll maintain this position for the duration of the exercise. Your shoulders should be relaxed and your gaze straight ahead. To

prepare, breathe in. As you exhale, draw your navel back to your spine and stabilize your balance in the position.

Modification: If you have trouble reaching your ankles with straight legs, simply bend the knees and hold underneath the knees with the lower legs parallel with the floor. With each repetition, try to straighten your legs more, until eventually your legs are straight and you can clasp your ankles.

2. Inhale again and rock backward smoothly on your spine, with control, just up to the base of the neck, taking care not to let the back of your head touch the mat.
3. Immediately rock forward and back up as you exhale, using your abdominal muscles to return your body to the starting position, where you will hold your balance for a count of three, lifting taller, deepening your abdominals, and perfecting the posture.
4. Then repeat. If you have trouble keeping your knees straight, that's okay. In time, this exercise will help you to stretch your hamstrings and you'll be rocking and rolling with straight legs like a circus performer.
5. Repeat five to seven times.

Saw

The Saw is a breathing exercise above and beyond its other benefits! It strengthens the lungs and increases overall lung capacity, which aids in healing breathing challenges, like asthma, even as it reinforces the postural muscles of the back and powerhouse and makes the spine more fluid and flexible. It specifically increases the range of motion in the twisting plane.

1. Sitting up tall, extend your legs in front of you, slightly wider than hip-width apart, and flex your feet strongly.
2. Extend your arms out to the sides of your body at shoulder height, and

feel the crown of your head reaching up to the ceiling as you draw the navel to the spine, coming into perfect posture. Squeeze your buttocks to give you an extra boost up.

3. Inhale as deeply as you can, puffing out your chest—you should feel almost barrel-chested from the prodigious intake of air. Hold the breath as you twist your torso to face your right leg, bringing your left arm across your body, in front of you, over the right leg, and the right arm behind you.
4. As you exhale, drop your chin to your chest and bend forward over the right leg, pulling your abdominals up and in, and rounding the spine slightly into a deep C shape, using the back of your left hand as if to saw off the pinky toe on the right foot—push your left hand past your right foot, as the right arm reaches up behind you in the air, palm facing your body.
5. In the forward bend, as you are "sawing off" the right pinky toe, stay in the position long enough to empty your lungs completely. Feel as though you are twisting and exhaling so deeply that you become the physical incarnation of wringing out a wet towel, expelling any stagnant chi and detoxing your lungs right there and then.
6. Inhale as you rise up, bringing your torso back to the center starting position, and lifting tall through the spine, accompanied by the arms in the same swift motion, which will once again reach out from the shoulders to the sides of the body, where they will be ready to repeat the same sequence on the left side.
7. Repeat for a total six sets (right and left make one set).

Single-Leg Kick

The Single-Leg Kick strengthens the muscles of the back and the glutes, inner thighs, and abdominals and teaches you more than most exercises about how to defy gravity. It gives the abdominals and the spine a chance to stretch in extension (as opposed to the flexion, which is

Pilates

Hundred

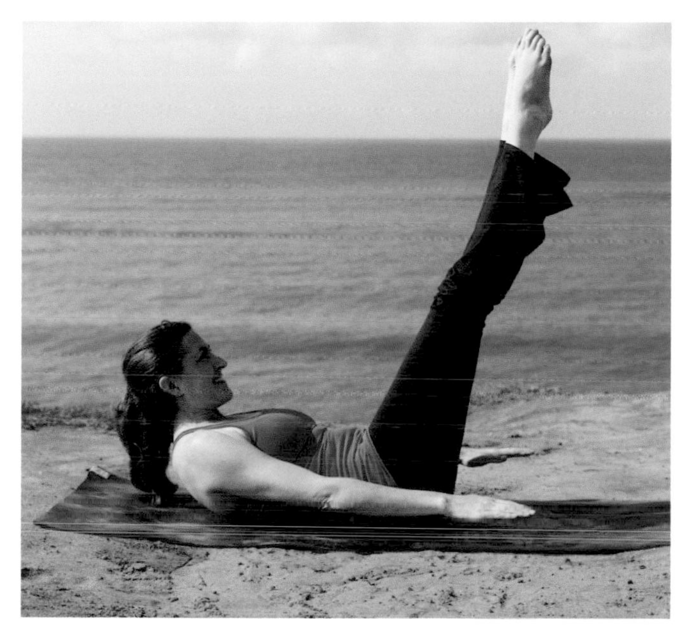

Rollup

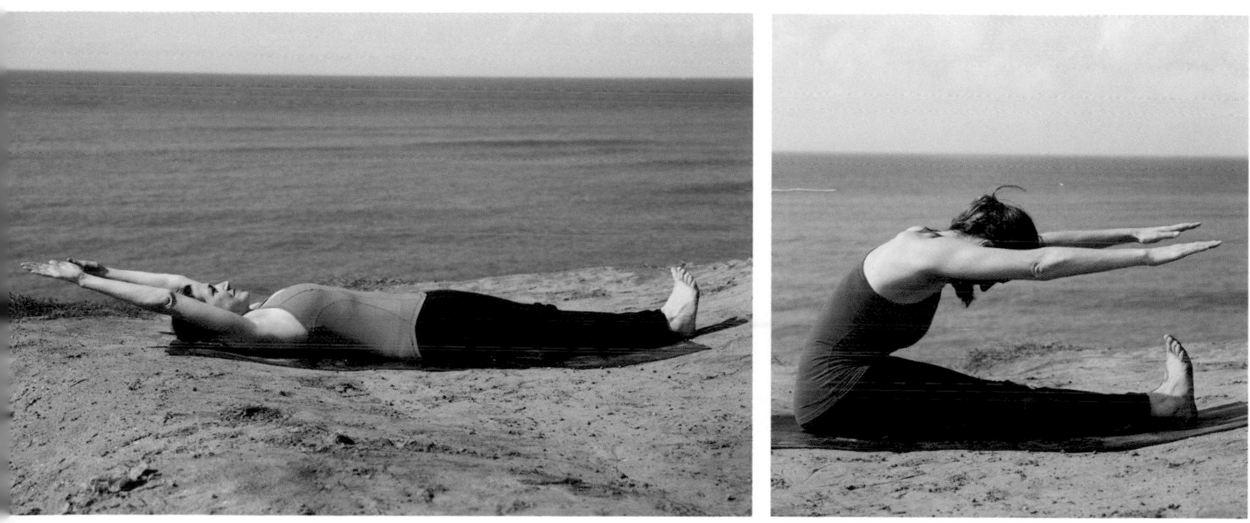

Rolling like a Ball

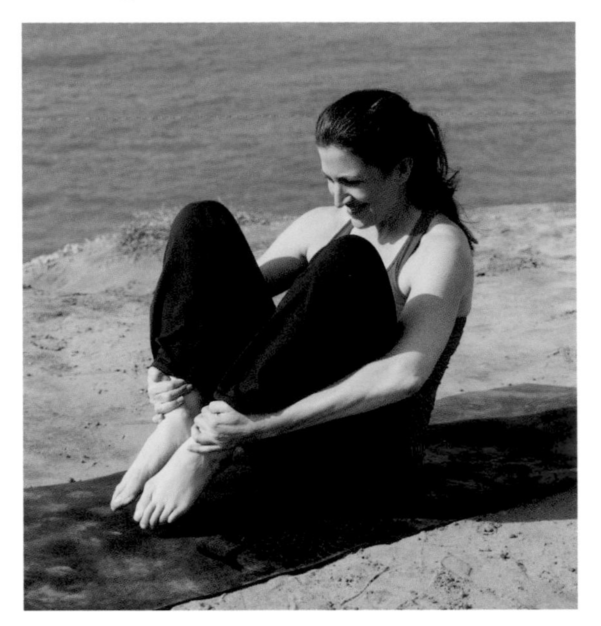

Single-Leg Pull

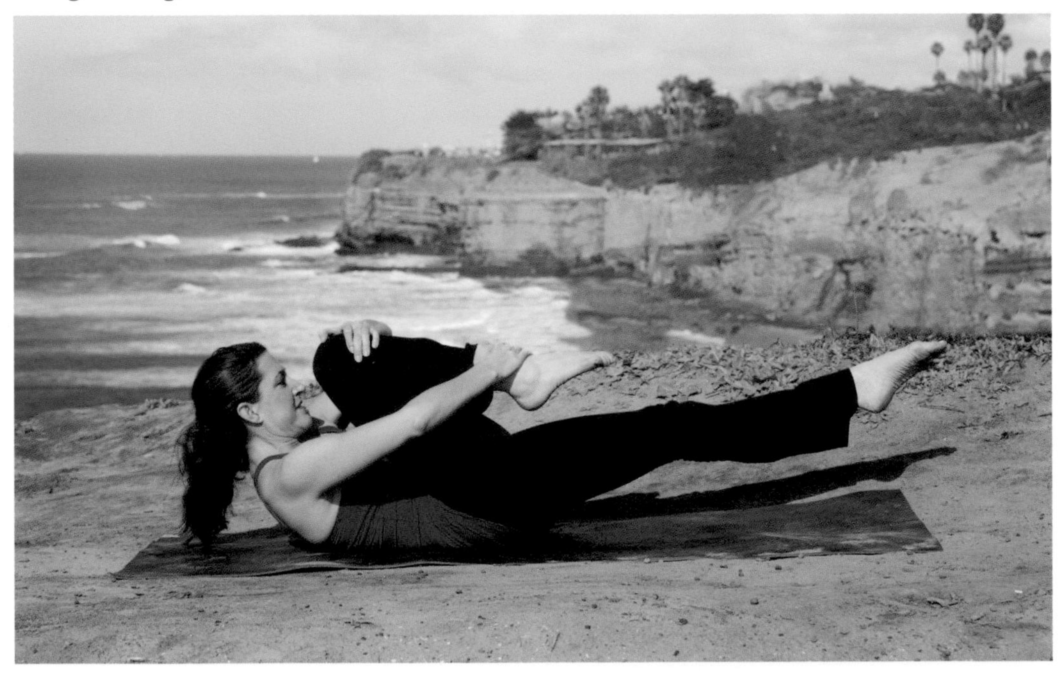

Spine Stretch Forward

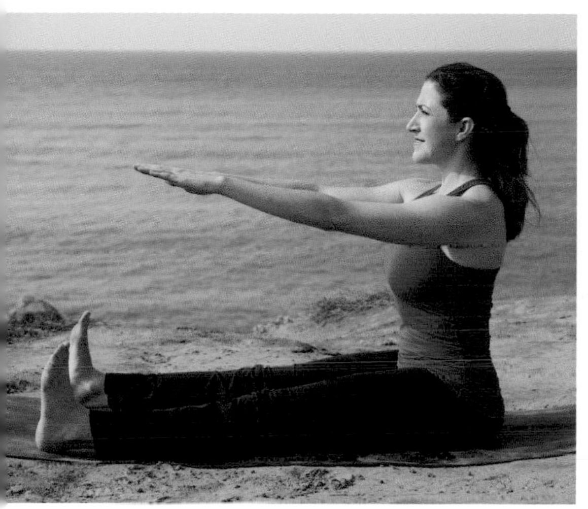

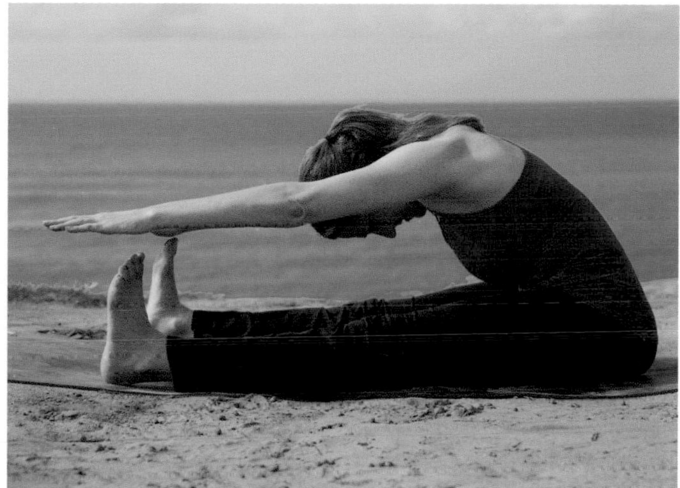

Open-Leg Rocker

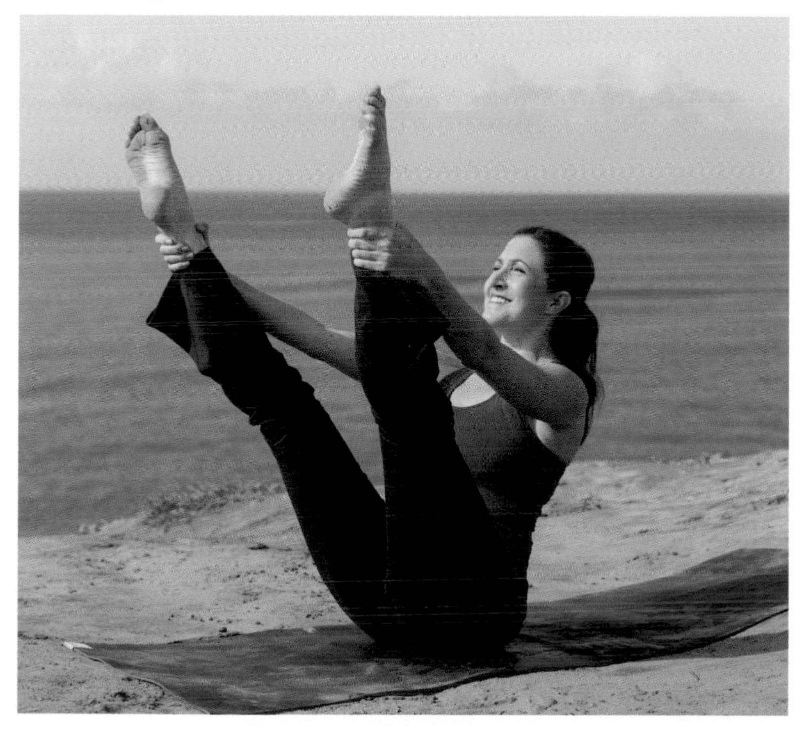

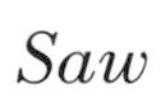

Saw

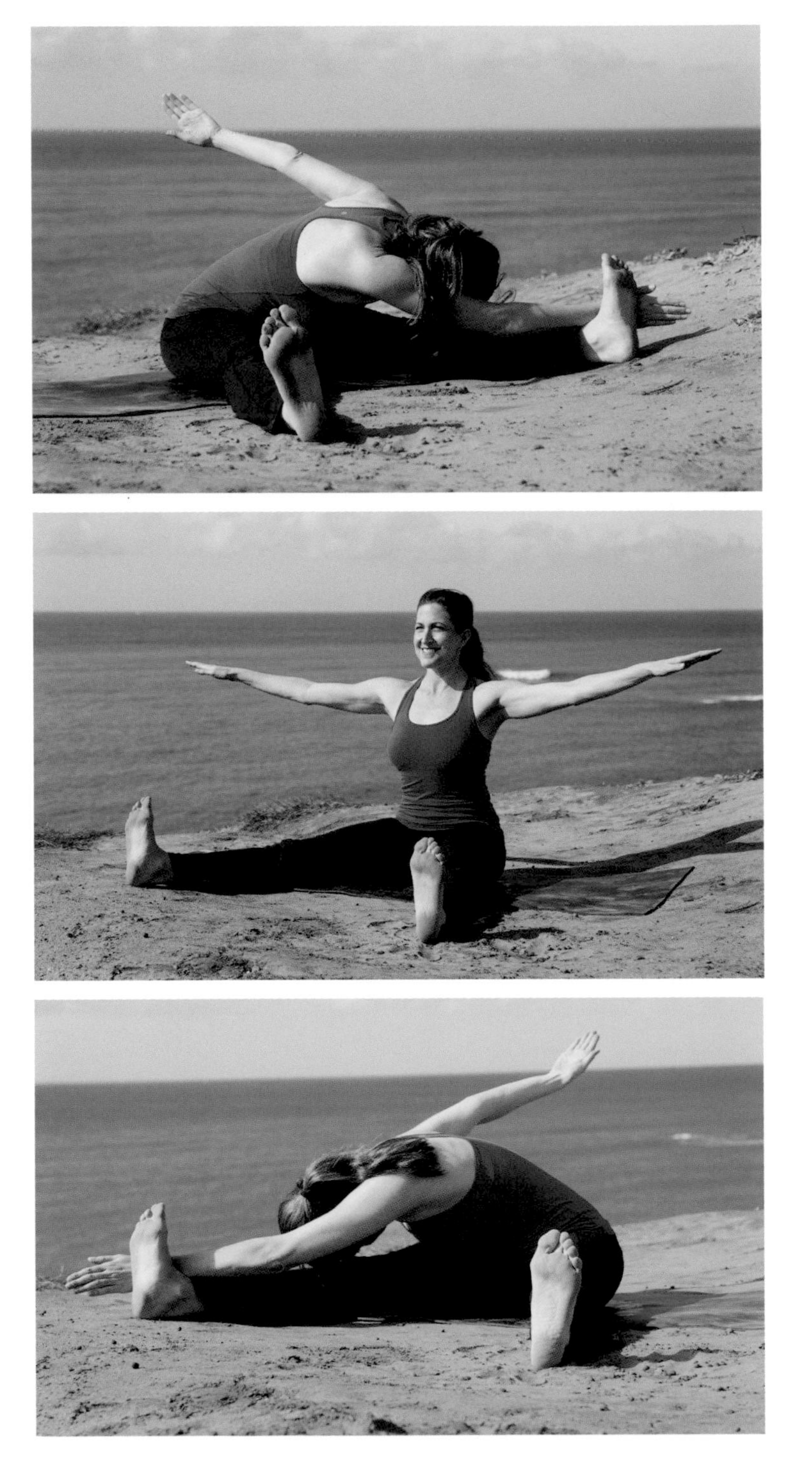

Single-Leg Kick

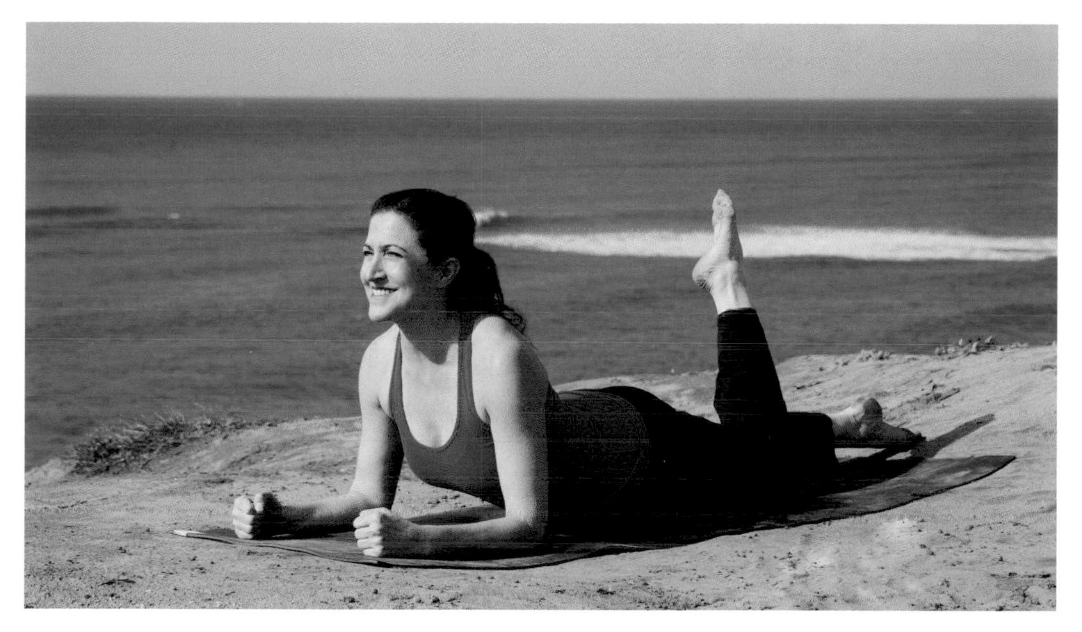

Pendulum

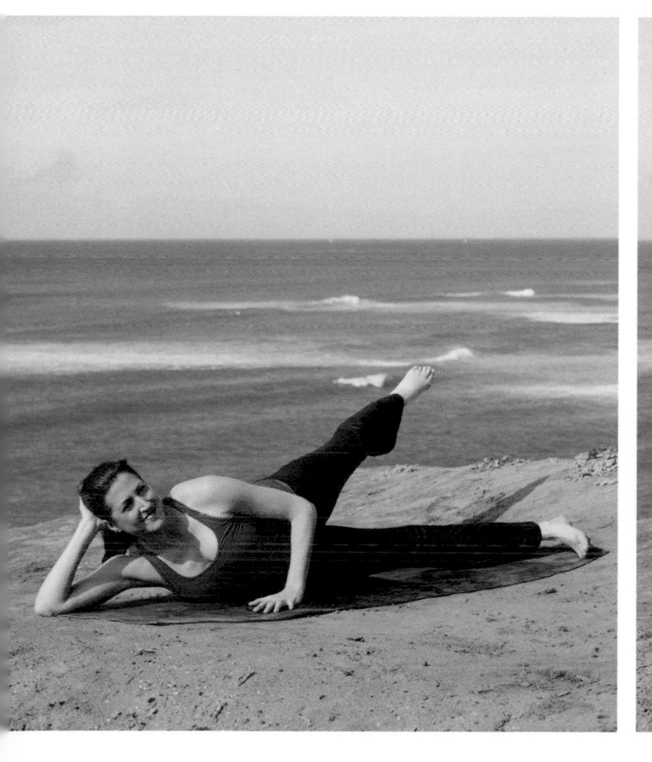

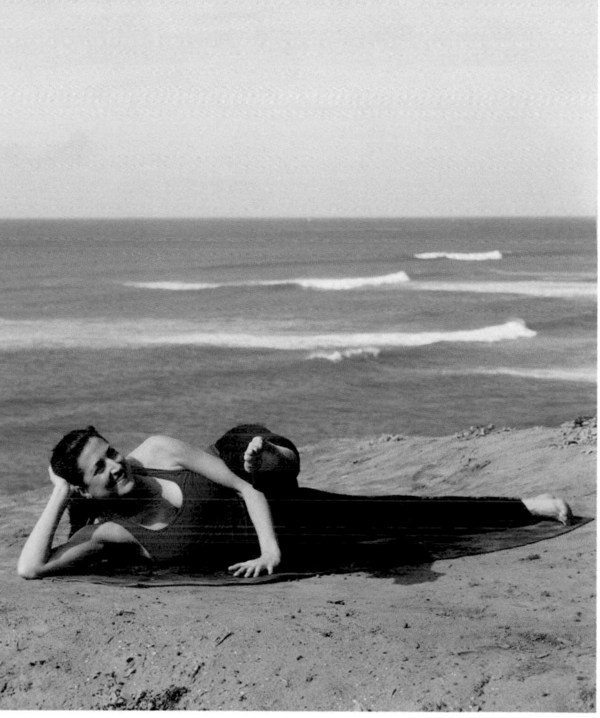

Classic Teaser

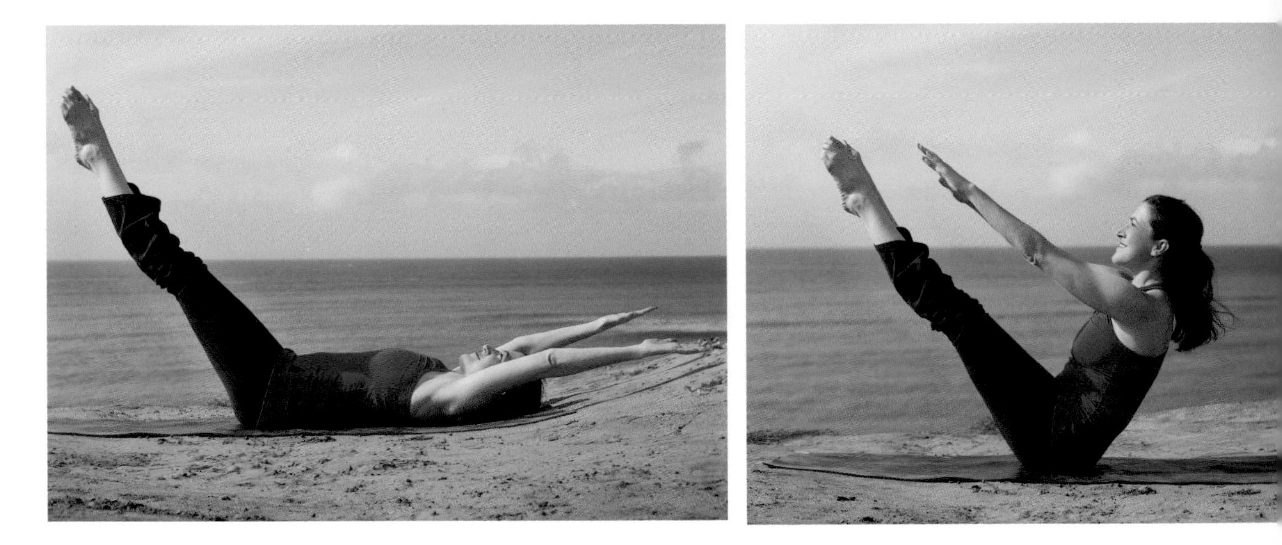

Swimming

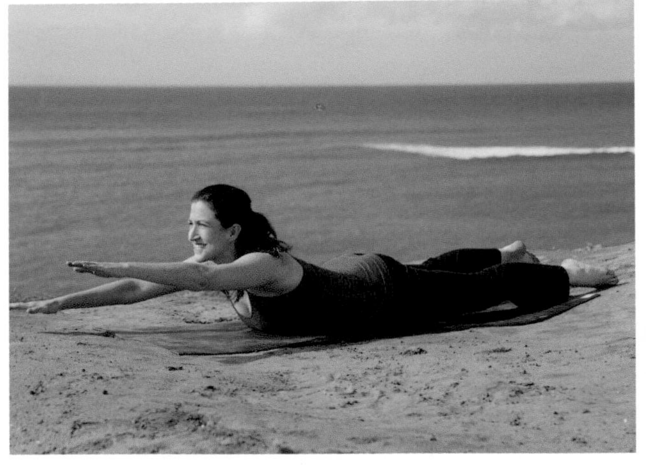

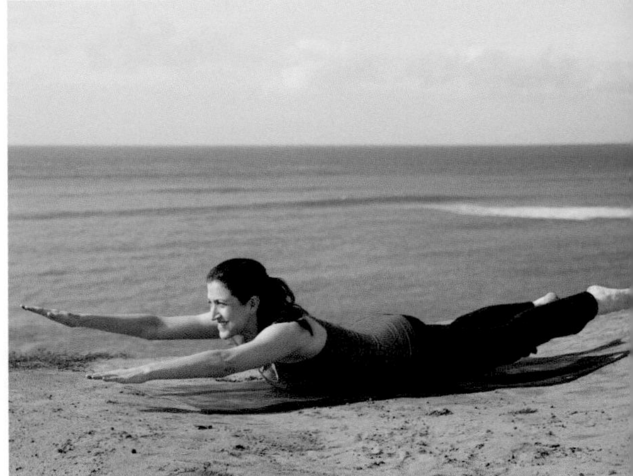

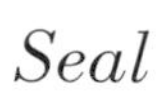

Seal

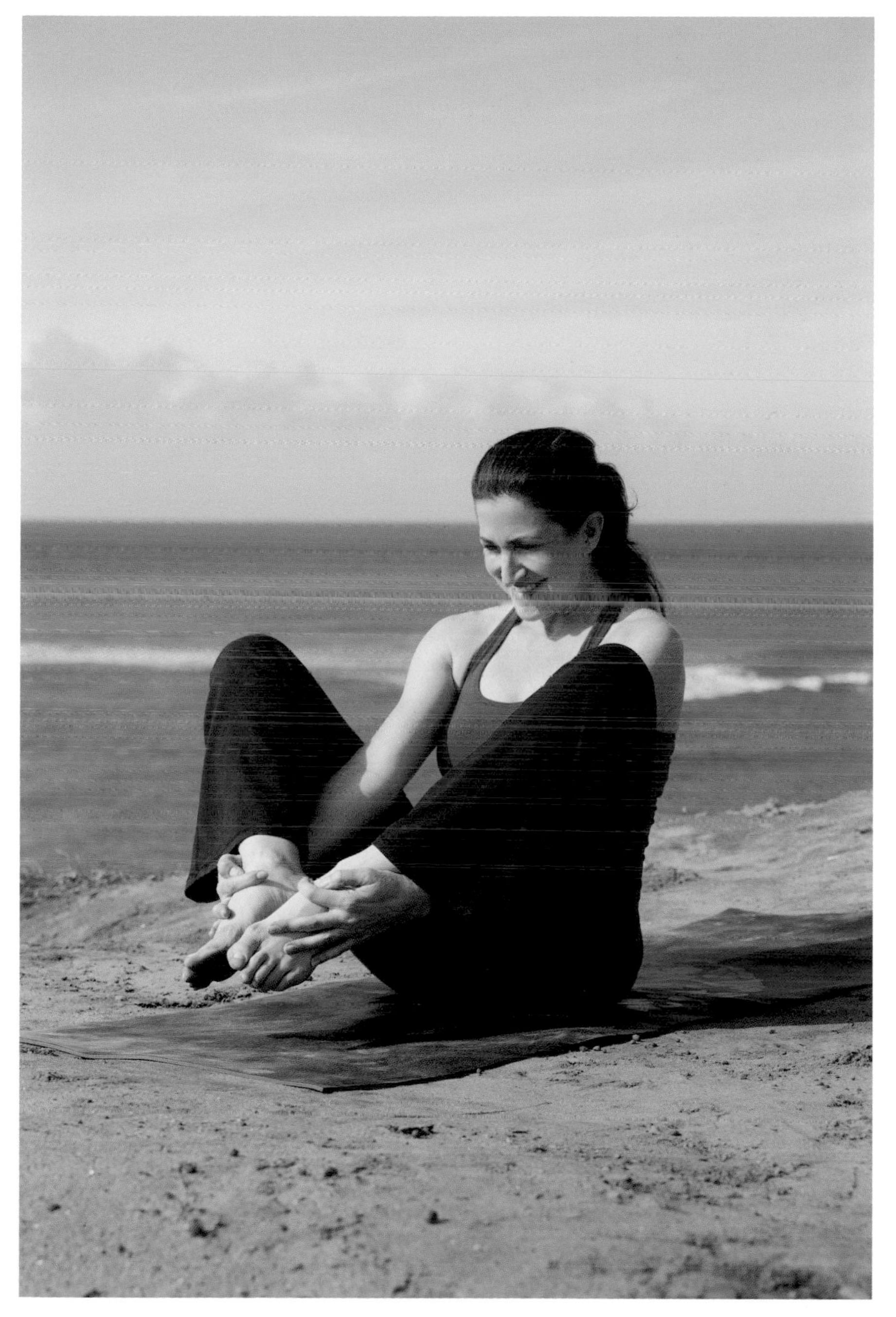

Yin Yoga

Meridians

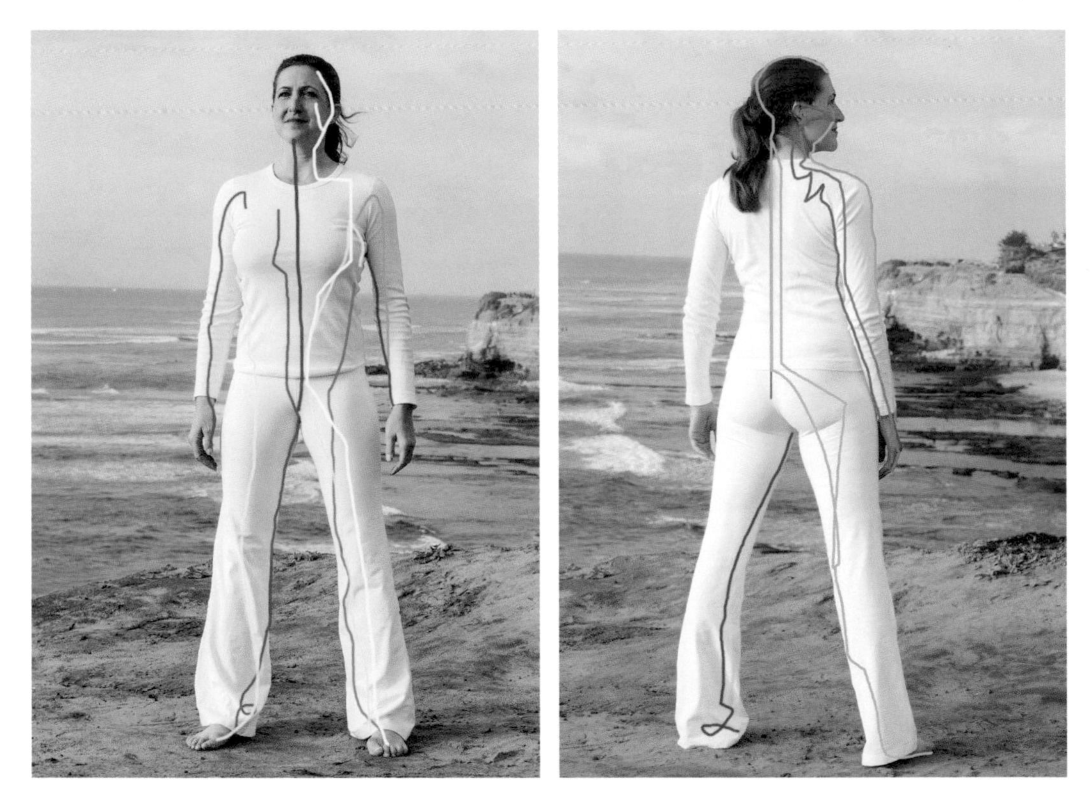

Child's Pose

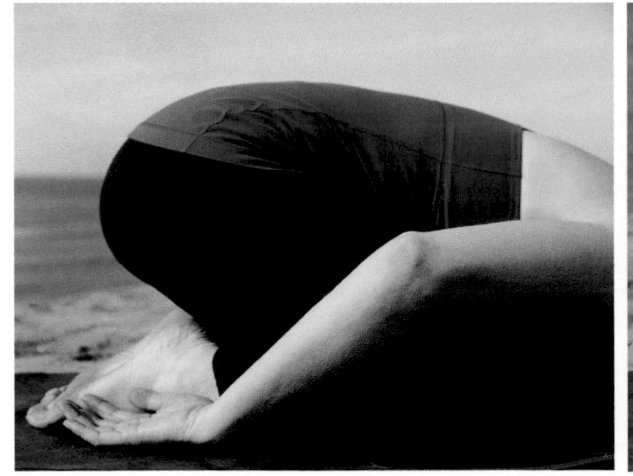

Butterfly

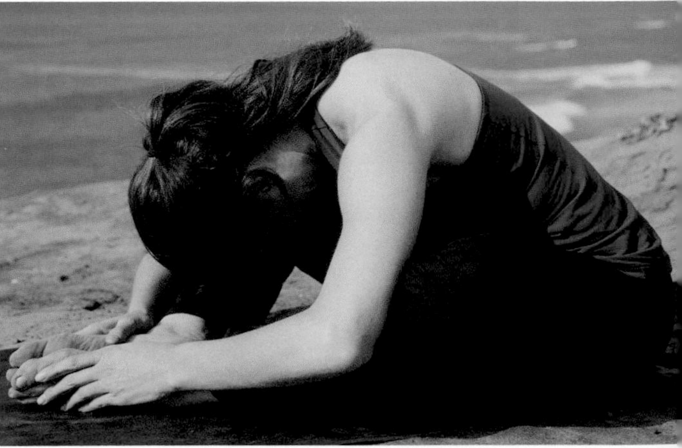

Dragonfly

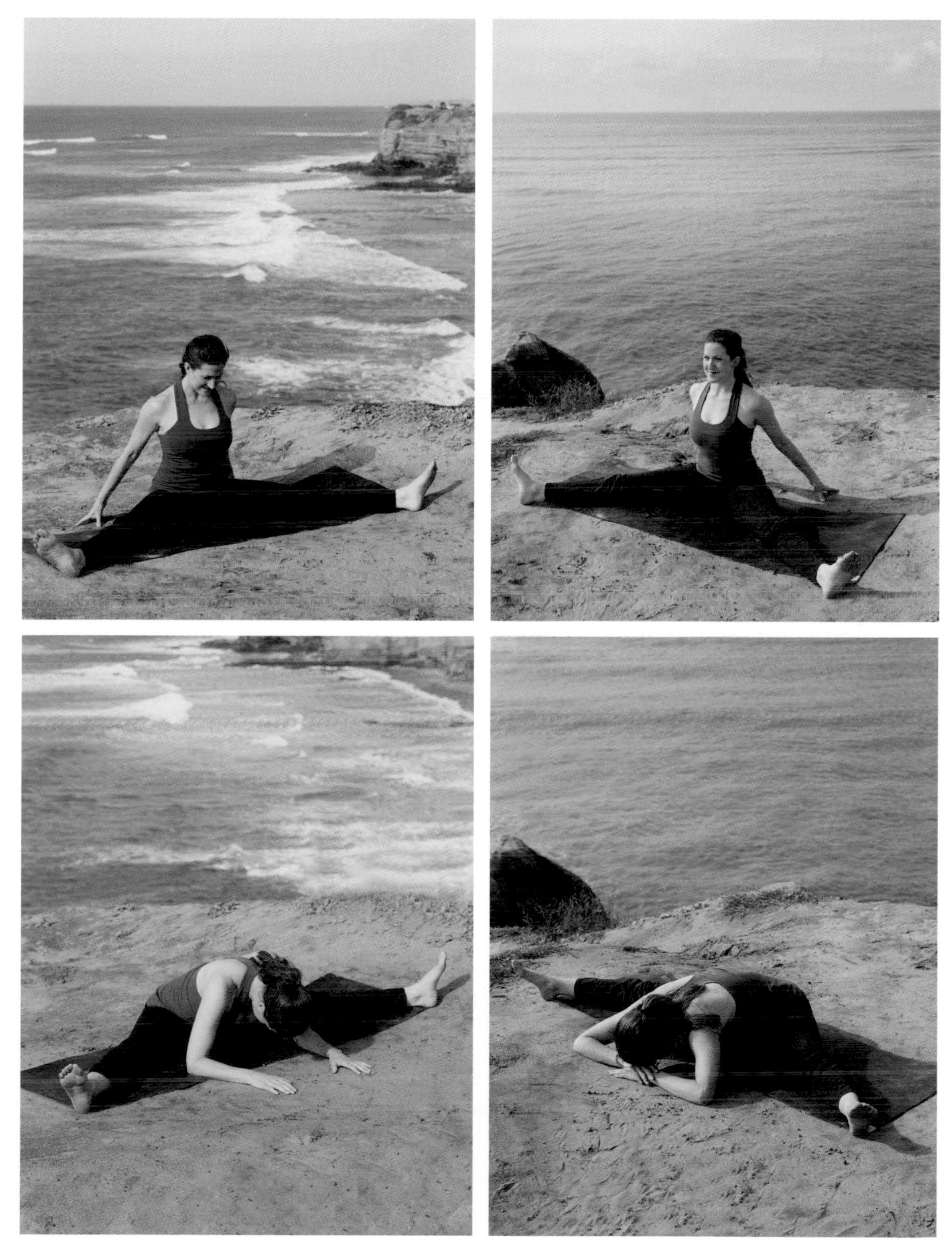

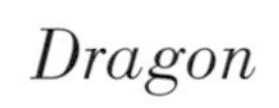

Dragon

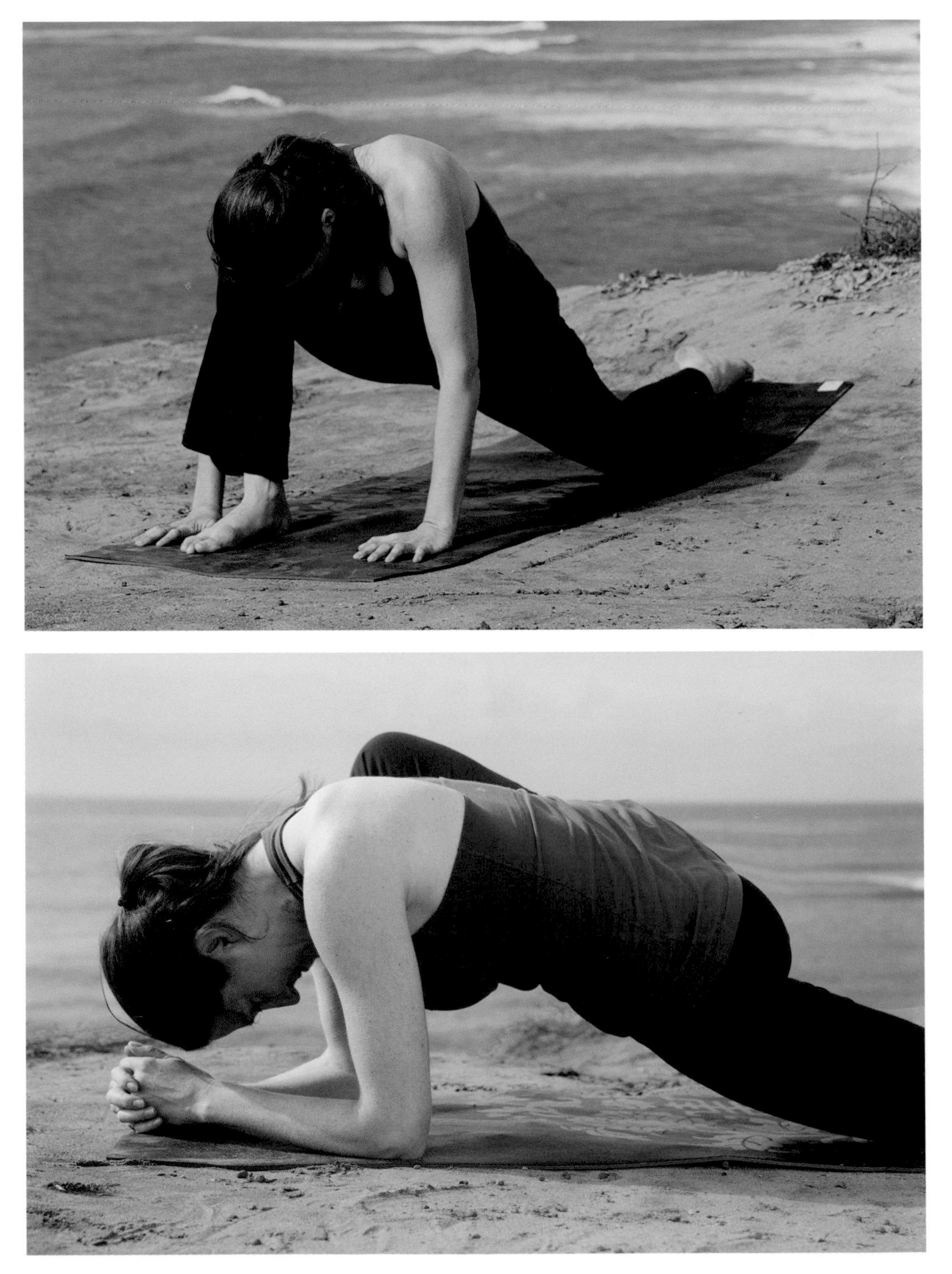

Forward Bend

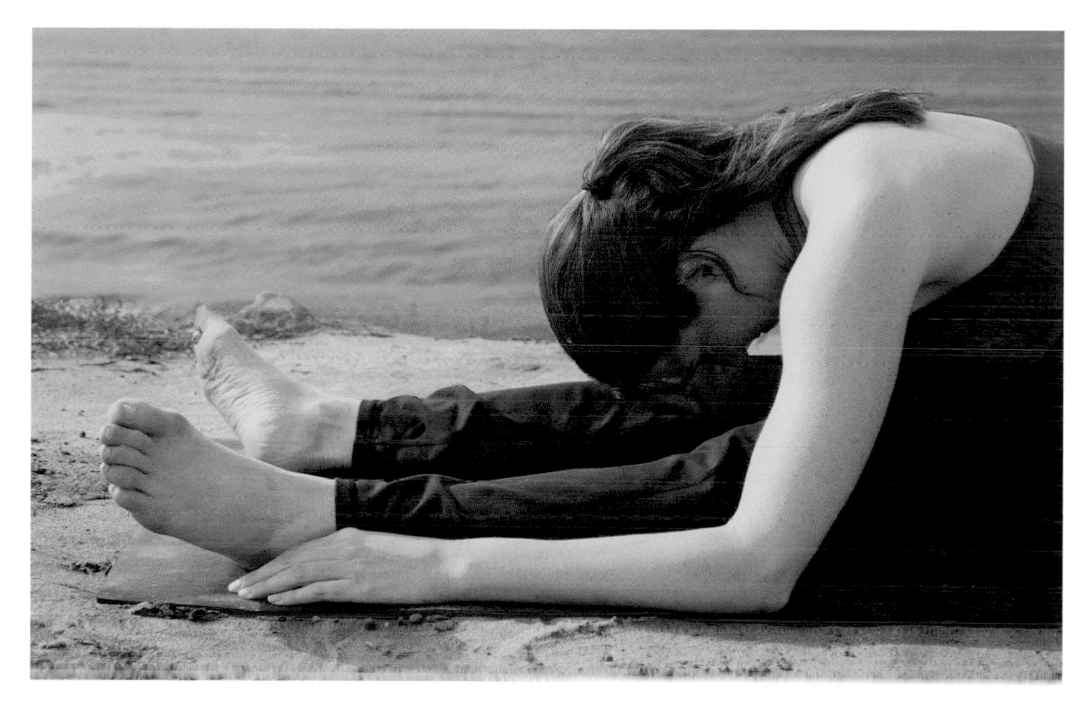

Half Saddle

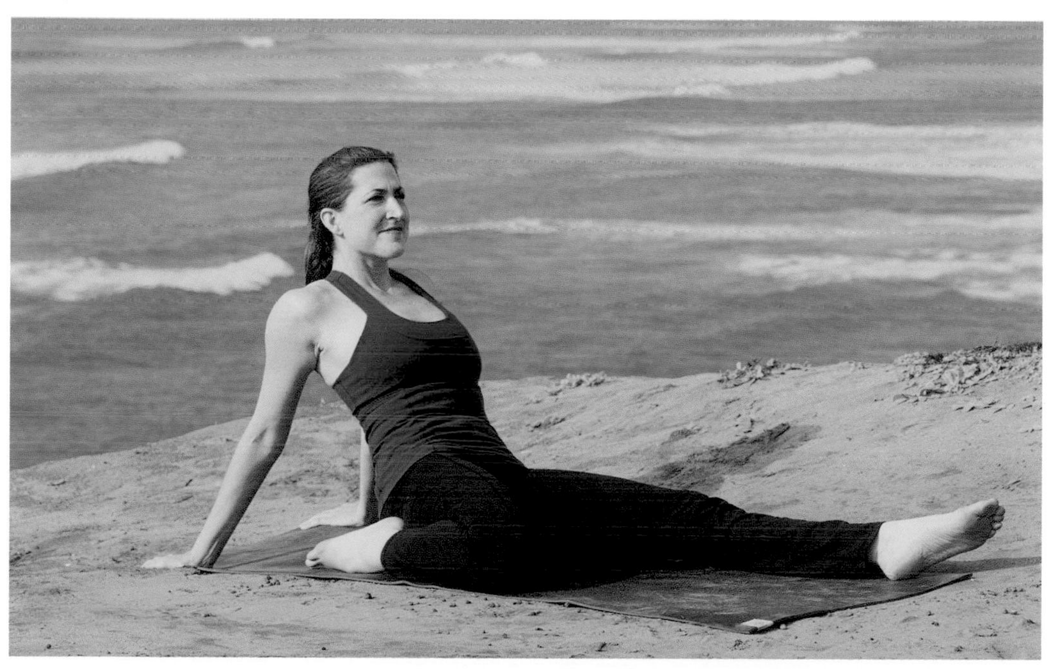

Sleeping Swan

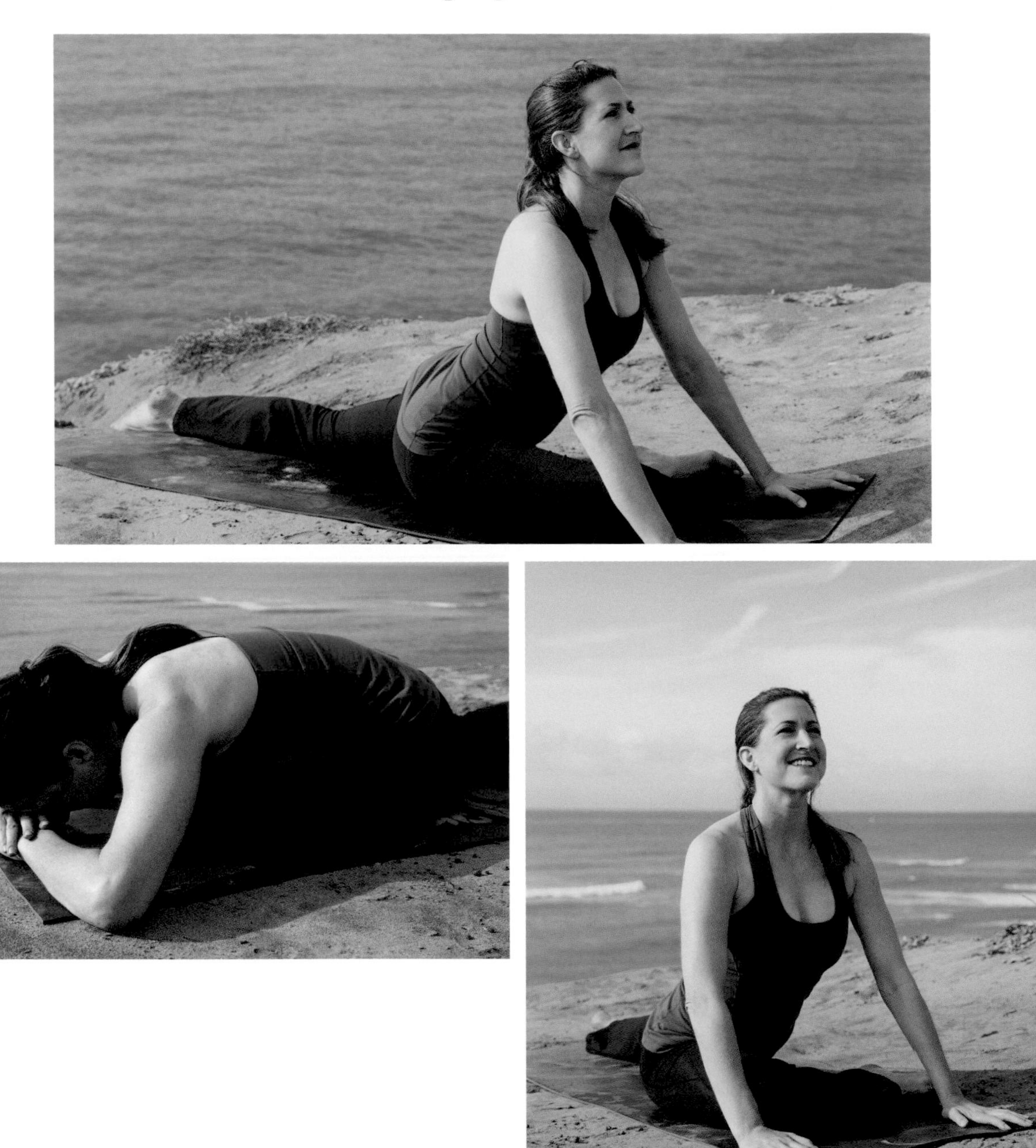

Quarter Dog

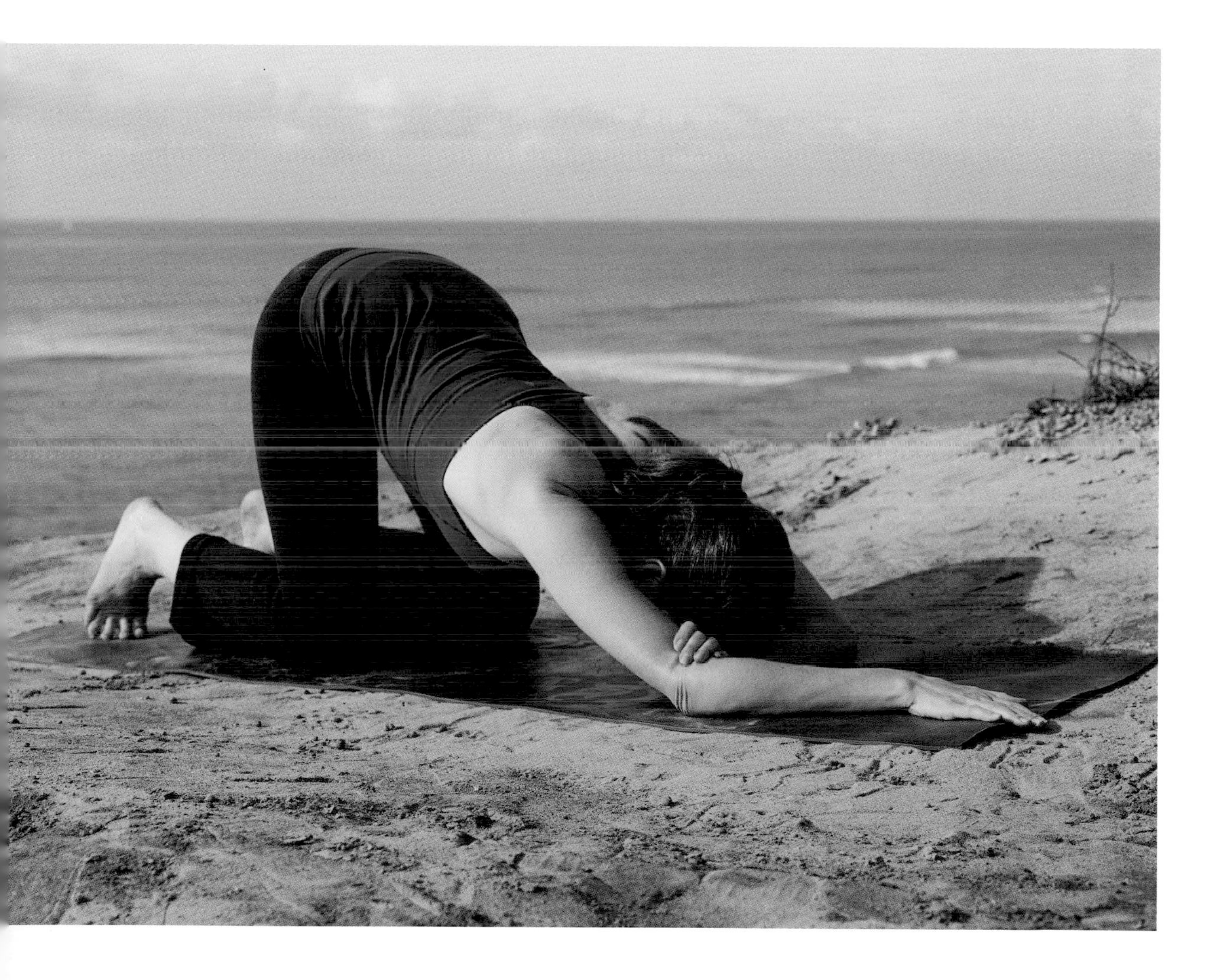

Eye of the Needle

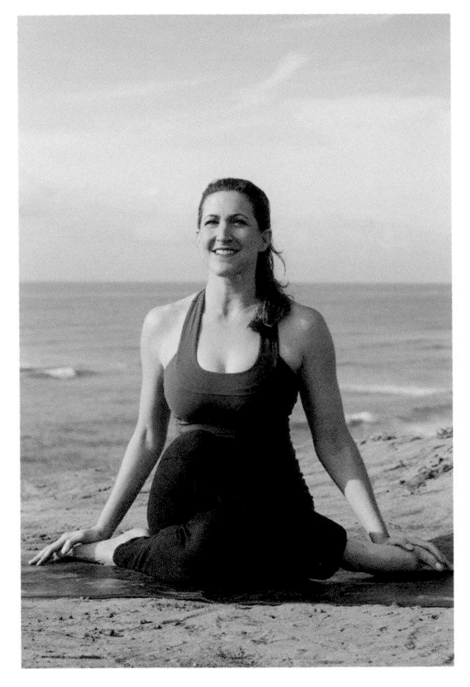

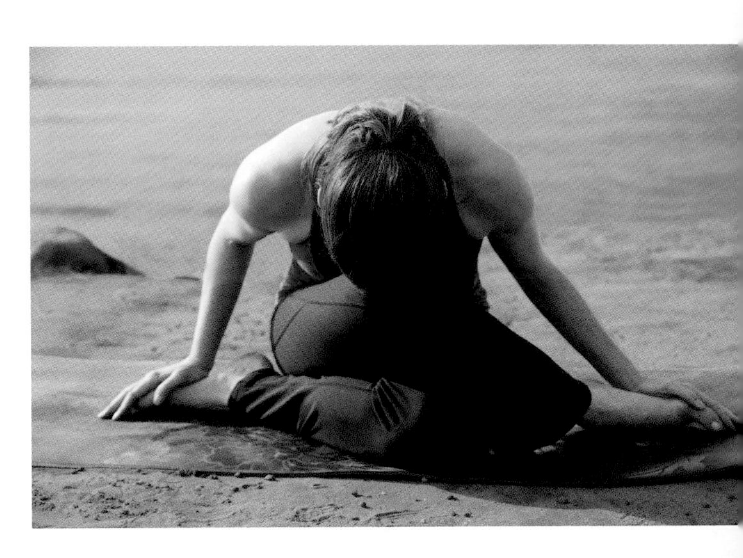

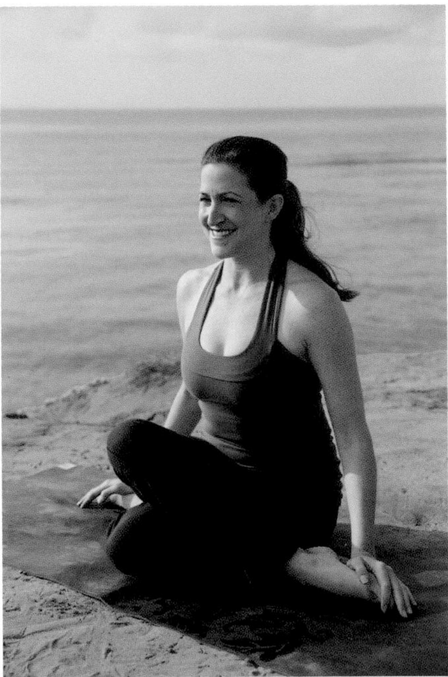

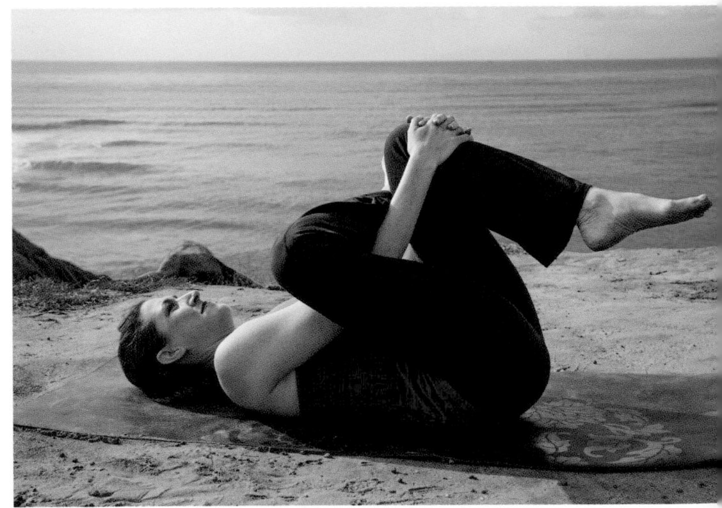

Spinal Twist

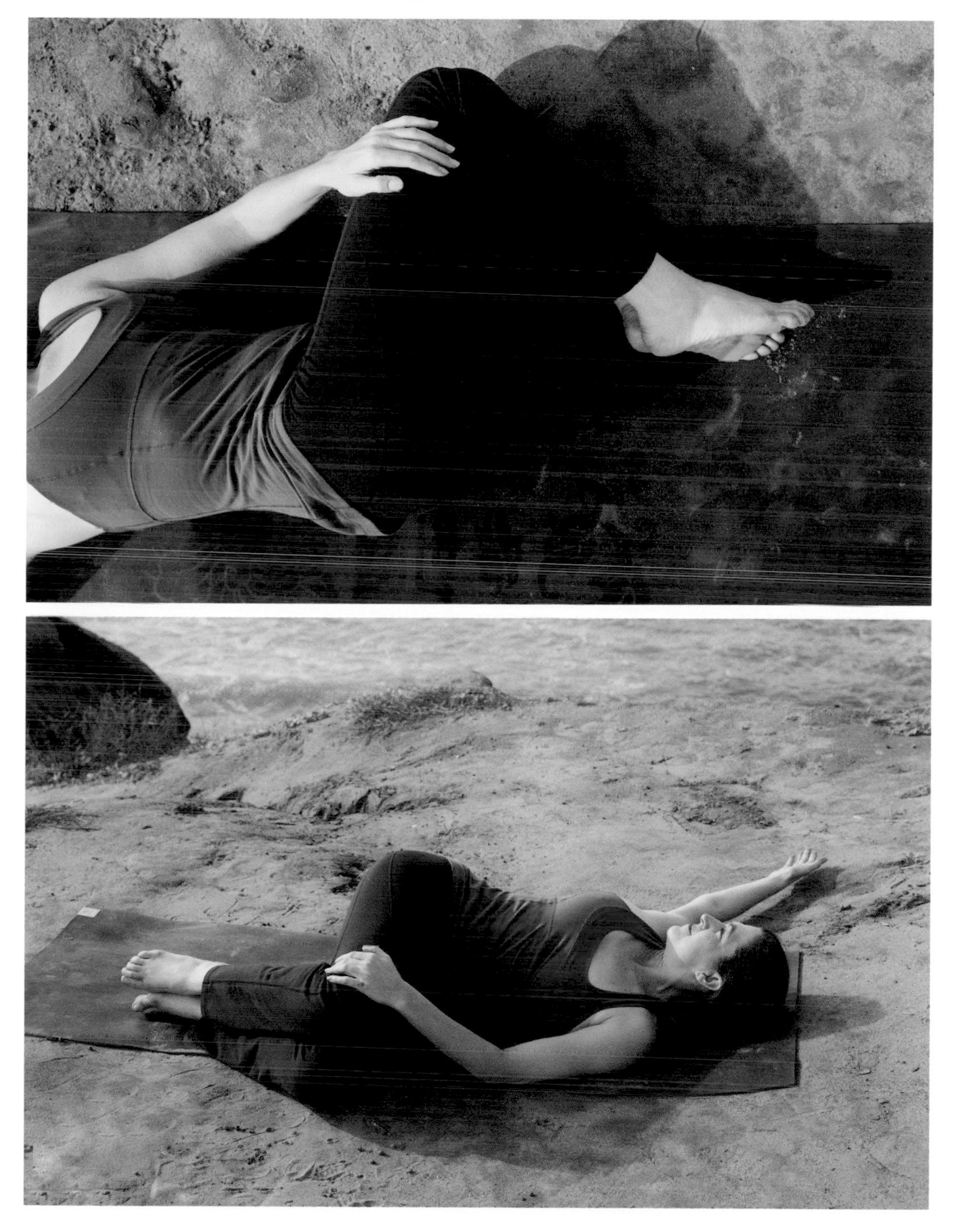

Sphinx and Seal

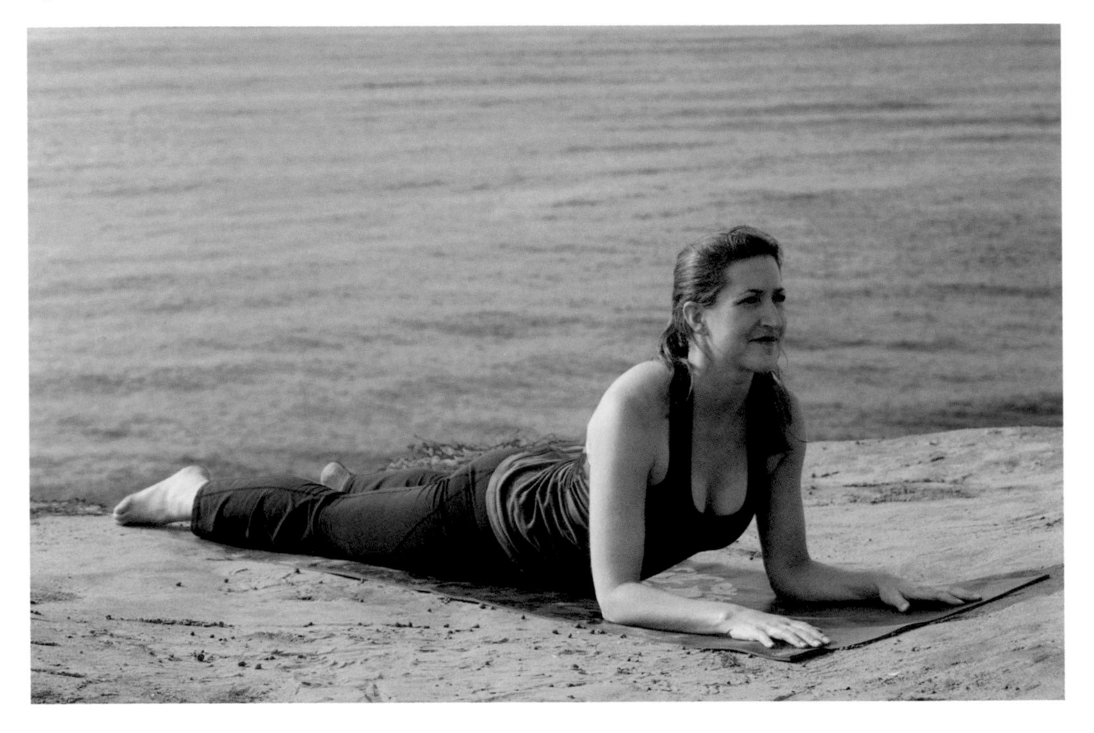

Corpse Pose

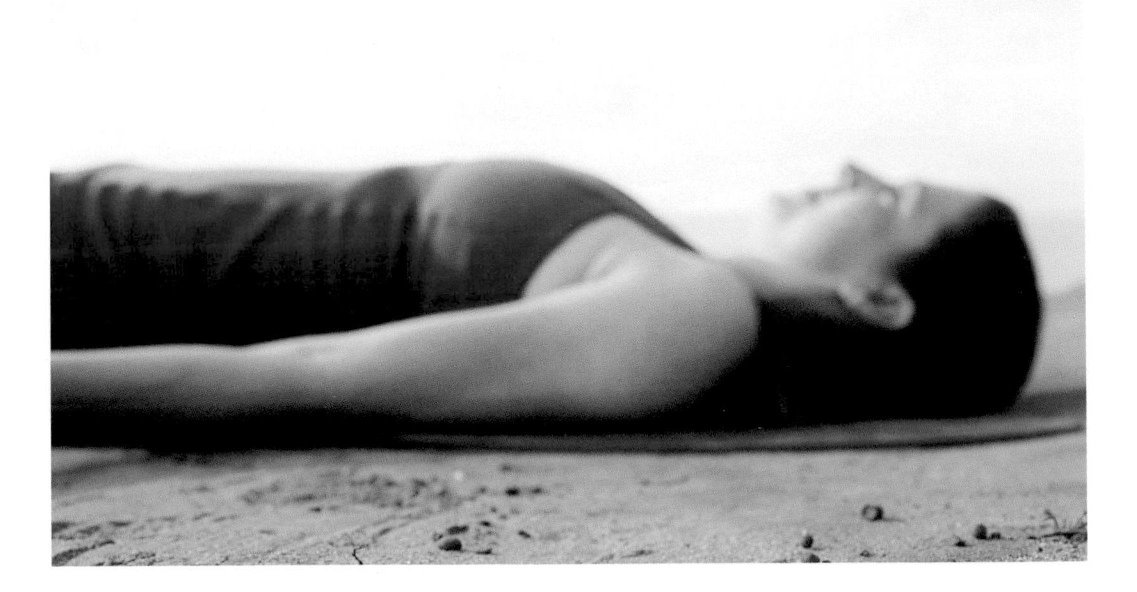

what you've been doing a great deal of in all the exercises preceding this one).

1. Lying on your stomach, legs lengthening down behind you, press your body up so that you come into a sphinx position, with your fists extended, forearms flat on the floor in front of you, and the elbow points directly under your shoulders.
2. Draw your shoulders down and back away from your ears, and almost feel as though you are dragging your body forward in space because the muscles of your upper body are so activated and primed. Feel your shoulder blades pressing together as you lift your upper body proudly, like an Egyptian sphinx, lifting your gaze slightly above the horizon line.
3. Bring your heels together with the tops of the feet lengthening down into the floor in a long, soft point and squeeze your buttocks, lifting tall out of the crown of the head as you pull the navel up into the spine.
4. Bend the right knee, making sure that as you do, you keep the knees pressed together to activate the inner thighs. Pointing the right foot strongly, kick the right heel toward the right buttock twice quickly and concisely as you inhale in tandem with the movement. Remember to continue to push the floor away with your elbows and fists as you perform the kicking motion. Extend the left leg longer as the right leg works.
5. Switch immediately to the left side and kick the left heel toward the left glute twice as you lift taller toward the ceiling, pushing the floor away with elbows and fists. It's easy to forget about the abdominals while you concentrate on the legs, but since you want to protect your lower back you must engage your powerhouse effectively by splitting your attention between your upper body and your legs. Focusing on your breathing in tandem with the movement of the legs as you push the floor away and lifting through the crown of the head will help you to execute this exercise beautifully. Of

course, don't forget to keep your knees squeezing tightly together throughout!

6. Repeat for a total of eight sets (right and left make one set).

Pendulum

The Pendulum is a side-lying exercise. Side exercises reinforce core stabilization, improve coordination and balance, and strengthen the postural muscles and abdominals—with a focus on the obliques—as they lengthen and tone the muscles of the buttocks, legs, and feet. You'll apply the principle of opposition in the side-lying lateral plane and experience it in an entirely different way than you did when you were on your back or stomach.

1. Lie on your right side, with your right arm extended toward to the top of the mat, palm down, right ear resting on right arm, and elongate your body. Turn your right palm up, bend your elbow, bring your hand up toward your head, and rest your head on your right palm. Align the length of your back with your elbow.
2. Place your left hand, palm down, in front of your chest for greater stability on the mat.
3. Lengthen your legs and set them at a slight angle in front of you, aiming toward the lower left front corner of your mat, so that the legs are perfectly stacked and aligned one on top of the other.
4. Lift your chin and chest so that you are gazing directly ahead of you. It should be almost as if you are trying to imitate your optimal standing posture in this side-lying position on the mat. Remember not to look down at your working leg and foot to check that they are behaving! Trust your body and continue to look straight ahead in order to reinforce proper posture, keeping your eyes on the prize of a taller, longer, more powerful you!
5. Flex your right foot, making sure that the pinky-toe edge of the foot is pressing firmly into the mat. Mind you, this is not the easiest thing

to do, so take a moment and make sure that you have achieved this position. You'll have to maintain some of your focus here while you are multitasking and splitting your concentration, dedicating some of it to reaching in opposition and working the left leg with the utmost precision.

6. Lengthen your left foot into a long point as you draw the navel deeply in toward the spine to prepare, and reach tall through the crown of your head. Employing opposition is the key to preventing your torso from rocking forward and backward when the leg moves front and back in the next steps.
7. Externally rotate the left leg in the hip socket, and then, as you inhale, kick the left leg forward toward your nose in a long stroke followed immediately after by another little kick, so that the feeling is "KICK-kick." As you're doing this, press the left hand into the mat for greater stability and lift your chin and chest to maintain optimal side-lying posture.
8. Then, without so much as a second's pause, KICK-kick the left leg behind you, maintaining the same plane of motion (moving the leg neither higher nor lower). The leg is swinging back into the position dancer's call an arabesque, reaching long through the leg with a pointed foot. Squeeze the buttocks firmly as you kick backward.
9. Repeat for a total of eight sets (front and back make one set).

Classic Teaser

The Classic Teaser challenges what you thought you knew about yourself and reveals new levels of patience and capability. It builds extraordinary integrated abdominal and back strength, strengthens the quads, lengthens the hamstrings, and improves overall coordination, balance, and stamina.

1. Lying on your back, draw your knees into your chest and reach your arms long overhead, holding them six inches above the floor behind you.
2. Extend your legs straight up to the ceiling, and then come into the

heels-together-toes-apart position, externally rotating your legs in your hip sockets while squeezing your inner thighs together. Even as you establish your balance here, you'll already be working very hard, so to lighten the load, imagine that you are shooting sparks through your fingertips and toes, trying to send those sparks as far away from your core body as possible.

3. Drawing your navel deeply into your spine, lower your legs as far down to your point of control (the point where your abdominals are engaged and your lower back is securely rooted into the floor). Keeping the legs exactly where they are, in your established point of control, you will use the power of opposition to roll up.
4. Reaching with equal and opposite energy and strength through your fingertips and toes, inhale to prepare. Then immediately exhale and lift your arms toward your toes, peeling your body off the mat one vertebra at a time without letting your legs move. Do your best here, and if it's too much, bend your knees slightly as a modification.
5. Come up as high as you can, with control, and then, at the height of the movement, with your arms reaching forward slightly above shoulder height, inhale.
6. Exhale as you roll back down to the mat, keeping your legs strong and straight, moving sequentially through the spine, one bone at a time, until you return to the starting position.
7. Keep the legs extended and do not rest between repetitions. As soon as you reach the starting position, begin again. With your arms energized overhead, inhale to prepare, and then exhale, peeling the body up and off the mat to come into the V position once again.
8. Repeat three times. Then rest before trying another set.

Swimming

Swimming—on dry land—strengthens the entire back body, encompassing the arms, shoulders, buttocks, legs, and feet, as it enhances coordination and builds stamina. It reinforces muscular cross-patterning, which can rehabilitate chronic back pain by strengthening the oppositional muscular corridors in the back body (for example, by reaching away with the right arm as the left leg lifts). As a bonus, like all the Pilates mat work exercises, it beautifully sculpts and tones your body, in this case with a specific focus on the back, buttocks, and legs.

1. Lying on your stomach with your forehead resting on the mat, extend your arms as far in front of you as possible, shoulder-width apart. Do the same with your legs, which should be hip-width apart.
2. Inhale to prepare, and then lift the right arm off the floor as you lift the left leg, engaging your abdominals and defying gravity. Exhale, pulling the navel up into the spine as you simultaneously lift your eyes, chin, and chest off the mat.
3. Lift and lengthen beyond your capacity, really feeling the oppositional forces of isometric resistance at work. Take pride in the strength you may feel vibrating or shaking in your body to lift yourself off the mat in this extension.
4. Breathe naturally now and switch sides, lifting your left arm and right leg and again reaching as far away from your core body as possible. Then lower those limbs and lift both arms and both legs up off the mat as high as you can.
5. Gaze straight ahead and lengthen your neck, relaxing your shoulders down and back. Start to beat the opposite arms and legs up and down in midair quickly and with great control and determination. Continue to inhale and exhale naturally, but deeply.
6. Continue swimming powerfully for eight sets of eight counts as you breathe with your entire body, maximizing the extension of your spine, working the arms and legs as you maintain your strong core.
7. Then stop the action of arms and legs, and stretch all limbs as long and as high as you can. Then rest, releasing your body to the floor. Pull back into the Child's Pose for a few breaths.

Seal

The Seal is your reward for all your hard work up to this point. It massages the spine as it continues to build abdominal strength, core awareness, balance, and coordination. This is a playful exercise that reflects Joseph Pilates's love of nature and the effortless, organic expression of animals' wisdom. He admired their flowing, economical movements. Even though it's simple and straightforward, the Seal is a culmination exercise. Like the Classic Teaser, it serves as a wonderful example of everything you have done up to this point. Revel in your accomplishments!

1. Sitting slightly behind your tailbone, round your spine, pull your knees to your chest, shoulder-width apart, and plant your feet six inches in front of you.
2. Bring your palms to touch in front of your heart in Prayer Position, and then point your fingers down between your knees and straighten your arms, so the outer elbows are touching the inner knees. Open your hands, reach around the outside of the calves, and grab the outside of the ankles.
3. Lifting your feet off the floor, bring your heels together with your toes apart and balance on your buttocks with your toes pointed down toward the floor. Press the elbows into the knees and the knees against the arms with equal force, so that you have constructed an inner circle of self-imposed isometric resistance.
4. Drop your gaze to your navel center as you inhale and rock back onto your spine. Go just to the base of the neck and balance there for a few seconds, then "clap, clap, clap" the feet together three times, making contact with the heels while maintaining the position of the feet you established in the beginning.
5. As you exhale, rock back up to the starting position and clap the feet together three more times while holding your balance on your tail-

bone. Focus your eyes straight ahead and pull the navel to the spine. Also make sure to check in with your shoulders and relax any compensatory action you are engaging in there.

6. As you continue to rock, clap, and roll, remind yourself to breathe deeply. Pull the navel into the spine as you allow your body to grow heavier and softer so as to amplify the compression of the body rolling against the floor, stimulating the nerves that run along the spine to derive maximum benefit.
7. Repeat six to eight times.

Transition: On your final few repetitions of the Seal, you'll build momentum. Provided you have no knee issues, use your final rocking up and forward to stand up without using your hands.

8. On the final rocking forward, instead of clapping your feet together, disengage your hands from your legs. Reach them forward and up to facilitate the forward motion of your body in space as you use your powerhouse, legs, and the force of opposition to rise up to your final Pilates tripod stance, where your heels are together and your toes are slightly apart, established at your natural external rotation.
9. Once you're erect, bring your heels together with toes slightly apart. Place your arms behind you, locking the thumbs together, pointing the fingers down to the floor, and rolling your shoulders open and down. Lift your chin and chest so you are standing even taller. Lift your eyes slightly above the horizon line, as you squeeze your buttocks and inner thighs together. Feel your legs working collaboratively with your powerhouse to make you feel invincible, taller, stronger, and more confident and capable than ever!
10. After a few breaths in your Pilates stance, release your hands and grow even another inch taller as you feel your feet pressing into the floor and your head spiraling up to the ceiling and beyond. Breathe

in a deep sense of satisfaction. Feel the pride that comes from honoring your miraculous physical machine and also turning back the clock of aging by making your spine more fluid and flexible and stimulating and lubricating your life-force center. Revel in the boundless energy you've generated on your mat. Standing tall, take a deep breath and enjoy the sensations of the energy that's circulating in your body.

8

go deep, open, and energize: yin yoga

One sunny afternoon at Alan Finger's studio, Be Yoga, on 19th Street and Fifth Avenue in Manhattan, I had just finished a dynamic vinyasa practice taught by one of my favorite teachers. I should have been looking forward to my reward for working so hard, and what is always my favorite part of any yoga class—final relaxation in *savasana*. Instead, as my eyes swept over the rainbow of yoga mats, watching a sea of thirty-plus sweaty bodies contentedly cozying in for their dessert, I braced for the inevitable. For months, my lower back had been plaguing me. I was worried. I'd been seeing massage and physical therapists without much relief, and even acupuncture didn't help as it always had. On some days, it got so bad that I couldn't even bend down to tie my own shoes.

The airy studio, with its soaring ceilings and ornate crown molding, in one of my favorite buildings in the Flatiron district, had always been my refuge, the place I could count on to right my world. But lately it only served as a reminder of how hopeless I had started to feel.

The sunlight streamed in through the grand, arched windows, and the third chime of the bell signaled perfect quiet. It should have been the cue to my body that it was time to rest and receive, but instead of being able to let go, I was bearing up against the overwhelming frustration—silencing a primal scream. As I started to extend my legs along the floor, the pain was so intense that I nearly started to cry. Looking up to the ceiling through gritted teeth, I whispered desperately, *How could this be happening to me?*

I'd been successful at keeping my lower-back issue a secret while I was performing, but when the music stopped and I was confronted by deep stillness, I couldn't pull off the simplest of pedestrian movements without being in absolutely torturous pain, and I had no idea why. When I could no longer "push" and muscle through as I was accustomed to, in those moments of quiet when my body was supposed to be supporting me in relaxing and releasing, I felt as though it was betraying me. Little did I know that it was trying desperately to be heard.

After class, my eyes caught a flyer on the announcement board advertising a "Yin/Yang Workshop," which offered long-held "cooling balancing poses" after a vigorous "heating" practice. I was intrigued. Somehow, it seemed the answer to my prayers. And I needed a miracle. I was in the midst of producing, choreographing, and performing in a large-scale production at Lincoln Center. My show was less than a month away from opening, and I couldn't afford to let anyone know how much I was suffering. The show had to go on! So I did what every good performer does and what I'd been practicing daily for most of my life: I put on a brave face, and I stuffed that painful secret down.

Surfer God

I showed up at the Yin/Yang Workshop to find that it was being led by no mere mortal, but by a tall, obscenely handsome guy with a bright white smile and sun-kissed skin, who looked as though he'd just emerged from the ocean, jogging up on a California beach with a long board under his arm. As Surfer God launched into his class, he warned us that we would be holding poses longer than usual and, as a result, feeling things more deeply than we did in a vinyasa practice. As someone who maintained control over my inner feelings, I found this idea disconcerting. I habitually wrestled every emotion to the ground, keeping the leviathans safely locked inside. When he explained that we might cry in the poses, I didn't really believe him. For years I had equated expressing my emotions with a loss of control and humiliation—it was dangerous. Nobody was going to see me in such a weak and compromised state. I was a consummate professional. I was in control.

The practice began with the Dragon, the yin yoga pose that had apparently started it all for our instructor—the one, he said, that had "cracked him wide open." It didn't sound appealing. Regardless, I dutifully moved into a long, low lunge with one leg behind me. I had done this pose a thousand times before in vinyasa yoga practices, but had flowed through it, holding it for five breaths at the most. Now, as I held the pose and the minutes ticked by, I started to feel . . . angry.

I realized that I was working on my left side, the site of my hip injury from years earlier. I started to feel as if my body wasn't big enough to contain the sensations that were rising up inside me. I needed to find the exit sign and get the hell out of there—out of the pose, out of the room, out of my body!

Suddenly I felt a wave, a literal *whoosh* of energy sweep over the entire length of my back and within seconds, the tears came. I began crying uncontrollably. Quietly, of course, because there was no way I was going to cry in front of anyone. I was stronger than that. Desperately hoping that no one would see me, shocked that this torrent of emotion was pouring out, there I was, feeling precisely what I was dreading—out of control, embarrassed, and exposed.

And just when I started to beat myself up for getting emotional, it got much worse. Surfer God was coming over. As he approached, I turned my face away, confident that I was sending a clear signal that I preferred to be left alone. But he wasn't having it.

He knelt beside me, his head just a breath away from mine, and, leaning in, he said, "You know, the same thing happened to me the first time. What's happening to you right now is a gift like nothing else you've ever felt, trust me. Cry. It's okay. You're going to feel like a new person after the practice. Celebrate your tears! Welcome to the first day of your new life."

I didn't believe him. Not even a little bit. I was in the midst of what felt like just the opposite of something to celebrate. Head bowed, incredulous, I watched the tears spill onto my mat. With each new pose, they kept coming. Slowly, I found myself giving in to it all, something I'd never done. I was surrendering to my fear and vulnerability—to this opening and releasing, purging the pain of the past from my body, memory, and spirit.

The true test came when we reached my once favorite moment. I started to lie back in *savasana,* bracing myself for the devastating disappointment I had grown accustomed to. Extending my right leg out, barely breathing, I felt . . . no pain. Incredible. Taking a deep breath to recover from the surprise, I braced myself again, lengthening my left leg down to join the right, allowing my legs to relax and fall apart. Nothing. No pain! Not an ounce of it. How was this possible?

Liberated from a lifetime of pressure, I felt as though the ten-ton boulder I'd been pushing uphill had just disappeared in a poof. The angst so big my body couldn't seem to contain it just one hour before had morphed into a relief so deep that it overtook my senses, exploding into an ecstasy of the soul that challenged me to breathe. As if I had just broken through the surface of an icy pond, barely making it to air again, my body sucked in oxygen, knowing exactly what it needed. Like a thunderclap, I started crying again.

Wave upon wave of overwhelming euphoria pulsed and billowed through me. What was this feeling? This extraordinary, internal billowing, this new thrill traveling up my spine? *It was energy moving!* It was so different from anything I had ever experienced before. I was emptied of my troubles, but also full, as in recharged, and somehow grounded! I felt delirious and giddy—I wanted to *live* in this new state. Flooded with the deepest relief and calm I had ever known, in gratitude I started to sob, and I no longer cared who saw me. After only two hours of this practice called yin yoga, *savasana,* a pose that had become impossible for me, became my refuge once more. Something miraculous had happened. I rose from my mat that day reborn.

I hope you find the same exhilarating freedom.

Let There Be Yin

Yin yoga was my first deep taste of hope. In that first yin practice, in the actual poses I did, I was *sent* into the very places inside that, unbeknownst to me at the time, were the centers of my pain, upset, confusion, and feelings of being powerless and overwhelmed in my life. Before then, I'd never been given the opportunity to physically "go into" what I would come to understand as *unconscious energy,* hidden pockets of unresolved trauma and pain that become lodged in the body. Yin yoga gave me the tools to change my inner dialogue and the energy that had manifested itself around it, inviting me to acknowledge the inextricable interconnectedness of mind and body and to create the life I wanted.

During that first yin session and over the course of months of practice, as I went deeper into the poses, I was surprised to realize that the more I surrendered, the better I felt at the end of them. The slower I allowed myself to go and the more fully and completely I breathed, the deeper the release and the greater the reward—new energy flowing through me. Yin yoga is what helped me know, in the deepest part of who I am, that the only way out is *through*, and that if I could make significant changes on my mat, I could expect to be able to do the same in my life.

The practice became a kind of training ground, a place where instead of meeting the difficulty and resistance I encountered in my body with judgment and condemnation, I learned to respond with gentleness and kindness. With each practice I did, I began to believe that I really did have the power to change my life, that I was worthy of love and kindness, and that I didn't have to face the idea of being stuck anywhere I didn't want to be—ever again.

This process of realizing my own power and the change I experienced in the practice wasn't gradual; it was rapid. Within the span of seconds, not even minutes, yin helped me know that anger could turn into sadness, which then could become relief and happiness, even joy! Yin yoga taught me that the path to liberation and finding your essential aliveness start with awakening the energy of love within your own being and that truly nobody can love you the way you can.

The "Unworkout"

Yin yoga involves deep breathing and total mind-body intention, leading to an ever deepening awareness of your inner landscape and the return to a more natural rhythm. It is a cooling, gathering, meditative "unworkout" that will calm and ground your energy at the beginning of your day, so you can get off to a steady start, or help you to slow down at day's end, preparing you for a restful night's sleep. Based on the same ancient principles as acupuncture, yin yoga is a needle-less modality that will enable you to gain access to some of your most deeply held, powerful, long-lasting energy.

Yin yoga's long-held, deeply transformative stretching poses target the deeper, interior, supportive structures of the body, the connective tissue known as *fascia.* The poses stimulate and open the meridian channels, the rarely accessed subtle energy pathways that run through it, encouraging prana to flow freely, helping you to restore otherwise unattainable youthful joint health and mobility. As you release tension, you quietly activate and gather your prana, harmonizing your body and mind and recharging your batteries.

Because our emotions are stored in the connective tissues and muscles in our bodies, as we send our conscious breath to those areas of restriction or pain, we experience a sense of physical freedom and flexibility we never thought possible. Repressed emotions are finally released for an incredible catharsis and an unparalleled feeling of tranquility.

This deeply energized calm doesn't just disappear after the practice concludes. Each session builds on the one before it, so the more you do it, the calmer and more flexible and energized you feel. By moving slowly and mindfully, you build your energy resources, increase your resilience, and improve your capacity to cope with the stresses and demands of your daily life.

What a gift, really, to be able to sit still, stop time, and return to the breath, to the pulse of perfect rhythm that exists in each one of us. It's a gift of balance and harmony we give ourselves when we listen to our inner voice. And it can be most easily heard when we surrender to the stillness of yin, which quiets the mind and heals the body, opening the door to infinite possibility.

Juicing the Joints

Our fascia has different preferences than muscle. Fascia is dense, fibrous tissue that does not respond to intense, dynamic, rhythmic contractions the way muscle does. Because of its innately more "stubborn" nature, it prefers to be stretched gently, like taffy. Think slow-motion movie sequences when you are deepening into a yin pose. Nowhere more than in the yin practice does the concept of *effortless effort* come into play; in order to properly, fully, and safely stretch your connective tissue, you must be as relaxed as possible as you move in and out of poses and hang out in poses with as little muscular effort as possible.

It's not muscular issues that ultimately impede our ability to run and jump and squat and fly as we age; it's our joints. One of the most incredible benefits of the yin practice is how it gently stretches, massages, rehabilitates, and reinvigorates the tissue that connects our joints. The joints of the spine, knees, hips, and shoulders, which become prone to injury after years of use and abuse, are lubricated, restored, and opened—made more flexible.

Yin poses "juice" the joints. They reconstitute the naturally occurring "fluids of youth" in our joint capsules—the synovial fluid and hyaluronic acid responsible for joint lubrication—which diminish as we age. This all-important "juice" is replenished by the practice, ensuring the smooth glide of our tendons and ligaments. In addition to making bones and cartilage glide smoothly through the joints, hydration provides our entire skeletal system with a kind of cushioning; this cushioning is akin to applying WD40 to machine parts to make them respond more efficiently and interact smoothly with the other aspects of the overall machine or system.

By placing the body in positions that challenge the range of motion of the fascia and as we appropriately stretch and put pressure on it, a slight degree of inflammation occurs that encourages the body's healing responses to kick in. Nerve signals from the body stimulate the brain to dampen pain by releasing natural feel-good opiates, encouraging the natural sedation of the fight-or-flight response, which calms the central nervous system, lowering our blood pressure and encouraging blood to flow optimally throughout the body. Signals from the brain travel through the connective tissue, stimulating growth and repair processes in our cells and rehydrating the tissues and joints.

Energy Delivery

Yin yoga poses unblock and flush out our meridians, restoring overall physical and emotional balance. The movement of muscles, the stretching of connective tissues, and the pressure exerted upon bone tissue in yin poses generate bioelectrical activity in the meridians in much the same way that acupuncture needles do. The stimulus of the needle magnetizes, attracts, and concentrates energy, activating the collagen that comprises the connective tissues by sending signals along the route of the meridians to landmarks along the way. Through a similar process, yin poses transmit energy throughout the musculoskeletal system, sending signals to cells like osteoblasts, which manufacture our bone tissues, and fibroblasts, which synthesize the collagen that our connective tissues are made of.

The meridians and the nadis conduct a reciprocal relationship with the chakras that run along the *sushumna nadi,* our central energy channel. The chakras, like the engines for our subtle body, gather, transform, and then distribute energy through the nadis. This energy feeds into our organs, ensuring proper nurturing of prana throughout our whole being.

Because the meridians rule specific geography in the body, when prana flows smoothly through them, ample energy is delivered to our organs and we feel emotionally balanced. When a meridian is blocked for some reason, prana is prevented from reaching the specific area it is supposed to nurture and stagnates, like a pond with algae overgrowth. The result is that the cells, tissue, or organs in the affected area suffer, as do the corresponding emotional qualities the organs themselves hold; as a result, emotions fall out of balance and express themselves as either too much of a good thing, *excess*, or not enough, *deficiency*.

The Art of Receiving

Trusting the simple and elegant work of the poses themselves is a miraculous cocreative process that occurs breath by breath. Meridians are being activated and harmonized, balancing the emotional content of the organs and the chakras, helping you to create new space through which powerful life energy can flow. Rising above all the noise of the mind and the internal protests, this new internal freedom, this life force, trumps everything, and what remains is pure clarity—the energy reserves and willpower not only to make better choices, but also to honor them.

Most yang endeavors like dance, Pilates, and even vinyasa yoga, have a kind of rigid, driving pulse that demands focus, control, timing, and coordination, all tasks that are performed under a kind of pressure; they emphasize dynamic, rhythmic movement and muscular contraction. Though phenomenally beneficial in their own right, they demand a high level of energy from you first before you receive their reciprocal energy.

Yin yoga is the opposite, inviting you to show up just as you are without striving for perfection. It entices you to release control and turn inward, open, and explore what has been hiding in your emotional being. In utter stillness, it helps you to create the space to transform the tensions and troubling feelings that live beneath the surface of your consciousness.

Yin offers a deeper, slow-burning, energized calm and a deep sense of confidence in your body's ability to regenerate itself. It's the kind of energy I imagine Mahatma Gandhi must have possessed—the energy of tremendous depth, patience, and honoring, the kind of energy that makes you know you have more than enough reserves to go around and allocate to every aspect of your life.

The Impala's Heart: Energy Intelligence

Animals in the wild provide us with a standard for health and vigor. . . . They offer us a precious glimpse of how we might function if our responses were purely instinctual. Animals are our teachers, exemplifying nature in balance.

—Peter Levine

Years ago, around the time that I signed up for my first yin yoga class without suspecting the impact it would have on my life, on one of my many visits to East West Books, I discovered author Peter Levine, and yin yoga would never be the same. As I was wandering through the aisles, somewhere between the sections on metaphysics and aromatherapy, I found his book *Waking the Tiger.* When I opened it, I happened upon the epigraph to the introduction: "If you bring forth what is within you, what you bring forth will save you. If you do not bring forth what is within you, what you do not bring forth will destroy you" (from the *Gospel of Thomas*). When I read those words, they stopped me dead in my tracks. Right there, in a bookshop that had become the magic portal to my future, yet another road to my healing and empowerment was revealed to me.

Ever since the sea change I experienced in my first yin yoga class, I understood its significance on some deep, intuitive level, but it wasn't until I found Levine's book that I understood why it worked so well. I wanted to shout from the rooftops the news about the pivotal dots that I had connected. I couldn't believe my good fortune: I'd finally found someone who understood what I'd been suffering from and was able to tell me how I could free myself. In my early twenties, after having miraculously survived severe depression and a dramatic swing into mania followed by a relentless cycle of death-defying panic attacks, I felt as though I had exited hell without an explanation. But there was no guarantee that I wouldn't just wind up there again.

One section of *Waking the Tiger* was particularly illuminating. In it, Levine says that when wild animals are confronted by danger, they have the same fight-or-flight response that we do. Unlike humans, however, they then have the innate ability to *discharge* their trauma and fear. He uses the example of an impala being chased by a cheetah, which can run up to seventy miles per hour. Faced with imminent death, knowing that it can't outrun the cheetah, the impala suddenly chooses to play dead. Although from the outside the impala appears motionless, on the inside the impala's energy is whirring through its entire system, its heart is beating wildly, and its nervous system is supercharged, flooded with energy. When the cheetah, thinking the impala is dead, becomes disinterested and wanders away, the impala, sensing the coast is clear, mobilizes and runs off the trauma, giving the energy an outlet and restoring homeostasis.

According to Levine, a threatened human (or impala) must discharge all the energy mobilized to negotiate a threat or risk becoming a victim of trauma. This residual energy does not simply go away. It persists in the body and often causes the formation of a wide variety of symptoms, like anxiety, depression, and psychosomatic and behavioral problems.

That animals know instinctively to discharge the stress that results from the fight-or-flight mechanism and we humans don't (despite allegedly being endowed with the gift of conscious thought) is proof of our alienation from both nature and our biological rhythms. In the ancient past, people were more connected than we are to the natural heartbeat of the earth and the cycles of the moon and more reverent toward the cosmos than we are today. Somewhere along the way, with the advent of societal "improvements," we distanced ourselves from nature and from our own true nature; we *unlearned* how to give trauma an outlet. If we are to cultivate own energy intelligence, we must turn to nature as our teacher, emulating our animal counterparts and recreating for ourselves what the impala knows to do instinctively. Only then can we live in harmony with our world and wake up the energy that is waiting there inside us.

As humans, however, we do not best discharge trauma by running it off, unless we do it while consciously acknowledging and processing our reaction to it. We discharge the nervous energy of our trauma most effectively by moving slowly and mindfully—by engaging in practices that afford us the space and time to experience our feelings.

Unreleased trauma quickly finds a place to settle in the body, where it disrupts the flow of chi. Wherever chi is obstructed, stagnation occurs, leading to disharmony and imbalance; that area can then become a chronic seat of pain and/or, ultimately, even disease.

The Waking Energy Way is the antidote, but the yin yoga practice in particular is especially effective, because its languorous rhythm encourages introspection. It's your chance to be the impala and discharge your trauma—but not by running away from it. You do it by getting still, going deep, opening, and investigating. Although you may feel a certain anticipatory anxiety about the thoughts and feelings that could arise, it is the *allowing* of what reveals itself to you that makes metamorphosis and waking your energy possible.

The Lion and the Lamb

Time records itself in the deep connective tissue of the body, where traumatic physical and emotional experiences find a home. When engaging in a yin practice, it isn't at all uncommon (and in fact is both natural and desirable) to release emotions that accompanied an original trauma. We can become angry, anxious, or frustrated and start to express powerful emotions through laughter or tears. This somato-emotional releasing is remarkably cathartic and therapeutic, physically and emotionally, and perhaps the most extraordinary benefit of the yin practice.

In the practice, what may appear at the onset to be a relatively innocuous pose, a sweet little lamb, can very quickly become a lion, roaring at you with a deafening, undeniable rush of sound. What you'll do is pay attention. You won't try to ignore the lion's roar. Heed any voice or primordial instinct you have, showing it kindness and adjusting your body accordingly, so that it can be your very best waking-energy partner.

We're taught to move away from discomfort, to mask it, hide it, to *shush* it away. Yin asks us to do just the opposite. It invites us not just to move toward discomfort, but to go inside it. Yin proves that whatever you anticipate isn't as scary as you thought it would be; on the contrary, unexpected relief and surges of energy flood your entire being when you lean into the poses and invite the "flames" of your emotional fire to consume you. Yin asks you to befriend what you perceive as a predator—not only to hold out your hand to the ferocious lion, but to feed it, pet it, and then lie down with it like a trusting lamb.

When you relax and allow sensations to come up in the physical postures without trying to mitigate or fix them, a magical alchemy takes place. Mind and body unite in peace and calm. When you can start to accept as truth that there is no good or bad, just energy, then you can experience the unfolding, releasing, and rising of stuck prana, bringing everything back to a place of equilibrium, where new energy awakens.

The emotional life of the body is central to yin. The visceral correspondence of organs and emotions and how we perceive this connection lie at the heart of the practice. For me, because of this vital aspect, yin yoga became *the* vehicle, along with therapy, for healing my personal pain. I learned that trauma needs to be discharged from the body and that healing is predicated on the confluence of our ability to find an outlet and our desire to become whole again, to initiate our own healing and reclaim parts of ourselves that got buried or lost along the way. This is the true gift of waking yin energy and what inspired me to want to reclaim myself—hope.

the go deep, open, and energize practice

TIME OF DAY: Morning or evening

QUALITY: Yin

SUBTLE ENERGY: Opens, activates, and harmonizes the meridian system.

BENEFITS: Relieves chronic holding patterns as it generates a deeply grounding, energized calm, a sense of well-being, and a lightness of spirit.

PROPS: Yoga mat, blocks, blankets, and bolsters

The Practice:

Child's Pose
Butterfly
Dragonfly
Dragon
Forward Bend
Half Saddle
Sleeping Swan
Quarter Dog
Eye of the Needle
Sphinx and Seal
Spinal Twist
Corpse Pose (*Savasana*)

Before You Begin

Make sure that you have the necessary props on hand: a yoga mat, at least two yoga blankets, a bolster, two yoga blocks, a yoga strap, and an eye pillow (optional). These props, although they cost a bit up front, are really an investment in you. They will soon come to be your favorite companions because of the self-love they signify, and they will serve you well for years to come. We all have varying degrees of flexibility in our overall musculature, which is based on genetics, lifestyle, and physical conditioning, so before you embark on your yin journey, know that this practice is yours, and it is up to you to be respectful of the miraculous machine you are inhabiting, the one that is serving you in this life, your best friend and greatest ally: your body.

Even if you are suffering from an acute injury, like the back injury I had when I started my yin practice, you can safely embark on a yin journey, and regular practice will go a long way toward helping you convalesce and rehabilitate. Compromising issues, such as restrictions caused by repetitive stress, trauma, or inactivity, are easily addressed with the use of props. You can achieve an ideal starting position that creates the appropriate amount of pressure to encourage the flow of prana, yielding the same kind of amazing benefits that someone with no issues or special considerations can achieve. Regardless of your age, health, or fitness level, yin yoga is deeply restorative and rehabilitative and can be tailored to your individual needs.

In the descriptions that follow, I'll start by explaining the ideal pose and give modifications with props, so that you can make the pose more accessible to your body and situate yourself in the most advantageous starting position to derive the greatest benefits.

The Meridian–Organ Pairs: Anatomy, Related Chakras, and Emotions

As you develop friendships with the individual poses, you'll enter them knowing their meridian and organ associations, and on some occasions you may choose to follow a sequence of poses designed to alleviate certain issues in the domain of a specific meridian–organ pair. The most important part of becoming familiar with the emotional energies of the organs is that you'll be able to link them in your mind to those of the chakras, balancing them and consciously transforming your own energy, raising its vibration from the shadow to the light, literally converting it into usable prana for your health and your life.

Let's get better acquainted with our chakras and how they specifically relate to the organs and their corresponding meridian pairs for our yin practice:

Root (*muladhara*): Kidney, urinary bladder, and small-intestine meridians (relating to elimination)
Sacral (*svadishthana*): Kidney, urinary bladder, and small-intestine meridians (relating to sexual and reproductive function)
Solar Plexus (*manipura*): Stomach, spleen, liver, and gallbladder meridians (relating to digestion)
Heart (*anahata*): Heart and pericardium meridians
Throat (*visshudha*): Lung and large-intestine meridians (relating to respiration and energy and physical elimination)
Third Eye (*ajna*): Governing Vessel and urinary bladder meridians
Crown (*sahasara*): Connected to the Conception Vessel and all meridians

Note that in each of the upcoming descriptions for your meridians, there are two bilateral branches of each (whether a single-entity organ like the liver or a double entity like your kidneys) that mirror one another running along the right and left sides of the body.

Lung (Yin), Large Intestine (Yang)

Chakra: Throat (*visshudha*)
In balance: Happiness, courage
Shadow emotions: Sadness, grief

The lung meridian starts in the center of the body and travels down into the large intestine before making an upward turn, running directly through the diaphragm and into the lungs, across the front of the clavicle on the same side of your body, down the inner arm, and terminating at the tip of the thumb on each side of the body.

The large-intestine meridian starts at the tip of the index finger, travels up the back of one of your arms to the shoulder, where one branch runs through the neck and mouth to the side of the nose on that same side; and the second branch travels down into the lung on that side of your body, the diaphragm, and your large intestine.

Kidney (Yin), Urinary Bladder (Yang)

Chakras: Root (*muladhara*) and Sacral (*svadhishthana*)
In balance: Wisdom, courage
Shadow emotion: Fear

The kidney meridian starts at the tip of the fifth toe of each foot, running through the Bubbling Spring Point (kidney 1 point) in the upper section of the sole (in the divet just below the pad of the foot), through the arch and up the inside of the knees and inner thighs, entering the torso near the tailbone. Moving up the longitudinal ligaments of the lower spine, it connects internally with the actual bladder and one of your kidneys.

The bladder meridian starts at the inner corner of each eye, travels up across the forehead and to the crown, entering the brain. From there it runs down the back of the body on either side of the spinal column, with an inner branch going to the lumbar spine, connecting to one of the kidneys and bladder, and an outer branch running down the entire length of the backs of the legs and terminating at the tip of the fifth toe on the foot on that same side of your body.

Liver (Yin), Gallbladder (Yang)

Chakra: Solar Plexus (*manipura*)
In balance: Compassion, peace, love
Shadow emotions: Anger, frustration, stress

The liver meridian starts at the tip of the big toe and runs up the length of the inner leg just above and adjacent to the kidney meridian. Entering the torso through the groin, it travels through the liver and gallbladder, into the lungs, up through the throat, and into the head, circling around the lips and moving into the eyes themselves.

The gallbladder meridian starts at the outermost corner of the eye and moves down the lateral side of the body through the outer hip, down over the outside of the knee, and terminating in the tip of the fourth toe of the foot on that side of the body. The gallbladder meridian also has an internal branch that runs through the neck and chest directly into the liver and gallbladder.

Spleen (Yin), Stomach (Yang)

Chakra: Solar Plexus (*manipura*)
In balance: Trust, openness, contentment
Shadow emotions: Anxiety, worry

Immediately adjacent to the liver channel, the spleen meridian starts at the medial side of the big toe, runs up along the inside of the legs, through the inner thighs, and into the groin, and enters the stomach and spleen, moving then through the diaphragm, chest, and heart, terminating at the root of the tongue.

The stomach meridian starts as two branches, in the shape of a tuning fork, on either side of the nose and bifurcates as it travels down through the diaphragm, into the stomach and spleen; finally it moves down through the quadriceps muscles on the tops of your thighs, the insides of the knees, and terminates at the tip of the second toe.

Heart (Yin), Small Intestine (Yang)

Chakras: Heart (*anahata*) and Root (*muladhara*)
In balance: Love, joy
Shadow emotions: Depression, anger

The heart meridian has three branches, all starting in the heart itself. The first branch runs down through the diaphragm into the small intestine. The second branch runs up through the throat and tongue into the eye. The third branch runs across the chest, travels down the inner arm, and terminates at the tip of the fifth finger.

The small-intestine meridian starts at the tip of the fifth finger of either hand and travels up the outer arm to the shoulder, where it divides into two paths, one running down into the heart, diaphragm, stomach, and small intestine and the other running up into the face, across the eye, and terminating in the ear on the same side of the body.

How to Go Deep, Open, and Energize

Once you've created the perfect environment for yourself and assembled your props, come to your mat, and let's talk about exactly how you are going to collect the jewels of the yin practice.

You'll approach every new pose the same way, following a sequence of seven steps. You will *establish the pose, greet the pose, go deep, surrender, honor, open and energize,* and *rise and return.*

Step 1: Establish the Pose

As the first step for every yin yoga pose in the series, you'll *establish the pose,* which means to physically set up the pose with your body, moving to a range where you feel a significant stretch. This is one that walks a fine line between intense challenge and acceptable discomfort. If you're unsure of what is acceptable discomfort, move gently into the position. As you become more familiar with the sensations of your body over time and with practice, you'll understand better how to find the right initial stretch for you—and you'll be able to go deeper after you've held that position for several rounds of breath.

As you establish the pose, tune in to how you are feeling on that specific day, in that very hour and moment. Decide where you want to begin, cultivating empathy for yourself on the spot, so that you can give yourself exactly what you need. Staying open and listening to your inner wisdom are at the heart of the practice.

For the duration of the practice, make a point to keep your array of props close at hand. As I give the instructions for each specific pose during the setup, I'll recommend which props to use, but if you need even more support than I'm suggesting, feel free to avail yourself of as many props as you require. Consider your props your best friends. Rely on them to make your position as comfortable as possible before you go on to Step 2. The building of your pose should be whatever you need it to be. Every pose is meant to be designed around your own unique personal needs, so feel free to plump up your "nest," as it were, before you really settle in.

I can't emphasize enough just how important this part of your practice is. In order to feel safe enough to surrender and go within, you need to establish yourself in an optimal starting position. The level of challenged comfort you feel in the positioning of your body, either with or without props, is what sets the stage and makes this possible.

Once you establish your pose and after you do any "housekeeping," such as prop adjustment and general futzing around (which is really resistance in disguise), try to stay true to your initial position. Even if you've done everything in your power to ensure your maximum comfort before you begin, if you still feel challenged (not in pain, but pushed beyond your comfort zone), stay with it, committing to your position and trying it out for just a breath or two before you make any other decisions that are likely to be informed by anticipatory anxiety and not led by what you are truly capable of. You won't know until you try, until you breathe and start to "go deep," so take a leap of faith and allow yourself to be surprised at how well you are able to settle into the pose. You'll feel greater comfort after you start to breathe into it. You want your initial position to be tolerable, so here is where you can test the waters, checking in with your breathing to guide you and reinforce that you are pleased with your decision. If for any reason you are not, this is the ideal opportunity to make adjustments.

Of course, your body and your props are yours to do with as you please. Your position can be adjusted at any time, if necessary—it's not considered cheating, but self-honoring. Congratulate yourself when you've heeded your body's wisdom and acted upon it. It's an act of self-love and self-care.

Step 2: Greet the Pose

The next step, before you surrender to gravity and start the melting process, is to introduce yourself to the pose and vice versa. There are a few versions, or "expressions," of any given pose. Each is just as valid and effective as the others, and which one is right for you can change from day to day. On some days, you'll come into the practice feeling good already. You'll likely feel more fluid and flexible to begin with and be able to move to a greater range from the start of a pose.

Alternatively, there will be days when you know you need a yin practice as a stress reliever (so badly, perhaps, that you're making a choice between yin and Xanax), and your body will feel tighter and more restricted. If this is a day when you feel more tension than usual, you'll want to practice being your own gentle lover, moving slowly and even more mindfully into your initial range of motion.

On those days, you'll likely come to your mat keyed up, perhaps under duress, battling many protestations and wrestling the Bacchae in your head to the ground (those are the sirens of the vine calling out to you to have a few glasses of red wine instead of practicing yoga). If you've won that battle, I congratulate you, because you'll feel a million times better. And afterward you can reward yourself with a nice glass of merlot if you still crave it. Enjoy the best of both worlds, I say! Truth is, you may feel so good that you'll no longer want the wine.

To *greet the pose,* you'll start by engaging the muscular sheath of your body, firming and flexing your muscles in a yang way as a kind of contrasting opening exercise. To illustrate what I've described, let's take the Dragonfly as an example. To establish the pose, you'll sit tall and place your arms behind you, using them to support your spine and leverage your legs, bringing them as wide apart as they will naturally go. Then you'll flex strongly into your legs and feet to feel the muscular effort, the contrast. You'll likely feel a stretch in the groin already, but you won't know yet whether you'll need or want props until you greet the pose by relaxing your legs and feet, letting them go completely soft and limp against the floor, and dropping your head down, even bringing your hands down in front of you to increase the depth of the stretch.

When you greet a pose, you're getting your first taste of the true yin expression of the position, meaning a place where you've allowed yourself to release all muscular effort and accurately experience what your true range of motion is as well as the level of sensation you feel. It's only then that you'll understand where this is all going and determine whether you need to stay upright and keep your hands behind you for a few breaths or progress by bringing your hands forward and keeping your arms straight as supports for your spine. In both cases, you'll then drop your head and feel the intensity of the deeper layers of your body stretching.

Part of greeting a pose is making initial adjustments. After your contrasting moment, as you progress to dropping your head down, you may need a block on its highest setting to support your head as you start to melt and open. If, on the other hand, you're more open from the onset, you might want to use the block for a few breaths and then, because your muscles have released a bit, you might be able to drop down onto your elbows. All these are options for you in each and every pose.

Adjustments made for a healthy body are *variations.* Adjustments made for injuries or physical limitations are *modifications.* You'll find descriptions for both in the instructions. Once you've greeted a few of the poses, you'll know how to work with all the poses because they are all very similar.

The true start of your yin practice happens when you close your eyes and begin breathing deeply into the position you've committed to. When you enter a yin pose, particularly if it is especially challenging, you can expect a few things, starting with a struggle in which you try to figure out how not to be in the pose. Once you make the decision to yield, your surrender is likely to result in a valuable somato-emotional release, meaning you'll cry, laugh, or cough. Here you officially start the journey inward, giving yourself over to gravity, and moving your body to a greater range so that you can feel the greatest sensation of stretch in the pose. This is where you'll move your focus past the exterior sheath of your muscles to the fascia underneath, contacting the sensations you find there.

I can guarantee that this will be a "Holy sh-t, what have I done?!" moment, when you can't believe that you've actually signed up for this. Now you'll need to decide on your optimal position. Choose one where you don't feel scared or overwhelmed, for example, by a stretch in your outer hip, but are sufficiently intrigued; let's say that you're suddenly alert and attuned. (I say this with a compassionate smile.) The sensations you'll feel in the yin practice are surprisingly intense and will, without question, demand that you give your full attention to what is going on inside your own body. What "wakes us up" also awakens our energy.

Breathe deeply into the sensation that's arising, and do it gently and lovingly. Do it without judgment, so that you can appease that rude awakening, which is a singular combination of your own natural reaction of shock and awe at just *how much* such a simple pose can elicit and, of course, the nervous tension that inevitably will ensue when you first come into the pose.

While your muscles are starting to release, breathe directly into the specific body areas being stretched in the pose. Know that if you just allow yourself to breathe into what you are feeling and allow your body to start to become heavy, sink, and befriend gravity, rather than resisting or fighting it, tension will melt away. Sensations that were so intense just seconds earlier will dissipate. The more you allow yourself to let go, taking comfort in the idea that the earth supports you, the faster your body's wisdom will take over. Before you know it, you'll start to trust, and your muscles and fascia will respond. Your subtle body will start to celebrate and do what it knows how to do best and the meridians, organs, and chakras will all start to flow, sing, and spin beautifully under your guidance and care.

Step 3: Go Deep

After you've acclimated yourself to the pose, your mind starts to slow, and you've come to understand and accept where you are and that getting into this position was in fact a voluntary act, you'll *go deep,* the next step in our yin sequence. Going deep or dropping down (allowing your body to melt into the floor) happens sixty seconds to two minutes into the pose, when you've really started to connect to your breath and the way it flows into your body as well as to the sensations you are feeling. Here, you'll start to feel willingly seduced by the idea of giving over to gravity and begin to believe that maybe this is a good thing.

You'll continue to direct your breath into the areas of greatest sensation in the body, knowing that as you breathe into them, just like the weather, they will change. You'll be here for a minute at least. Each time you inhale, breathe new life and energy into your body. As you exhale, let go of holding and tension. Offer what you no longer need to the earth below you. Tune in to your body using your intuitive listening skills. If your muscles and fascia are starting to melt and open, you can increase your range of motion ever so gently and slowly by making adjustments in how far away from the floor you hold yourself, either with your body or with props.

Give your weight over as much as possible to the props and to gravity. As you do, you'll create the space to release even more, and the intensity of sensation will likely increase when you adjust your position, but in a way that is palatable. Remember, you're the one in control, titrating how much you feel.

After you've moved into the deeper expression of the pose, use your breath to do a body scan, seeking out new areas of greatest sensation or discomfort and deliberately breathing into them. Your body scan will lead you to the first of a few proverbial forks in the road—one of several you'll encounter over the duration of any given pose. At this juncture, if you feel that your body is capable of going beyond the range of motion your prop affords you and you are ready to accept greater sensation, make some strategic physical adjustments to facilitate a deepening of the pose. You can turn the block under your head to a lower height or remove it entirely; you can shift a blanket or bolster out from underneath your hip (or move it farther away from you) or drop down onto your elbows. Do whatever you feel you need to do to allow your body to release further and move, without straining, into a greater range of motion.

If, on the other hand, you feel at this juncture that you've gone beyond the range of motion that you thought you could handle when you were greeting the pose, you can bring a prop back to its original height or replace a blanket or bolster. If you've dropped down onto your elbows and feel as though it's too much, you can lift up and return to straight arms.

Step 4: Surrender

As your body continues to open, what lies underneath the surface of your consciousness will now be revealed, like an iceberg with only a quarter of its mass above water. Emotions that are out of balance will inevitably arise. Your next step, *surrender,* occurs when your entire body is willingly partnering with you and there is very little holding or tension remaining, in the sense of protective guarding or muscular armor. This is when you really start to physically, mentally, and emotionally let go and you open to the sensations and feelings that arise, instead of recoiling from them in fear.

Surrender means accepting what is. It means accepting what is already here and giving up the fight that keeps you in limbo, struggling against what cannot be controlled, so that you can invite peace into your being. It involves trusting that your breath will carry you through to a place where you begin to unblock your energy pathways, liberate holding patterns in your tissues, transform your emotions, and take back your power. Simply stated, surrender doesn't mean losing a fight; it means finding the courage to know when to yield—all in the spirit of self-love and self-preservation. It means trusting your body's wisdom to reveal your purest life force.

By this point in any given pose you'll be at around minute three or four. As you continue breathing and surrendering to gravity, when you encounter challenging sensations that bring up uncomfortable feelings, each time you exhale, here is where you'll want to really start relying upon your mantra: "I am letting go of anything I no longer need" or "I am letting go of anything that no longer serves me."

It is very important that, as you speak the mantra in your mind, you visualize stagnant energy leaving your body and going down into the earth, where it will be recycled. Rely on your breath here and remember that it's the most powerful transformation vehicle you have.

After repeating the mantra several times, you may find that your body responds by opening more than you anticipated, like a thirsty plant when it finally gets watered. If you sense that your range of motion has shifted and exceeded what your props or body affords you, here is another opportunity to make adjustments that will take you deeper in the pose.

Repeat your mantra. Then simply melt.

Step 5: Honor

Aligning with our overarching theme for the practice, the next step in your progression, *honor*, follows on the heels of surrender. As you continue to sink into the earth and stretch even more deeply, encountering sensations and emotions that run the gamut, do your best to honor the feelings that arise. If surrender means accepting what is, honoring is the next evolution of surrendering and signifies consciously acknowledging the gift of your new awareness—paying homage, offering reverence for this shift in thought, which has a directly positive impact on your physical being and energy.

Honoring emotions, thoughts, and memories is akin to showing gratitude for them. Your body feels this and celebrates your mind's expansion by leaping for joy internally. When you've surrendered to what is, you give up the story of whatever was tormenting you as well as the accompanying sensations or emotions; and when you honor your decision to be in the present, you liberate yourself—you feel free and energized!

Harkening back to our Dragonfly example, it's possible that at this point you'll experience the shadow side of your emotions, feelings that you would prefer to deny. Every pose affects specific meridian channels as well as the corresponding "shadow" and "in balance" emotional states I have listed for you in my instructions. Simply by virtue of moving through the pose, you'll be contacting the shadow and transforming it into balance and energy with your intention and breath.

For instance, you may feel an emotional imbalance corresponding to the liver-gallbladder meridian pair as frustration, stress, or anger. To honor it, simply breathe deliberately into your arising emotions and into the organs that are targeted by the pose you're in. Then you'll use your breath and focused intention to bring them into a higher vibrational state by infusing them with the matching balanced emotion. In this way, your breath, like a glowing pipe cleaner, goes plunging through your meridians, whisking away the detritus from accumulated stress in your tissues, organs, and chakras, and you'll bring your shadow emotions into balance, transforming them into the higher, positive vibration that results in new energy.

As you continue to melt and breathe, allow the feelings to come up without becoming attached to them or judging them. Breathe into them, honoring them with your attention. On your exhalations, repeat your mantra and let these emotions and mind states go. Let them exit your body. Then allow yourself to go even deeper into the pose with as little effort as possible. Let yourself sink deeper into the floor—or if you are challenged to your capacity with the stretch you are feeling, stay exactly where you are and just continue to focus on your breath.

Step 6: Open and Energize

Around minute five, you'll move into the deepest expression of the pose. Although you've actually been opening your meridians ever since you took your first breath in the pose, after spending several minutes in the pose you are ready to maximize your earlier investment of effort to remove stagnation and unblock your energy pathways by moving into the greatest range of motion your body affords you in that moment. You'll consciously continue to *open* your heart, your body, and your mind so that the best of your transformational efforts may occur.

To *energize,* you'll now breathe balancing emotions into your meridians, tissues, and organs. On this step, you'll harmonize your energy by replacing out-of-balance emotions with purely positive emotions and mind states, bringing more light into the body. Energizing is a kind of cathartic, etheric cellular reprogramming process in which you literally change the internal dialogue that has been running in your head and contributing to held tension in your body. This is when you take your power back once again.

You'll purposefully breathe the in-balance emotions associated with the meridian pair your pose is targeting, including compassion, peace, and love through your meridian channels and into your every cell as you continue to melt and release. Each time you exhale, you'll let go of anger, stress, and tension, and everything else you no longer need, in a process comparable to clearing clutter from your shelves. The key difference is that new prana will begin to circulate throughout your body at this point, and you can harness it intentionally to reprogram your cells for optimal wellness. Just continue to consciously breathe the higher vibration of balanced emotions into your meridians, organs, and chakras.

With each breath, as you replace the old with the new, the shadow with the light, you'll have created greater balance in your body and mind, and you'll experience the harmony of waking energy! In this last segment of the pose, you'll want to tune into your subtle body and feel the sensations of the fresh prana flowing. Even if you don't feel anything special the first time you practice, after a few sessions, you will.

Step 7: Rise and Return

When you're ready, you'll perform your final step, *rise and return*. After a good minute or more spent energizing your body, you'll exit the pose very carefully, with as little muscular effort as possible. Before you do, however, take a moment to observe the changes that have occurred in your body while you held the pose. Simply tune in to how you are feeling now compared to how you felt when you first started.

Of course, what you perceive may be subtle or significant. Moving in and out of a pose is just as important as surrendering in one. Every transition needs to be done with extreme presence and care, so move slowly and listen to your body. Treat yourself like a newborn baby, an emerging being who needs love, attention, and tenderness. Slowly disengage from the pose, moving as if you were asleep, keeping your eyes closed and making sure that that your head is the last thing to rise—always exerting minimal muscular effort. Unless otherwise indicated in my instructions, once you've risen out of a pose, you'll come into the Child's Pose, returning "home" where you can rest and consciously gather all the prana you awakened in the pose, harnessing and directing this energy into your kidneys and adrenal glands to replenish and restore them.

Rise and return is the step where you have the option, if you feel the need to bring life back into your limbs before moving into the Child's Pose, to do a little self-massage. You may use the fist-thumping technique from the Door-of-Life Love Tap exercise in Chapter 4.

After rising from any pose, slowly and gently extend your legs in front of you. To move prana down to your feet and restore your circulation, you're going to "beat yourself up" with a little love. Rub your palms together vigorously and then clap them three times fast and hard to dispel any negative energy. Then bring your hands into fists and gently, but firmly, rap on your legs. Strike your fists along the outer legs in a rhythmic fashion, moving from the upper thighs down to the lower shins, and then work your way back up the inner legs. Do a Horse Breath or two as you do this.

Then, as though you were brushing lint off your favorite black pants, work your way down the full length of the legs. Bounce your legs against the floor for a few moments and then make windshield-wiping movements with your feet and legs.

Once your circulation is restored, return home by moving into the Child's Pose, where you'll rest and recharge for several breaths before moving on to your next pose.

Now for the practice. Go forth—go deep, open, and energize!

The Practice

Child's Pose

Meridian pair: Kidney and urinary bladder

IN BALANCE: **Wisdom, courage**

Shadow emotion: Fear

Just as with all the yin poses, when you enter into a shape, you balance the associated meridians that are targeted by the architecture of the pose, appease the shadow emotion, and call forth the optimal balanced state.

Before we move on to the more active of the yin poses, I'd like to begin by welcoming you home. With the Child's Pose, we revisit our beginnings, assuming the same shape we took in the womb, and allow ourselves to receive nurturing feelings of safety and peace. In this enfolding embrace, we commune with Mother Nature.

The Child's Pose gives us a taste of what we're ultimately moving toward at the end of the practice session, *savasana* (Corpse Pose). *Savasana* is the final relaxation and the ultimate surrender, helping us to cull all the healing benefits of the practice and completely let go. In the Child's Pose, we sample deep rest while still consciously directing our energy to our organs. When it's used to transition from one pose to the next, not only does it give us a chance to absorb the healing benefits of our practice thus far; it also serves as an opportunity to harness the bounteous prana we've liberated in the preceding pose, directing it into the prenatal bank account—our kidneys and adrenal glands.

On the scale of challenge, the Child's Pose sits at the lighter end, so for most of us it will be a refuge from the other yin poses that stretch and exert pressure on the tissues. Like all forward-bending poses, it brings you into an introspective state of mind. It's a chance to experience the contrast between the relief and relaxation you feel here and the adversity that arises after navigating the often challenging moments of opening your meridians and calling up the emotions that connect to them in the more demanding poses. Comparatively speaking, it doesn't ask a lot. It simply invites us to rest and recharge. You'll appreciate the relief that the Child's Pose offers, especially after doing the first side of the Dragon or the Sleeping Swan. For all these reasons and more, you'll find yourself looking forward to it. Every time you exit a pose and "come home," you'll feel the change and you'll feel better.

With the first Child's Pose of the practice, take your time and treat it as you would any other pose, staying in it for between three and five minutes. After that, as you move through the other poses in the practice, you'll stay in the Child's Pose for two to three minutes at most, as you are moving more rapidly through the sequence.

Caution: If you have knee issues or chronic lower-back pain, you should ease into the Child's Pose or perhaps avoid it altogether. With my own back pain, the Child's Pose actually felt like a relief, but trust your own body's voice and adjust accordingly. You are always welcome to come into a comfortable cross-legged pose or any other position that suits you in which you can relax.

1. On your hands and knees, press your hips back so that you are sitting on your heels with your big toes together and knees shoulder-width apart. Extend your arms straight out in front of you and bend forward so your upper body is resting on your thighs. Allow your forehead to rest on the floor. Stretch your arms out in front of you, palms down, and then bring the arms back beside your hips with your palms facing up.
2. Consciously connect to your breath, breathing more deeply into your chest and your belly. Allow yourself to settle into the pose by sending the breath into your entire body and particularly into the areas where any specific sensations arise. Tell yourself that you can now relax—no more work, no more navigating, no more output. It's time to receive and recharge.

Modifications. If your knees are tender, you can place a blanket underneath them for more cushioning. Or experiment to see if you get more relief by rolling up a blanket and placing it behind your knees before you try folding forward.

Butterfly

Meridian pair: Kidney and urinary bladder

IN BALANCE: Wisdom, courage

Shadow emotion: Fear

At the official start of our yin yoga practice is the pose that best personifies transformation, the Butterfly. You have my permission to play a little and be curious, like a child; sneak in an assessment after even thirty seconds of conscious breathing. You'll be able to gauge a palpable difference and will likely be very surprised at how far you've come in that short time.

Caution: If you suffer from lower-back pain, sciatica, or spinal issues of any kind, be careful as you come into this or any of the other forward-bending poses in the practice. If, after a few breaths, a pose doesn't feel right for any reason, trust your inner wisdom and either opt to do a reclining version of the Butterfly (you lie back instead of bending forward) or bypass it altogether, replacing it with a modification or an alternate pose that better suits your body once you have cycled through the full collection of poses and can choose what feels best.

1. Sitting on your mat, bring the knees toward the chest and then spread them open. Bring the soles of your feet together, forming a diamond shape resembling butterfly wings with your legs. Your feet should be about a foot away from your groin, with their outer edges resting on the floor.
2. Bring your hands behind you and extend your fingertips long into the floor, so that they're facing away from you and your shoulders are rolled open and back. Energize your fingertips and arms as you push the floor away, using your hands to leverage your spine so that you can sit tall. Reach the crown of your head toward the ceiling in opposition as you expand your chest.
3. Drop your head gently forward and soften your spine so that you start to relax your torso, rounding as far as you can go forward without straining. Wherever you meet resistance is where you are meant to begin. If you feel excessive restriction when you try to round forward, then leave your hands behind you at least for the first few breaths to serve as support for your spine. If your body naturally rounds forward without issue, then bring your hands in front of you.

4. Stay where you are for a few breaths and sense how you feel. Inhale deeply, and then exhale all the stale air from your lungs. Feel your spine melting forward toward the floor, as your body releases and gets heavier. Breathe into your shoulders, arms, and hands. As you exhale, feel the weight of the world sliding off your shoulders and releasing into the earth. Feel that when you breathe into your arms and then exhale, you're sending any of the discomfort you experience in your spine, neck, or shoulders out through the exit points that are your fingertips into the earth.
5. After moving through the full sequence of the pose, slowly rise up through the spine, stretch your legs out in front of you and make your way into the Child's Pose.

Dragonfly

Meridian pair: Liver and gallbladder

IN BALANCE: **Decisiveness, action**

Shadow emotion: Anger

The Dragonfly offers you a bonus gift. Not only does it target the liver and gallbladder meridian; it also stimulates and opens the spleen and stomach meridian and the kidney and urinary bladder meridian, which run up the inside of the legs and over the back. Come with me now on the delicate wings of the Dragonfly for a flight you won't soon forget!

1. Sitting on your mat, open your straight legs as wide as they will naturally go; this is called straddle position. To be confident that you've found your proper starting point, you should already feel a good deal of sensation in the inner thigh and groin. Lift the crown of your head

toward the ceiling and lengthen your spine by placing your hands behind you, fingertips pointing away from your body, and actively pressing your fingertips into the floor. As you inhale, engage the quadriceps muscles in your thighs and flex your feet strongly, activating the muscular sheath of your body.

2. Now, to really feel the contrast between muscular engagement and passive release, inhale deeply. As you exhale, let your legs and feet go completely soft and limp against the floor. Stop holding and let the floor support you. Allow your body weight to drop down into the earth as you greet the pose with your conscious breath and relax. Drop your head gently forward and breathe. Tune in to the degree of sensation you are feeling, especially in your groin. This is the moment of truth in which you'll decide where best to go from here; you are at a crucial point where it is essential to calibrate how far you can safely go into the stretch.

   If you find that you are sufficiently flexible—meaning you feel a healthy stretch, but not so much sensation that you are in discomfort—go deeper. Bring your hands in front of your body, placing your palms on the floor, and drop your head forward, allowing your upper back to melt toward the floor, coming into a deeper, fuller expression of the pose. At your starting point, your arms may be straight, with palms on the floor, or perhaps your elbows will be bent and your head quite close to the floor. Remember that you can always come back from your edge if the sensation is too intense.

3. Now that you've found your ideal starting position, allow your body to adjust into this new shape, and with your head heavy and your legs and feet completely relaxed, give your full body weight to the floor beneath you. Feel fully supported by the earth. Breathe into the sensations you feel in your groin and upper thighs, and then, as you exhale, let go. In your mind, travel up to your head, neck, and shoulders,

and down through your spine, legs, and feet. Breathe generously into this entire expanse. As you exhale, feel your breath moving all the way down your arms and legs and out through your fingertips and toes into the earth below.

4. To come out of the pose, do your best to keep your eyes closed and preserve your new inner sight. Slowly walk your hands back toward your torso, using your arms to assist you in gently stacking your spine as you roll up to a fully erect posture.
5. Once you are sitting tall, inhale deeply and bring your arms behind you, extending your upper body, chest, and face up and back, moving into the slightest back bend as a counter stretch to the pose. You'll likely feel as if the muscles of your inner thighs have been stretched as never before, so move with caution!
6. Gently and slowly, draw your legs back together with your hands, bounce them out, and swing your legs back and forth like a windshield wiper a few times before coming into the Child's Pose.

Dragon

Meridian pair: Spleen and stomach

IN BALANCE: **Trust, openness, contentment**

Shadow emotions: Anxiety, worry

I would like to remind you that the Dragon is the pose that started it all for me. There's a reason I had a doozey of a somato-emotional release doing the Dragon in my first ever yin practice: the Dragon is one of the more intense yin poses. As soon as you get into it, you'll understand why. Although you can expect intensity from the onset, do something counterintuitive: instead of bracing yourself for something unpleasant, greet the pose with an open mind and welcome whatever you feel by *leaning in* to it. You'll find that the intensity diminishes, and in its wake is the gift of energy.

1. Starting on your hands and knees, step your right foot between your hands, coming into a low lunge, lining your toes up with your fingertips. Lengthen the left leg down and back away from you, keeping it slightly bent, allowing your pelvis to drop down toward the floor. As you come into the pose, you'll feel a significant stretch in your left hip flexor and in the muscles at the front of the left hip.
2. Breathe into any sensations you feel and allow the weight of your head to drop toward the floor. At this juncture, you have a few options. Experiment until you find the one that suits you best. You can stay exactly where you are now and see what comes up. As your tissues open and the restriction you feel eases, you may want to move on to one of the following variations.

   Variation 1: Grab a yoga block. Turn the toes of your right foot out to the side, coming into a slight external rotation in the right hip, and either place your palms flat on the floor inside the leg with straight arms or drop your elbows softly down on the block, dropping your head and continuing to melt into the pose from there.

   Variation 2: If you are more open and have a greater range of motion, you can forgo the block completely and drop down onto your elbows directly allowing your upper torso to ease down toward the floor, where you can come to rest your head on your cupped fists or by interlacing your hands into one fist. This last option is the most expanded, fullest expression of the pose.
3. Inhale and send a sweeping breath, like a soothing waterfall, all the way down the length of the back of the body, starting at the crown of the head and releasing it out through the back foot, and let go. Take another full-body breath in through the back foot and send it up the front

length of the body through the back thigh, hip, pelvis, belly, and chest. Let it move all the way into the face and out through the crown of your head. Let go completely, and let your head weight drop further. Feel like the Komodo dragon, a lizard that is at one with the earth. Allow its steady heartbeat to inform your grounded, measured movements.

4. Breathe into the areas of greatest sensation and let go of anything that no longer serves you. The Dragon, because it is the most intense of the poses you'll have done so far, will likely "stir the pot" almost immediately. It's entirely natural to feel the mind racing and strategizing, trying to figure out the best route for escape! You might need a Horse Breath right now. Do it! Take a deep, smooth breath into your busy brain, and when you exhale, let all concern cease and feel the release. Let it all go. Know that with each breath, you are clearing, activating, and harmonizing the energy pathways and creating the space for balance to thrive—for new life-giving energy to surge and bloom inside you.
5. With as little effort as possible, start to come out of the pose. Move carefully and slowly. Your hip ligaments are strong and will feel stiff when you try to move them to come out of the pose, since you've gone deep and stretched the body's canvases in ways they are not at all accustomed to. Breathe as you use your hands and upper body to take the weight out of your hips in order to shift them back and drag the right leg back toward the left, coming into the Child's Pose. Savor the buzz and flow of prana flowing through your body. Breathe gratitude into your belly and heart. Rest and let go.
6. Repeat the steps on the other side, stepping up with the left foot and lengthening the right leg behind you. This is the moment in my classes when I say, "Be happy you're not a millipede and have only two legs!" Each side is different because of how we use our bodies in life: our posture, our habits, our awareness. If one side is tighter than the other, it is already time to bring your breath and your compassion to your body in the first stage of the pose. Inhale into every area of greatest sensa-

tion in your body and then let it go. Repeat the entire journey on your left side, and afterwards, slowly and gently, come into the Child's Pose.

Forward Bend

Meridian pair: Kidney and urinary bladder

IN BALANCE: **Wisdom, courage**

Shadow emotion: Fear

After the intensity of the Dragon, the Forward Bend should prove especially soothing to your mind and bring you into an introspective state, where you can thoughtfully integrate the work you've done up to this point. Because it increases the range of motion in the hamstrings, which connect to the muscles of the lower back, this pose is especially beneficial for improving chronic lower-back conditions. A great stress reducer, it also improves digestion, relieves fatigue, and calms the mind.

1. Sit tall with your legs extended in front of you, hip-width apart. Place your arms behind you, fingertips facing away from your body, and press the floor away with your palms, reaching the crown of your head toward the ceiling in opposition. Breathe deeply into your chest and belly while you simultaneously strongly flex your feet and engage your quadriceps—this helps you to experience contrast in the pose before you greet it.
2. Now relax your legs and feet entirely, letting them go limp, allowing every other muscle in your body to soften at the same time. Take stock of what a relief it is not to have to "muscle" your way through anymore. Give yourself over to nondoing. Start to round your upper body forward, breathing deeply as you go, and bring your arms in front of your body by the sides of your hips. Wherever you naturally land—as far as your body rounds without effort is where you are meant to begin.

3. Wherever you are, with or without props, start to greet the pose with your breath. If your neck or upper back feels stiff, place a block on its higher side (so that it's standing at its tallest), underneath your forehead and rest it there, allowing your body to melt into it. Allow your head, neck, and shoulders to release down toward the floor. Breathe into your legs and feet and also let them sink into the floor. Breathe into your arms, allowing the breath to travel through your hands and out of your fingertips.
4. When you're ready to come out of the pose, slowly, with as little effort as possible, walk your hands toward your torso, stacking your spine until you've returned to a fully erect position. Use your hands, not the muscles of your back, to do the work. Allow the stacking process to take several breaths. As you gently transition into a new shape, ask the muscles that were resting in the pose to reengage.
5. After you are sitting straight up, with a tall spine, do a slight back bend. Expand your chest and lean back into your hands, keeping your arms straight and pressing your palms into the floor. Feel the contrast in your back and upper body as you breathe into this new shape. Feel the subtle energy flowing through your body. Breathe. Then slowly, mindfully, come into the Child's Pose and direct the prana you've harvested to your grateful kidneys and adrenal glands.

Half Saddle

Meridian pair: Spleen and stomach

IN BALANCE: Trust, openness, contentment

Shadow emotion: Anxiety

Not only does the Half Saddle improve digestion, but it targets the quadriceps and hip flexors as well as the psoas (a deeply internal postural muscle). Stretching these three muscles properly and consistently can alleviate chronic back pain. It's highly effective for people who do a lot of walking and running. If you allow your head to release back into a slight back bend while in the pose, the pose will also stimulate your thyroid gland.

Caution: If you have any knee issues, of if you experience any pain, please forgo Half Saddle and opt for the Quarter Dog instead, which also targets the stomach and spleen meridians.

1. From the Child's Pose, sit up and bring your hands behind you on the floor for stability. Lean to your right side and stretch your left leg straight out in front of you. Keep your right knee folded underneath you, internally rotated. In this position, your right shin should be facing the floor, and the sole of your right foot facing up to the ceiling, with your right ankle touching your buttock. Lean back into your hands, activating a stretch in the front of the thigh (the right quadriceps muscle). To experience contrast in the pose before you greet it, engage the top of your left thigh by straightening the knee fully and flexing the foot strongly as you sit up tall, using your hands behind you as leverage to press your spine forward and up as you expand the chest.
2. Inhale deeply and as you exhale, let the left leg and foot go entirely limp, and allow the leg to roll out to the side if it naturally goes there. Relax the shoulders and, even though the arms are supporting you, relax any pointed muscular effort to keep them perfectly straight. Breathe into the stretch you feel in the front of the right thigh, and tune in to the sensations you are feeling to assist you in making your decision as to where you want to go from here. You can either keep your arms straight behind you if you feel enough of a stretch and/or drop back onto your elbows to increase sensation.
3. Once you've chosen your preferred starting position, close your eyes and start to breathe into the areas of greatest sensation, such as your thigh and your neck and shoulders. As you exhale, release any related tension that may be arising in an effort to pull you out, up, and away from the intensity of the pose. Inhale fully, starting at the crown of

your head. As you exhale, allow your breath to sweep down the front of your body, through the active right thigh and out through the sole of the right foot. Allow your upper body to soften.

4. To come out of the pose, as with all others, move slowly and mindfully. With your eyes closed, keeping your left leg and upper body entirely relaxed, take care to move with delicacy as you bring your right knee out from underneath you, extending the leg straight out in front of you. Bounce the leg out and massage around the knee cap and surrounding muscles to release any stiffness you may feel. Good-bye, stagnation. Hello, waking energy!
5. Repeat the entire sequence on the left side, and then come into the Child's Pose.

Sleeping Swan

Meridian pair: Liver and gallbladder

IN BALANCE: **Action, decisiveness**

Shadow emotion: Anger

There is nothing sleepy about this swan. Not as intense as the Dragon, but pretty darn close, the Sleeping Swan always brings a wry smile to the lips of those who are familiar with its challenging character. Because we hold so much emotion in our lower bodies, particularly in the pelvis, this area is loaded, and this pose promises great sensation from the onset. If you can honor what comes up, it also promises some of the greatest relief and release of "stories" and held tensions (read: you may need a few tissues).

Caution: This pose can put strain on your knees. You'll want to set your pose up with the utmost care to find the best position that will help you to completely avoid any issues. If you ever feel a sudden, sharp pain, stop immediately, pull back to safety, and reassess. Either find a position that feels better or opt for an alternative. You'll want a yoga block nearby.

1. From your hands and knees, slide your right knee forward to your right wrist and fan the lower leg open so your right shin is parallel with the front of the mat and the right foot is in front of the left hip. Of course, stay within the parameters of your comfort and ability and know that everyone's range is different, so honor wherever your body wants to go without pushing it past its limits. This means that perhaps your shin may not line up with the front of the mat; it may be at more of a forty-five-degree or lesser angle.
2. With your arms pressing strong and straight in front of you to create a kind of leveraging framework and steering mechanism for your pelvis and legs, extend the left leg behind you, making sure that your hips are squared and centered. It helps to tuck the toes of the back foot under to direct it more efficiently into the center position. Ensure that the front of your chest and your hips are squared to the front of the mat. Flex your right foot to protect the knee, and then reach back through your left thigh as you draw your left hip forward. Your toes should still be curled up and underneath you, getting a healthy stretch for this set-up moment, and then once you greet the pose, you will soften both feet, releasing them into the floor.
3. As you are trying to establish your optimal position, you may find that because of restriction in your right hip, the hip doesn't easily reach the floor and you are tilting off your axis, perhaps listing to the left. You may also be feeling some discomfort in the knee. If you are askew or need to relieve some discomfort, grab a blanket. Either roll it up or fold it in such a way that it is high enough to provide you with ample cushioning and sufficient extra height to level your hips. Place the blanket underneath your right buttock, under the sitting bone, to level the pelvis. Once you reach a sufficient height, you'll find that you feel more comfortable.

4. Once you've established what feels like a good starting point, one in which you feel no pain, only a healthy stretch in the outer right hip and perhaps in the front of the left hip and upper thigh (the hip flexor), you may feel as if you want to come out of the pose even before you've begun melting. If this is true, welcome! You've arrived at your perfect point of departure—no, not to exit, but to greet your Sleeping Swan. On a discomfort scale from one to ten, with ten being the most intense, you want to start at a place that is a clear seven or eight—you're uncomfortable, but not in pain.
5. Now either grab a yoga block and, placing it on its lowest side, lengthwise in front of your bent right knee, come down onto the block with your elbows, or if you are more flexible and don't feel an overly intense stretch in the outer right hip, come directly into Sleeping Swan by releasing your entire upper body to the floor and extending your arms long in front of you.
6. Exhale and cease all proactive muscular engagement. Allow your back leg and foot to soften, releasing the foot to come flat on the floor. Start to relax and drop down into your chosen variation for the pose. Close your eyes and start to connect to your breath inside your body. Breathe into the area that is speaking the loudest to you—in this case, likely your outer right hip—and observe the sensations.
7. Before you come out of the pose, note that coming out of it is as much of an art as getting into it. Using as little effort as possible, start to bring your torso back to an upright position, and slowly roll onto the outside of your right hip. Stretch your legs out in front of you and bounce them out. Come into the Child's Pose.
8. Repeat the steps on the opposite side, and remind yourself that each side is unique, with a different range of motion and different considerations. Be compassionate, patient, and gentle. If you feel your left side is tighter, then ease into the pose with care and delicacy. If, on the other hand, your right side was tighter and your left is more open, then you can establish the pose with more alacrity, increasing the an-

gle of the lower leg by bringing the left foot closer to the right wrist to start, and allowing yourself to go deeper from the onset.

Quarter Dog

Meridian pairs: Lung and large intestine, heart and small intestine

IN BALANCE: **Love, joy**

Shadow emotions: Depression, anger

One of my favorite yin poses and not one that's as frequently taught in most classes, the Quarter Dog is a powerful heart opener as well as an immediately effective antidote for digestive distress and breathing issues. Because it is both a forward-bending pose and an inversion, it encourages introspection and settles the spirit, as it gives our internal organs a much-needed break from the stress of gravity.

1. Start on your hands and knees, with your legs hip-width apart, and walk your hands about a foot in front of your shoulders, ensuring that your hips remain stacked over your knees so that they form a right angle. Keep your right arm extended forward and bend your left elbow, bringing it to rest on the floor. Place your left hand on top of your right elbow crease. Then lean your forehead on the left forearm or on the back of the wrist as a cushion. If it feels more comfortable, place your forehead directly onto your mat, next to your left elbow. Bring your upper torso to the floor so that your chest is elongated and your back forms a deep arc or a hammock shape. You'll look like a dog doing its favorite arching stretch.
2. Relaxing your feet, knees, and pelvis, concentrate on lengthening your upper back, chest, and arms against the floor and come into as

deep a stretch as you can, without straining or pushing. To experience some muscular contrast, lengthen the fingertips of the right hand, deepen the belly by drawing the navel up toward the spine, and actively lengthen the back down and out along the floor.

Modifications: If you have shoulder issues, you can place a folded blanket underneath your head to elevate the upper body and ease tension on the shoulder joint. If you have sensitive knees, you can place a blanket underneath them for more padding.

3. The next time you inhale, release all muscular effort. As you exhale next, allow your body to give over to the floor completely. Your right arm should still be extended, but soft. Allow your upper chest and belly to release fully. Let your back passively drape down toward the floor and close your eyes. Breathe into your upper back, chest, and shoulders, especially the places where you're feeling restriction or discomfort. As you exhale, release your chest even farther toward the floor and release any holding or bracing you may have been engaging in unconsciously.
4. On your next inhalation, ever so slowly and carefully come out of the pose. Start to walk your hands back toward your torso and press yourself back into the Child's Pose directly, to recharge.
5. Repeat the entire sequence on the opposite side, and then come into the Child's Pose.

Eye of the Needle

Meridian pair: Liver and gallbladder

IN BALANCE: Compassion, peace, love

Shadow emotions: Anger, frustration, stress

Whenever I want a gentle hip opener that both relieves a feeling of muscular congestion in the pelvis and lower back and allows me to take a rest at the same time, I turn to the Eye of the Needle. It always reminds me to breathe into my back, which is not something I am always doing consciously. It has the same benefits as the more challenging hip openers, but is more accessible and a great preparation for deep relaxation and sleep.

1. Lying on your back, with your feet flat on the floor, knees bent, cross the right ankle on top of your left knee so that your right knee opens out to the side and the left leg is completely relaxed. Now thread your right arm between your legs and bring your left hand around the outside of the left leg to meet it. Interlace your fingers around the back of the left thigh, or if you're more flexible on top of your shin, creating a hammock for your legs. Ideally, your right ankle is positioned on top of your left thigh in such a way that you feel a good stretch in the right hip, but no pain in the knee; either have the ankle bone lining up with the middle of your left thigh or simply let the outer edge of the right foot rest on your thigh.
2. To experience contrast in the pose before you begin, flex your right foot strongly as you press your shoulders actively down against the floor. Then relax the foot, just making sure that it maintains its position crossed over the left knee.
3. Allow your arms, legs, and feet to soften completely. Close your eyes and breathe into your right hip and any other areas that are calling to you. Feel your body getting heavier and starting to melt into the floor. Lengthen your spine and release any compensatory tension in your shoulders or neck as you settle into the pose, allowing your chest and belly to soften as you give over to gravity.
4. To exit the pose, with eyes closed, slowly unwind your legs and send them up to the ceiling. Then begin the Monkey Dance, in which you lie on your back, extend your legs straight up to the ceiling, and shake them. Start shaking them slowly by just allowing the flesh on your legs to move, and then work up to a more vigorous pace that is quite intense, like real cardiovascular activity. It will look as though you're

having a temper tantrum on your back! You can then add your arms, shaking them as well. Once you work your way up to a vigorous pace, maintain it and know that you are moving stagnant prana out of your body and inviting new energy in. After a few rounds of breath, stop shaking, hug your knees into your chest, and breathe that buzz of new energy, the vibrating prana you surely feel into your brain, your heart, and your cells. Let it nourish and soothe your soul. Then with a substantial open-mouthed exhale, like a lion's roar, let it all go!

5. Repeat the steps on the opposite side. Then come into the Child's Pose.

Sphinx and Seal

Meridian pairs: Lungs and large intestine, heart and small intestine

IN BALANCE: **Love, joy**

Shadow emotions: Depression, anger

Because of the amount of time we spend hunching over computers and sitting in our cars, we need back-bending and extension of the spine more than ever. The Sphinx and the Seal (the more intense variation of Sphinx) restore the curve in our lower backs and invite us to send our healing energy in to reinvigorate all the tissues and nerves that connect to the spinal column. A flexible spine is a flexible mind, and although these poses may elicit cranky complaints from your back, they will ultimately inspire gratitude and appreciation.

1. Lying on your stomach, prop yourself up on your elbows and forearms, keeping them shoulder-width apart. Your palms can come down on the floor with your fingers spread wide apart, slightly in front of your shoulders. Extend your legs long behind you, hip-width

apart. Level your gaze so that you are looking straight ahead. Breathe into your chest and belly and feel your lower back releasing into the floor. Become a regal Egyptian sphinx—tall, serene, and proud.

2. To experience muscular contrast before we begin, squeeze your buttocks, point your toes, and draw your navel strongly toward your spine; draw your shoulders actively down and back away from your ears. Breathe deeply. Then, as you exhale, relax your feet, butt, shoulders, and belly completely.
3. If you would prefer to try something different with your arms and hands, but still remain upright on your elbows, you can draw your forearms closer together, bringing your palms to touch in Prayer Position in front of you so that the pinky fingers lie parallel against the floor.
4. If the Sphinx is an easy position for you to come into, you may want more of a challenge, in which case you can proceed to the Seal (but know that if you've been overzealous in your choice, you can return to the Sphinx at any time.) The Seal targets the kidney and urinary bladder meridians as well as the lungs and large intestine and heart and small intestine—a bonus. Move your arms slightly farther apart and straighten your arms, pushing the floor away with palms flat on the floor and slightly externally rotated, so that you feel as though you *are* a seal, supporting yourself on your strong flippers. Extend the spine taller toward the ceiling, deepening the curve of the lower back, and coming into a greater extension of the spine.

   Modification: If you feel lower-back tenderness in the Sphinx or Seal, you can place a folded or rolled blanket underneath your hips to create space in the lower back, which should provide instant relief.
5. Start to connect to the breath and see where it lives inside your body. Breathe into your head, neck, and shoulders and try to let go of any bracing up and away from the pose. Allow yourself to drop down and give in to gravity. If you've suffered from lower-back pain in the past or are currently dealing with issues there, you'll naturally feel ret-

icent about moving into this back bend. Trust yourself to know that if it's not okay right now, you'll press back into the Child's Pose and honor what your body is telling you. For now, though, breathe and let yourself go into what you are anticipating as the eye of the storm, and you'll learn that what you were protecting yourself from wasn't as bad as you imagined it would be. As you exhale, let go.

6. To exit the pose, with eyes closed, gently push back into the Child's Pose to stretch your lower back, with your arms extended forward on the floor in front of you or draped softly as your sides—your choice. Breathe deeply, relax, and relish the time you spend in your home position.

Spinal Twist

Meridian pairs: Spleen and stomach, kidney and urinary bladder

IN BALANCE: Contentment, courage

Shadow emotions: Anxiety, fear

The Spinal Twist can make us feel especially vulnerable, because the spine holds a lot of stagnant prana from our sedentary habits. It's natural to feel restricted or afraid when you first move more deeply into a twist, wringing out those feelings. The antidote to this anxiety is to remind yourself that you are fully supported by your body and the floor and trust that you can surrender to the sensations that are coming up. In addition to the two meridian pairs highlighted above, the Spinal Twist also targets the lung, heart, and intestine meridians by virtue of the upper-body opening it produces.

1. Lying on your back, draw your knees into your chest and give them a hug. Breathe deeply into the entire length of your spine. Extend

your arms out to the sides of the body in line with your shoulders, pressing your palms into the floor. Using your abdominals to control the movement and keeping your knees bent and stacked while you keep your upper body anchored to the floor, slowly allow your legs to drop over to the right side of your body and bring them to rest against the floor.

2. Rather than keeping your left arm extended directly out in line with your shoulder, raise the arm higher so that it forms a half V on the floor alongside your head. Turn your head to gaze toward your left arm or down toward your knees on the right side of your body, whichever position feels better. Remember that you can shift and change your head position if you wish, after you've started to melt in the pose.
3. If you'd like to open and direct prana into your middle and lower back, keep your knees tucked higher in toward your upper chest. If, on the other hand, you feel you need more opening and energy directed into your hips and sacrum, allow your legs to drop down beneath your hips or lower. You can keep the knees stacked, or if you are looking for a deeper twist and greater challenge, you can cross your left leg over your right and then drop the legs over to the right, placing your right hand on top of the legs to anchor them.
4. Once in your chosen starting position, experience a contrast before you start to melt. Stretch your left arm up away from your body and gently press your right hand on top of your knees and flex your feet strongly as you draw your navel into your spine. Inhale deeply and, as you exhale, let your body relax completely.
5. Slowly and mindfully come out of the pose. Move with delicacy as you unwind from the Spinal Twist, bringing both knees back to center and hugging them in toward your body, where you'll take several breaths to realign and center yourself. Then extend the legs straight up to the ceiling, and do a short Monkey Dance. After several minutes shaking your limbs, stop, draw your knees into your chest, close your eyes, and breathe into your brain the buzzy energy

you will surely feel. You'll feel a quiet surge of renewal with this one simple sequence.

6. Repeat the steps on the opposite side. When you're done, come into the Child's Pose.

Corpse Pose (Savasana)

Meridian pairs: All

IN BALANCE: **Peace, harmony**

Shadow emotion: Restlessness

Now it's time to meet the most important pose of the entire practice, the Corpse Pose, *savasana* (*sava* means "corpse" in Sanskrit), a pose that signifies ultimate stillness and surrender. In every practice I do, it's the moment I imagine what it will be like when I one day abandon myself to infinite surrender—when I let my life go. Although simple in appearance, *savasana* embodies the complex yogic teachings of surrender, nonattachment, and self-awareness more than any of the other yin poses. This is your golden opportunity to practice the "letting go" that is essential to receiving all the healing benefits from each and every pose we have done in the practice.

1. Lying on your back, bend your knees toward your chest and extend your arms down by your sides at a forty-five-degree angle away from your body, palms up. Inhale into your chest and belly, and feel the back of your body resting on the floor. Notice any excess tension. Breathe into your entire body and let it sink deeper into the floor as you exhale. Inhale and lift your hips slightly. As you exhale, start to lower your hips to the floor, incrementally lengthening your back and buttocks down toward your heels as you go, so that you create more space between your vertebrae as your back descends, rolling bone by

bone, to the floor. This promotes the distribution of prana that you've cultivated during your practice, sending it into your organs, chakras, and every other part of your body through the meridian channels. After your back settles into the floor, extend your legs along the floor one at a time, separating them slightly wider than hip-width apart.

Variation: If you feel that you would like extra grounding, place two or three blankets folded in half over your upper thighs and torso. With this, you'll instantly feel more secure and rooted to the earth.

Modification: If you feel lower-back tenderness when you extend your legs straight down on the floor, place a bolster underneath your knees for extra support.

2. After establishing your pose and before you officially begin, take a moment to experience contrast in the pose. As you inhale, squeeze your buttocks firmly and flex every muscle in your body, fully straightening your legs, pointing your toes, straightening your arms, and making fists with your hands, raising your arms slightly off the floor and contracting the muscles of your face as if you've just sucked on a lemon. Hold your breath as you exert this intense, full-body, muscular effort, and then, with eyes open wide and an opened-mouth exhalation, make a sound like a lion's roar or a really deep sigh, as the breath exits your body. Let your limbs fall gently against the floor, releasing your buttocks, belly, chest, head, and feet. Let the floor support you. Breathe and let go.
3. Close your eyes. Do a body scan from the crown of your head all the way down to the tips of your toes. Seek out any areas of held tension that may remain from your practice. Breathe into them and then let them go, giving your full body weight over to the floor. If thoughts come up, notice them, breathe into them, and then allow them to pass like clouds in the sky on a sunny day, returning to focus on your breath as it flows through your body and brings you deeper and deeper into relaxation.
4. Place your attention on the subtle sensation of your body relaxing and sinking into the floor. Let the earth receive you. Let your shoulders

and neck soften and open. Allow your thighs, hips, pelvis, and lower back to release. Bring your attention to your legs. Release the inner thighs away from each other and let your outer thighs drop toward the floor. Allow your legs to sink into the ground as if your thighs had heavy weights on them. Move your attention up to your pelvis and imagine your hip bones moving away from each other, allowing your pelvis and organs to release any last remnants of tension.

5. Release any remaining hold in your stomach or diaphragm, and now just allow your breath to breathe you. Let the backs of your arms sink into the floor and the muscles of your neck and shoulders relax, as you allow any last thoughts to spill out of your mind and into the earth below. As your upper body melts into the floor, soften your jaw and temples. Imagine that your brain recedes slightly away from your forehead and nestles inside the back of your skull. Feel your eyes grow heavier and softer underneath the lids, sinking into soothing, velvety darkness. This perfect quiet and stillness is where deepest healing can happen. Here you'll honor, open, and energize your body simply by letting go. Let your heart area softly blossom, opening like the beautiful flower it is, and be soft, receptive, and free. Now let go of time, of thought, of worry. Let go of your life. Breathe and surrender to the gift of this moment and these precious breaths of deepest conscious relaxation. Say yes and receive all the healing benefits of your practice.
6. After five to fifteen minutes—when you feel ready—slowly start to deepen your breath. Gently come back to an awakened, elevated, conscious awareness. Send your breath into your fingers and toes and start to bring quiet movement back into your body. Join your hands over your chest, interlacing your fingertips, and then invert your wrists and palms, bringing your arms up straight overhead to the wall behind you, as you would in a deep morning stretch. Alternately flex and point your feet. Then rotate your feet to open your ankles.
7. Bring your knees to your chest. Sweep your arms around your body and encircle your knees, hugging yourself. From this shape, depend-

ing upon what kind of energy you want to cultivate now, roll over either onto your right for greater energy (yang) or left side to manifest more calm (yin). Bend your upper arm and tuck it underneath your head like a pillow. Rest here on your side and breathe in the deep comfort and nourishment this side-lying Child's Pose offers you. Inhale this nutritive, loving energy into your heart and then exhale, letting go of anything you no longer need.

8. With as little effort as possible, keeping your eyes closed and using your hands to press up, come into a cross-legged position with your palms resting on your knees and your spine tall like a graceful oak tree. Meditate for a few breaths and bathe in the waters of deep, healing prana that you've cultivated with your practice. Feel bounteous new subtle energy flowing and rising gently inside you like the ocean's tides. Feel the magnitude of gratitude pulsing in your heart and soul—gratitude to the universe, gratitude for your body, for this chance to go deep, open, and energize. Say thank you for this new space, for this relief, this hope, and for all the exciting possibilities that await you: "Thank you for this new life flowing through me!"

Congratulations! You've gone deep, opened, and energized. You've surrendered and welcomed some of the deepest, nourishing healing energy into your being. These tools—your yin poses—for tending to your treasured life force will always be available to you when you make the choice to move into stillness, reminding yourself of your own heartbeat, the sound of the world that lies beneath the surface and keeps you alive. Your body thanks you. It is already rewarding your effortless efforts with new radiance that rises up from the depths, like the sun, for all to see, a new energized calm that shines out from your heart, yours anytime you call upon it.

9

the power of love: inner smile and cosmic healing sounds

I'll never forget the moment Master Chia started his lecture at his Asheville workshop in 2007.

"What's the main focus of life in the West?" he asked. "It's work. People are always being told to 'focus their minds on their jobs, on their performance.' Why not shift perspective? What would happen if we were all to turn that focus inside and actually concentrate on sending that energy into our bodies first? We're so concerned with building our actual bank accounts that we deplete our body's 'health' bank account. Then what happens? We're forced to spend the money we have worked so hard to earn to restore our health." He went on to say that we suffer from the ravaging effects of stress—indigestion, heart disease, back pain, to name just a few examples of inner imbalance—that all result because we move too fast and our focus is everywhere instead of where it should be: inside first.

He continued, "If you were a child with disharmony in the household, with your parents fighting, would you want to stay or would you want to run away and seek more peaceful pastures?" In Eastern philosophies, the "spirit" in your body is like the child. When you don't look after your inner household and there is disharmony, when you are at odds with yourself, scattering your focus, spreading yourself too thin, the spirit likes to wander; the child runs away to seek a calmer, more peaceful place to live and takes the energy with her.

"How do we get the spirit to stay with us and grow inner virtue?" he asked. "How do we 'grow the love' we can cultivate for ourselves? By quieting and focusing our minds on the place where love begins—in our hearts. We need to acknowledge our negative emotions, no matter how unpleasant, and then make the decision to 'delete' them, just like on a computer."

Very matter-of-factly, he said we needed to take that energy, which has been left to its own devices, and brazenly mount a "takeover." Master Chia's lectures were consistently peppered with military allusions because so much of qigong history is centered around preparing soldiers for battle; for example, the liver is said to be the "general of the army." He said that we needed to take control again, reroute the energy, transform it and distribute it to all our organs, so that they would work like a team, a united front to ward off disease and increase our immunity. "You have to organize and train your army!" he exclaimed. We had to engage in practices that fortified our immune defense, and in order to do that, we had to become intimately acquainted with our bodies, demonstrate reverence for them, and show them love. Only then could we enliven our spirits and tempt them back into their headquarters after taking our power back and establishing balance in the household.

As he spoke, everything fell into place for me. We were learning the Inner Smile, a Taoist inner-alchemy practice that focuses gratitude and joy on the internal organs to resolve the physical and mental tensions that can lead to illness. For me, it was the logical progression after yin yoga, which had opened and energized my energy pathways and introduced me to my organs and their emotional resonances. Now we were about to learn unequivocally that they had feelings and needed our love and attention. It all made sense; we have more than thirty-seven trillion cells in our body, and they all naturally seek balance. Possessing incalculable innate intelligence, these cells develop a positive imprint when they receive positive energy along with the healing power of specific sound currents. This instantly boosts the life of each cell, and they all join forces as a united front to ward off disease.

Master Chia told us that our focus naturally brings energy to the place our mind is directed toward. Energy follows intention. When you don't take the time to focus and generate your own inner chi, when you don't replenish the well, when you continually give it away, you are giving your power away. You keep using the energy you have "on reserve" inside, and then it runs out, and that stress makes it run out faster.

The solution was quite simple, he explained: clear out the negative emotions inside your actual organs and make them into a team that works for you. To manage stress, slow down, turn inward, and create your own calm. Focus your mind and look inward, to the heart, to the liver, the spleen, the lungs. "Sing to them their favorite song, which I will teach you, and they will be inspired to thrive within you. When they come together, they will be 'good soldiers,'" he said, "strengthening your inner resolve and serving you faithfully" as formidable opponents to life's vicissitudes.

He sat there with his eyes closed, and his hands, palm over palm, facing his own body, floating directly above his heart, "Delete anger, jealousy, impatience . . . breathe, let it go." Raising his palms to the sky, he inhaled deeply and then projected the sound for the heart, "*Hawwwwww,*" and his hands returned to the space just over his heart. "Believe that your mind has the power to bring love to your heart, radiate the joy, the love, the happiness into your heart and then take that growing love and now bring it into your liver," and his hands went down over his liver, the gallbladder, the small intestine, the spleen.

I followed his every movement, taking a peaceful, but deeply cathartic tour through my own body. With each sound I made according to the organ it was meant for, I intuitively felt my organs smiling back at me, making the decision to rally, to unite, because I was taking the time to focus my energy on each one, telling my kidneys, my liver, my heart that I appreciated their hard work and that I was working with them now, keenly aware of their existence. I was even learning new songs to sing to them and smiling at them the way I would smile at someone I liked. It paid off, and faster than I could have imagined. At the end of that weekend in North Carolina, I had truly learned the power of love, and my back pain was gone for good.

Even all those years ago in North Carolina when, as a group, we did the Inner Smile and Cosmic Healing Sounds together, it was fundamentally life-altering for me. Discovering that I had the ability to visit the inside of my own body and delve into to its inner workings, that I could actually smile to my organs and effect such significant change, was beyond empowering. And with Master Chia in person! I won't even try to pretend that I was calm about it! It was thrilling. I felt as though I was entering the inner sanctum of secrets and well on my way to starring in my own Indie version of *House of Flying Daggers*.

Although I had read about it for years, when Master Chia taught it in the flesh, it was utterly new. Watching him as he did the practice, witnessing such obvious satisfaction and pleasure on his face when he smiled to his heart and then released "evil wind" as a result—coupled with the notion that he wasn't just okay with doing such a thing in public, but that he was proud of it—was beyond liberating. It elicited such abundant nervous laughter from the entire group that I was excited the way a child would be if a grown-up had misbehaved and sung about it—if he had done something that was considered inappropriate and completely out of character, and oh was it a hit!

Such buoyant laughter, such fulfillment—we all felt it. We were not only being given permission to feel free about our bodily functions (collectively rebuking a long history of repressive habits that had been inculcated by society); we were being told in no uncertain terms that it was an accomplishment, that when we released "evil wind," we were removing stagnation and gathering chi! And the joy we all felt was so much more than just the smile we were giving to our organs; it was the entire in-the-round experience of watching our teacher practice and derive the benefits right before our eyes.

I marveled at Master Chia's childlike spirit, how heartily and unselfconsciously he laughed, how effortlessly he felled a tribe of men like trees in the forest with his otherworldly, centered, rooted strength. But nothing was as compelling as the radiance that filled the space around him when he laughed and practiced self-love. When I watched him perform his first healing sound, it was one of those slow-motion moments of truth when everything crystallizes in your brain and tectonic plates shift inside. I knew in that moment that I was witnessing in real time what the ancients knew. Their secrets were being revealed and made manifest before my very eyes. His act of smiling to his heart, merging with source energy, and harnessing universal chi (that clearly made him capable of superhuman feats) was a thing of such naturalness, power, and beauty.

It may sound funny to you that this little-known, esoteric practice left me dumbstruck, but it did. I was awestruck. I thought it was genius. I knew it was. It all made sense. I understood everything in that moment, that he and his masters before him were really on to something, and not just on to something, but on to *it,* the secret to living optimally. In that moment, I thought to myself, *There is a reason those secrets were guarded as long and as closely as they were, because the ancients figured out through these practices how to live their best lives and go beyond.*

All the practices they devoted themselves to helped them recapture the ease and flexibility of youth, which was made obvious just observing Mantak Chia for a few minutes. For them, however, although the physical aspects were hugely significant and imperative for reaching higher levels of evolution, on their scale these were the fringe benefits, for their eyes were on a higher prize. Keeping the body well-tuned and loved was how they would attain their ultimate goal of higher incarnations in future lives, and along the way they were able to boast glowing good health and extraordinary longevity.

At the core of the ancients' secret, in the eye of the tornado, the spiral (which you will soon learn how to do in the practice), there is total calm, and therein lies the key. All the practices were meant to help them recapture the spirit of youth. And they did this by nurturing their heart-mind and removing themselves as much as possible from the superfluous emotional machinations of life. They created the perfect conditions, perfect soil where flowers could blossom in the body and the mind, constituting the perfect container for the soul that would someday travel. How they accomplished this was by generating something called "inner virtue," and they achieved this not only through the physical practice we learned in Awaken and Play, but with the Inner Smile and Cosmic Healing Sounds.

They cleared their spiritual decks to make the way for purest energy cultivation. The mind is both our greatest ally and our greatest enemy. They figured out that if they could love and nurture the body, the mind would be at its best and primed to be "under their command," in the military jargon Master Chia uses frequently in his teachings. In order to achieve balance in the body and activate the mind for higher practice and then higher travel, one had to take care of business on earth first. I came to the conclusion that it all boiled down to one simple formula: gratitude, forgiveness, and love. This is what woke the child within, and with it the greatest joy and energy.

For me, as a dancer who had lived her life focusing entirely on what the body could do and how it could perform, this was a paradigm shift. The idea that a grown man was dedicating time to smiling and whispering sweet nothings to his organs—a man I esteemed so highly—was compelling. During those formative moments when I was watching him, in the montage reel that started playing in my mind, there was an immediate and dramatic refocus from macro to micro in an instant, and oh, so poignant an instant. The focus shifted from the scene in which I was only concerned with the externals, an unrelenting athletic coach tapping my foot on the ground and demanding that my body machine produce more, that it fly across the stage higher and higher and turn faster and faster, to a scene in which I as my present self was suddenly brought to my knees by being invited into the inner sanctum that was responsible for it all, into the flesh and beating-heart blood of it all, to bow my head in gratitude and acknowledgment and actually engage in a practice in which I thanked the body for everything it did.

And why was it so poignant? Maybe you can guess. It seemed like something that was long overdue. And though I didn't cry during the actual practice, that first night of the conference on a walk around the campus right after dinner, as I watched the sunset and thought of the healing rosy glow Master Chia taught us to use for cleansing the heart, I started to cry, and then sob, and then wail, right there with the mountains and evening songbirds as my witnesses. I cried for my sweet body and all the years I had taken it for granted.

The Inner Smile practice, just like the sequences in Awaken and Play, spoke to me, because I knew in my heart that it was the way that I would return to the beautiful, pure, joyful child I was before life happened. It was one of the greatest surprises of my life to be introduced to my body in a way that had nothing to do with how it performed on stage or for others. It was a simple, joyful loving acknowledgment of who I was inside and all that there was inside to love, just as I was, without any attachment to the outside world or who I was supposed to be to impress others, without trying to be someone other than who I truly, authentically was. Suddenly, there was no room for fear, fear of shining too brightly, fear of being too strong, fear of getting punished just for being happy. Who would have guessed that this extraordinary collection of practices would lead me to a place of such healing that I would rewrite my original, internal script, befriend myself in such a profound way that I would reparent myself, and love myself in a way I never dreamed possible, leading me to make sense of my place in the world, finally.

It is my guess that when you taste this Power of Love practice and try the Inner Smile, you will like it, perhaps even love it, and then start to laugh or cry or maybe even sob the way I did. And now that you've practiced yin yoga and are familiar with the idea of releasing held emotions, you won't think me a sadist if I tell you that I hope you do cry. I hope that you give yourself that gift of true liberty and freedom and that afterwards you allow yourself to celebrate the release, acknowledging the new flow, the very palpable flow of energy you will feel gently circulating inside your own body. It is your body's way of saying thank you, nodding and smiling itself, in deepest appreciation.

Waking Energy Pearls of Wisdom

When I think back to the 2007 workshop with Mantak Chia and the many extraordinary things I learned from him, I can say unreservedly that, aside from the bounty of the actual practices, these three pearls were among the most precious gifts he gave me: "Count your blessings," "Befriend your enemies," and "Train your army, because God doesn't care about germs." They not only sum up the entire Power of Love practice, but have become formative guiding lights in my life, as I continue to live my way into the answers, using these wise directives as my very own expansive lessons. These pearls, along with one of my other favorites of Master Chia's, "If you can't listen to your own body, how will you ever be able to listen to someone else?" offer an important perspective in the Waking Energy Way.

Inner Smile and Cosmic Healing Sounds

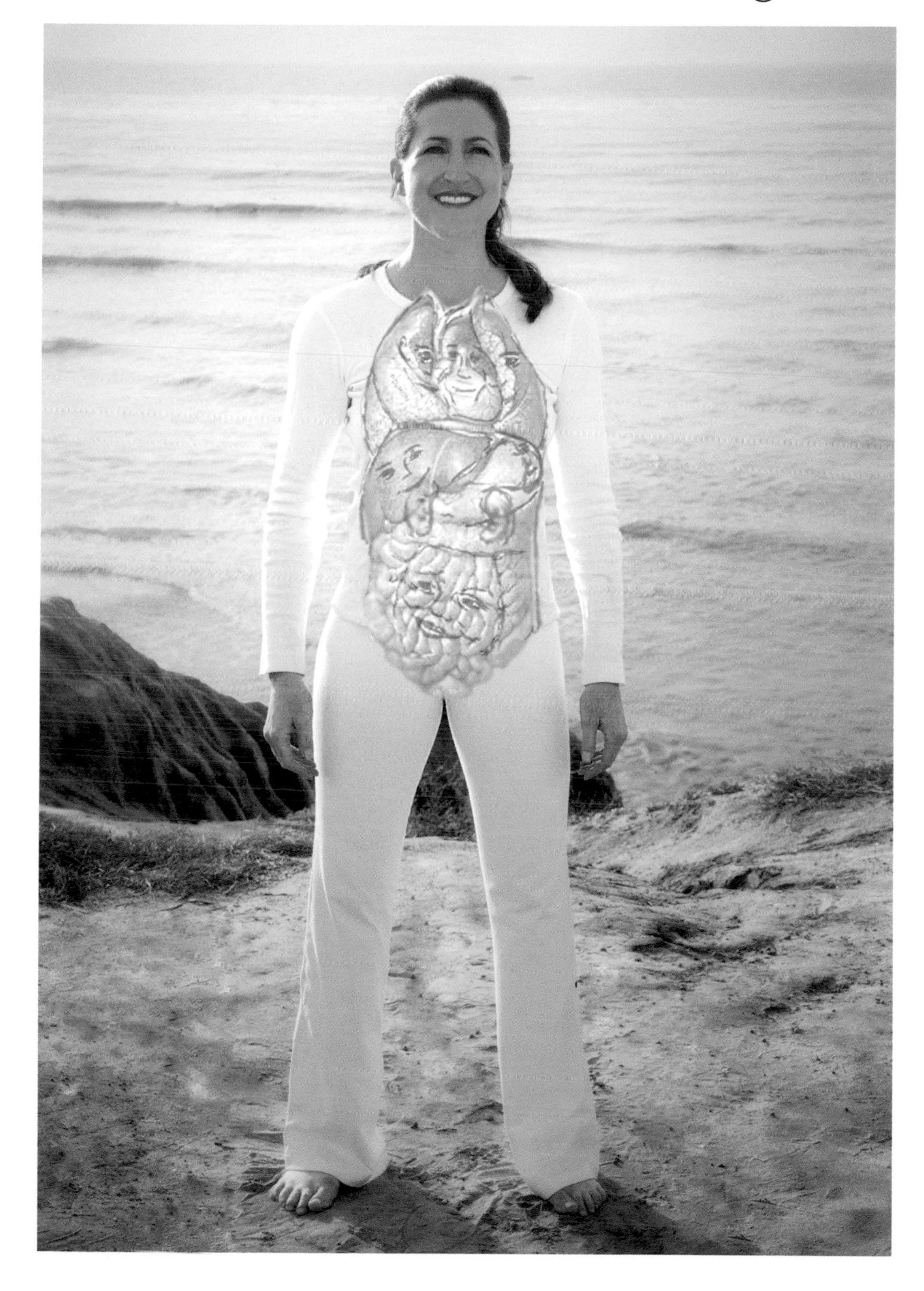

Cosmic Healing Sound for the Lungs

Cosmic Healing Sound for the Kidneys

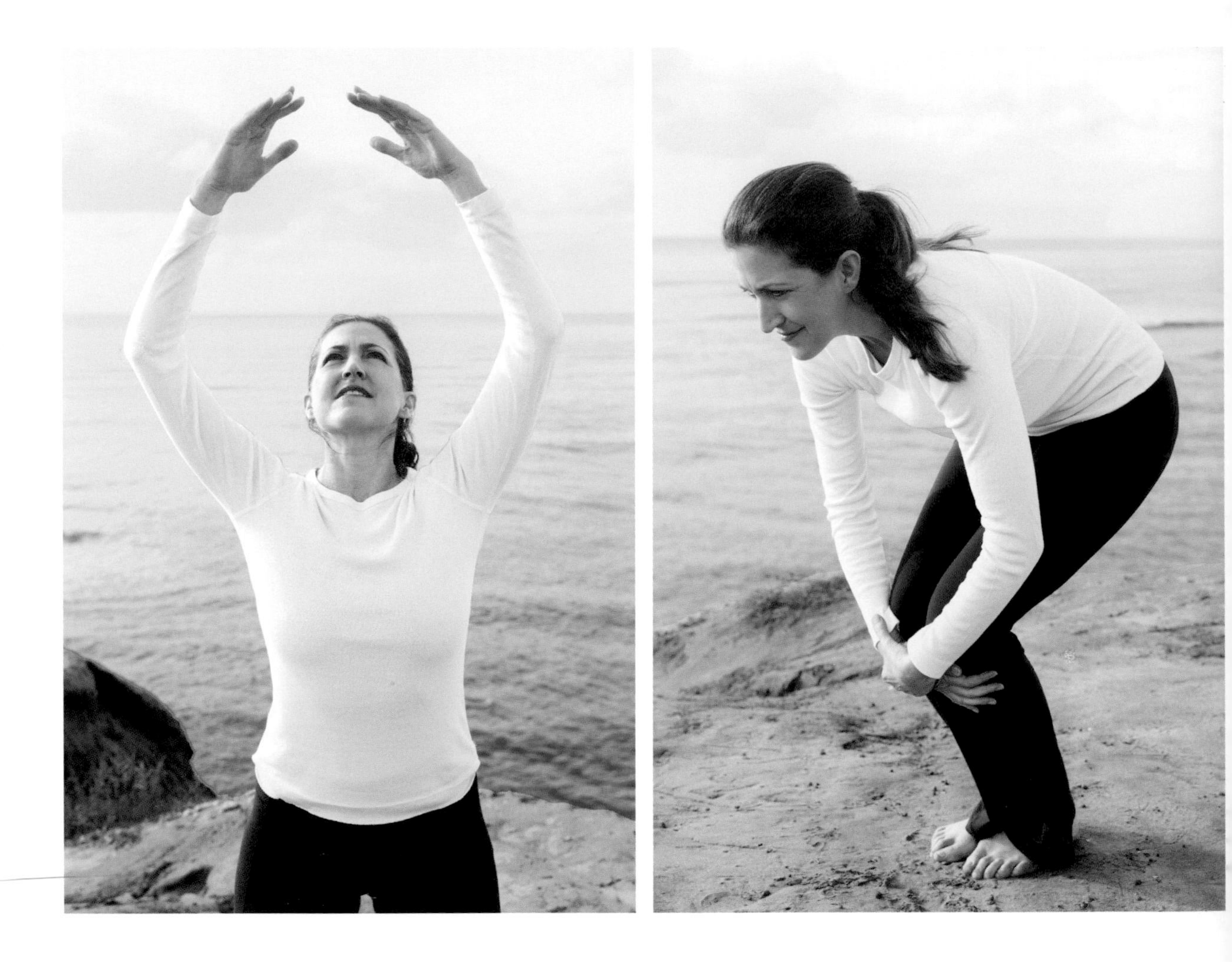

Cosmic Healing Sound for the Liver

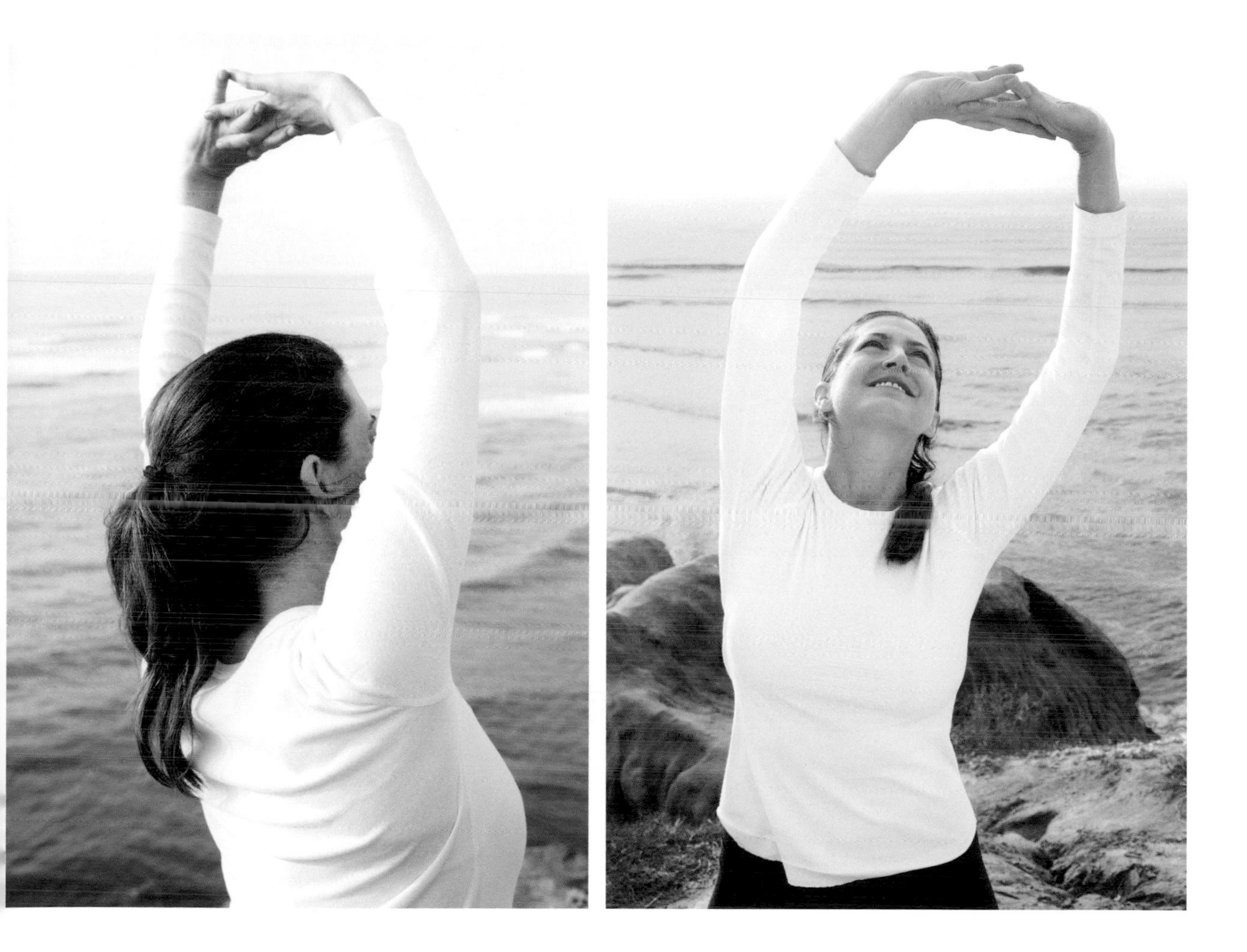

Cosmic Healing Sound for the Heart | *Cosmic Healing Sound for the Spleen*

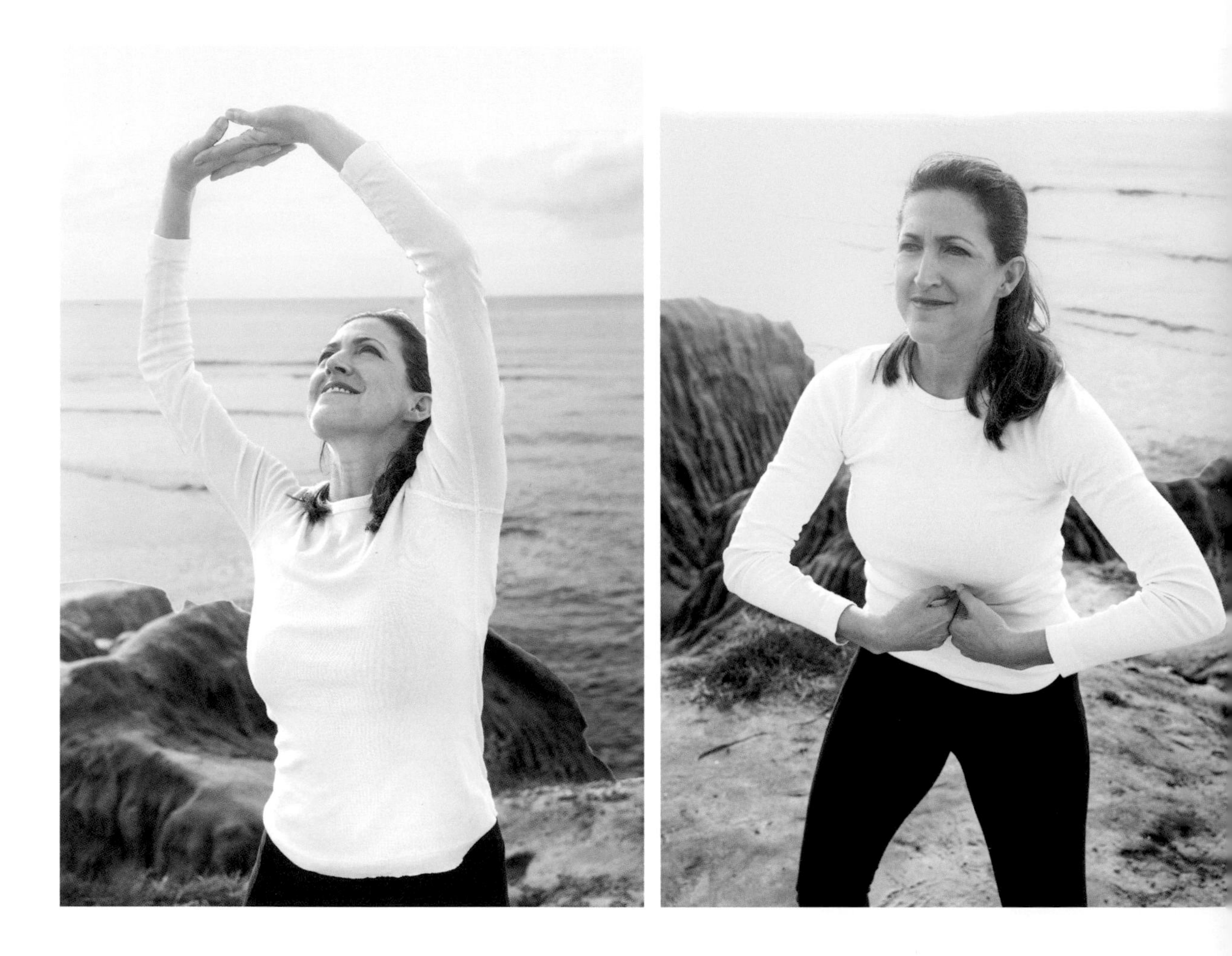

Cosmic Healing Sound for the Triple Warmer

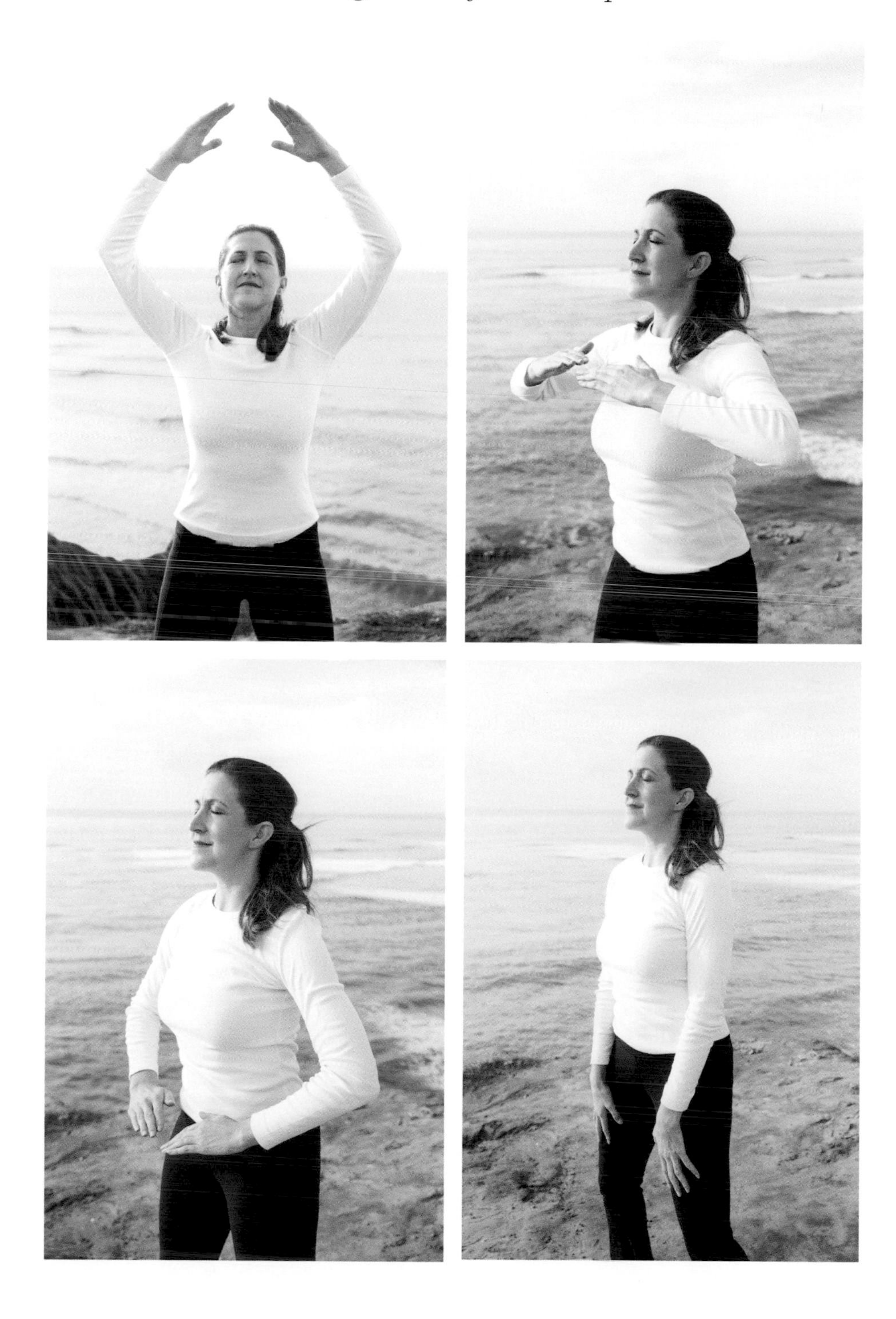

Meditation

Be a Tree

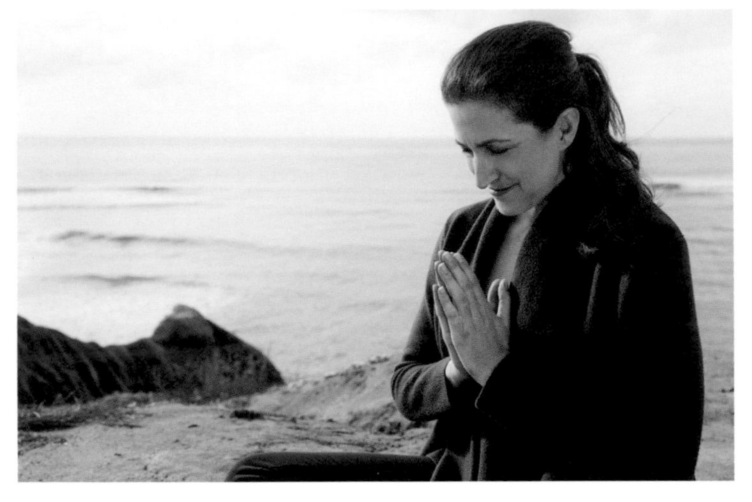

Surrender and Receive

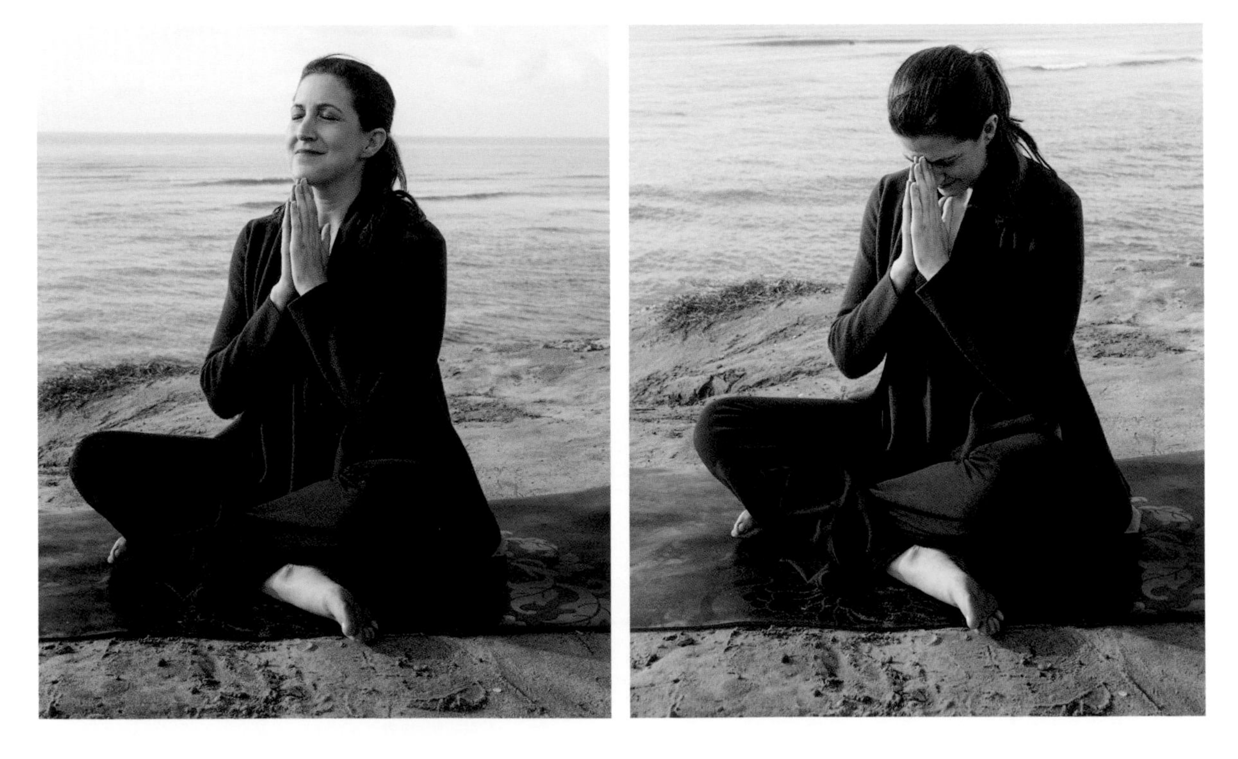

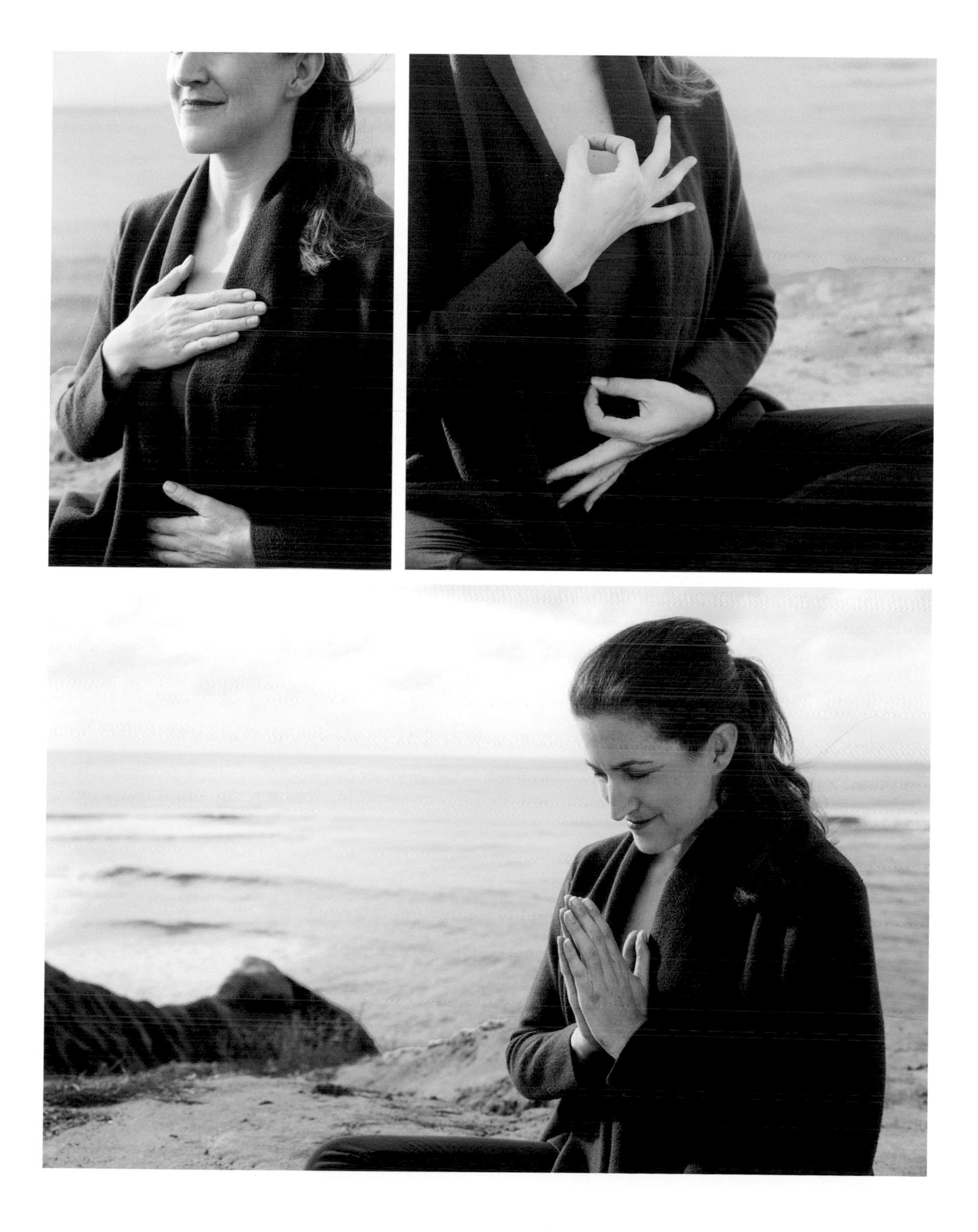

Blossoming Lotus

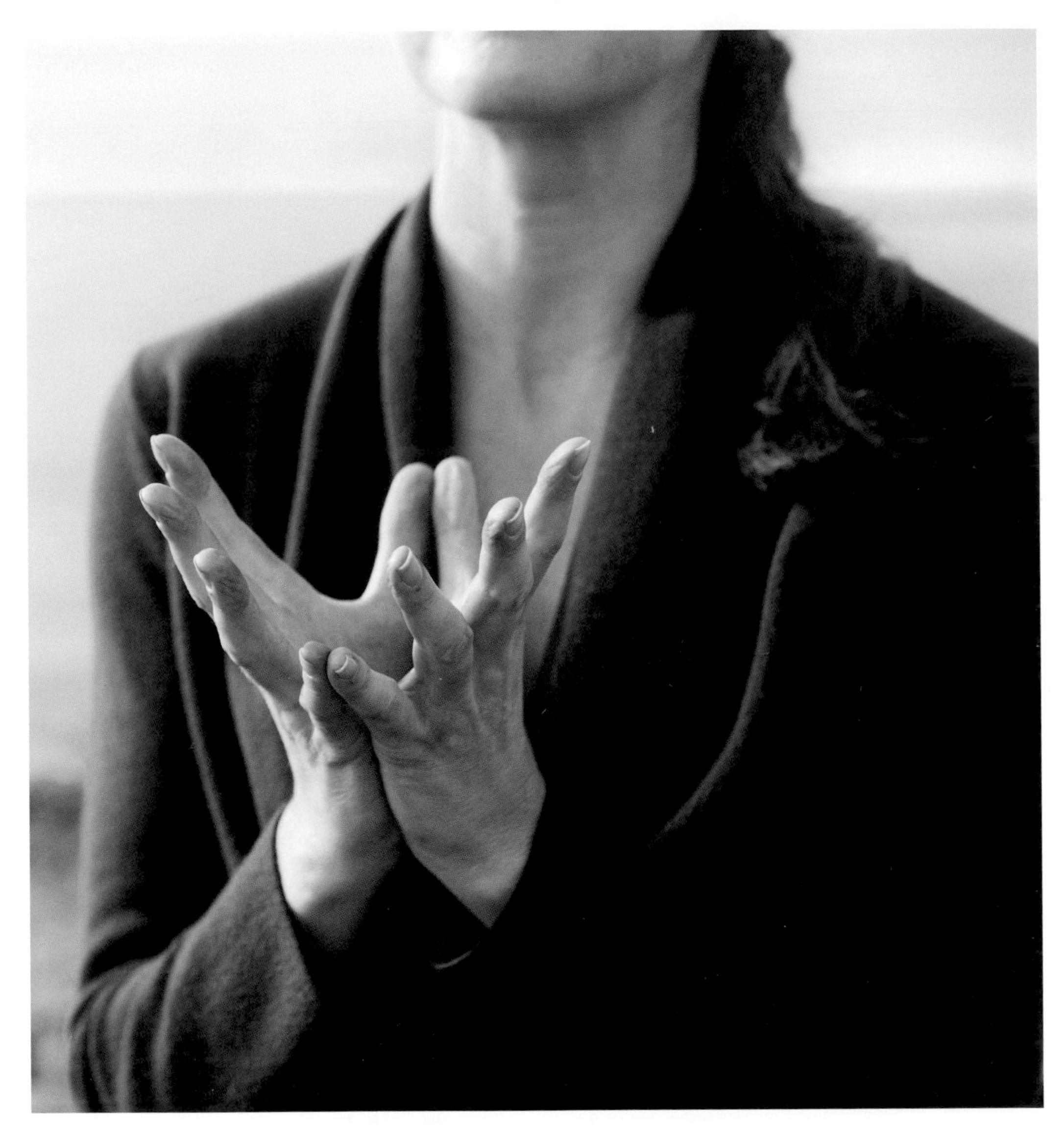

Count Your Blessings

The act of waking energy inside your own body, the Waking Energy Way, begins and ends with gratitude. There is no more effective gratitude or forgiveness exercise than the ritual of the Inner Smile. The Inner Smile shows you that the energy of love begins with you, right there, inside you. With the Power of Love practice, you come to know firsthand what love really feels like, because you are generating it within your own being first, for yourself, born out of the acknowledgment of who you are and all the gifts you have right there inside you.

Now that you have taken a tour of your inner topography with the yin yoga practice, *gone deep, opened,* and *energized,* and are more familiar with your organs and their associated emotions, we will actively experience what it means to "smile" at them and generate a deep appreciation for them and their role in our lives. Our organs are blessings, and once we start acknowledging them, it's easy to then experience the benefits of all that flows from them. When you feel grateful, when you take stock of the bounty in your life, you want for nothing.

The act of feeling gratitude activates the relaxation response in your central nervous system the same way a smile does, making every system in your body happier and better able to perform. When you acknowledge the gifts you possess and learn to love yourself first, you actually generate an abundance of love to give to your own organs, which are responsible for keeping you alive, and then you have more energy to give to others; this is how you do your small part to help to heal the world.

Befriend Your Enemies

After gratitude, the most powerful "delete" key to rid ourselves of accumulated emotional stress that we possess is forgiveness. Forgive, forget, and let go. Certainly, retaining the lessons of our suffering is valuable, but when we don't forget and hold on to anger, we deplete ourselves of vital life-force energy. Our current moment, with its digital devices and excessive multitasking, require more life force than ever before. When we are overexposed to emotional stress, a deleterious chain of stress responses is set in motion and our flight-or-flight response is triggered, which amps up the stress and creates excess inflammation in the body. And the antidote? In the face of such complexity, it is the simplest things that bring us back and restore peace in our inner kingdom: a smile and a "delete" key. It is only through self-directed loving-kindness that we can correct the internal imbalance and cultivate the wisdom and the strength to simplify our lives and redirect our energy to what really matters—befriending our enemies.

When you hold on to anger, who are you really hurting? Who actually suffers? In Buddha's words, "Holding on to anger is like drinking poison and expecting the other person to die." The person who suffers is you. And it doesn't do good things for your mental state, your body, or your immune system. When they talk about stress being the silent killer, they aren't kidding. Hating or resenting someone is the quickest way to challenge your immune system unnecessarily. Holding on to anger and resentment requires prodigious stores of energy. When you flip the switch to gratitude, anger doesn't have the room to squeeze in, to assert itself, to do its dirty work and wreak havoc on your psyche and then on your body. More often than not, this means looking inside, for the enemies are not always other people, but are there within our own psyche.

Gratitude erases anger, almost instantly. It's miraculous, actually. Try it right now. Feel grateful for just one thing in your life, and feel the instant and palpable change, the buoyancy that making that decision produces, the truly incredible lightness of being.

After the yin practice, where we have investigated and explored anger and shadow-side emotions and viscerally experienced where they take up residence in our fascia, now we're going further, pushing "delete," and taking a new neural pathway. Having lightened the load and exercised our neuroplasticity, we will come to "know our enemies all" and develop powerful inner defenses to protect ourselves from each and every one, making more energy available for productive purposes. And it all begins with your own consciousness and love.

Train Your Army

We mentioned counting your blessings and befriending your enemies; if you can do both, you are already way ahead of the game. Immune defense, good health, and energy actually start with you and how you manage your emotions. Like an astute general on the battlefield of life, picking and choosing your skirmishes with the greatest discernment translates into how well you love yourself and conserve your energy. The attention you devote to and the gratitude you feel for your body, what it holds, and how it hums and rattles and rolls for you determines the energy you have available to manifest positivity and abundance in your life. Taking the time to appreciate, enjoy, revere, and preserve the natural world you depend upon is the finest place to start. With this formula alone, you have awakened a great deal of energy already, and you have started to truly care for the temple.

You have also started to nurture and garner a powerful army. You would think that, with all this talk of love, nature, and the Garden of Eden that we create ourselves, there is no room for anything martial or defense-related. But here's where you're wrong. In order to really get to know some of the ancient philosophy that informs this book, you must understand that in life, to establish true balance and harmony, we must embrace the dark as well as the light. We must honor and cultivate our instincts, knowing intuitively when it is time to yield and when it is time to rally. Having strong immune defense, training your inner army, is anything but dark. It is necessary.

Because so much of qigong and related practices started as a form of martial training for soldiers going into battle, that same ideology and philosophy permeates the teachings. In every one of Mantak Chia's lectures, you will hear him talking about your meeting with the commanders and generals of your army and training the troops; with all due respect to religion, it is not God who will protect you from rogue viruses, but your own relationship with your body and your own immune defense, when the ideal environment is created for it to flourish and do its job. The Waking Energy Way wants us to be empowered, to live expansively, and asks us to take responsibility, honor ourselves, our vessels, take our health into our own hands, and live our strength.

It is your responsibility to take your own health into your hands, which is why it's so important to first and foremost know yourself, from the inside out, count your blessings, and befriend your enemies, so that you keep your army in tip-top shape. If you don't believe me now, you will soon experience it for yourself. The greatest defenses against illness are gratitude and forgiveness, which lead to the cultivation of peace of mind and a powerful army. This is why the Inner Smile practice is so immensely powerful in all its simple brilliance.

Waking the Child Within

Children react to life innocently. As children, we naturally interact using our true heart-mind instincts. When we mature and become grown-ups in this world, we unlearn the most important ways of being—how to simply express our feelings without censoring or judging them and how to greet the world with an open heart. We forget how to look through wide-open eyes that drink in the landscape with delight and surprise, taking nothing for granted, connecting to the natural world in the spirit of appreciation. Yes, we may learn how to be more discerning as the payoff for becoming adults, but at what price, if we can't preserve our childlike joy and enthusiasm alongside the cultivation of this skill?

The trick is to add that wisdom and discernment to your being without sacrificing that precious openness and effervescence. When you have both, you should want for nothing, because you're rich. You have real balance. Children share their smiles generously. Just think of a child's laughter; conjure it now. Think of what that babbling brook–like sound of joy does to you. This is the energy we want to learn to recapture and bring into our own lives. And the path back to this childhood purity and self-love is through is the body. By bringing this same sense of wonder and surprise to our own bodies, by smiling inwardly to our very selves and to the tender, brilliant, powerful, endlessly intelligent viscera that we possess, which are responsible for keeping us alive, we not only effect tremendous change within our own ecosystems, we wake up untold sleeping stores of energy.

Love's Smiles and Sounds

In the Waking Energy flow, we have now pulled back the curtain and revealed the shadow side of our organ-held emotions. By shining the light of love and attention on them, we have set the stage for what comes next. We have opened, harmonized, and energized the meridians that lead to our organs, and now it's time to get really intimate with them, to smile at them and sing them love songs.

The Inner Smile and Cosmic Healing Sounds exercises promote health, resilience, and vitality regardless of what is happening around us. They help us cultivate a new way of interacting with ourselves on a deep, internal level. They radically alter long-held, negative beliefs about ourselves and others that leach vital energy from our body's energy "bank account," replacing them with voices of compassion, empathy, patience, and understanding and leading to substantial energy cultivation and restoration and optimal health from the inside out. Just as receiving a kind smile from someone else activates our parasympathetic nervous system's relaxation response, our body appreciates a smile from the self no differently. It enhances every one of our body's functions, from our endocrine system to our circulation, respiration, and digestion; everything gets happy and, like someone whom motivation encourages, instantaneously functions better.

As you will soon see, this practice uses your own hands as *healing wands*. Charged with your own positive chi to bring new energy, light, and positive affirmation to your organs, your hands will hover above each organ in turn as you move through the sequence. Using the power of your loving smile, your "delete" key, and your gentle movements, you will change the emotional state and energy quality of each organ for the better. Through specific breath work and sounds that are enunciated subvocally (like a vibrational whisper), you will move in ways that immerse each organ in its favorite healing sound, repeated several times, until the body feels more fluid and less restricted, evidence that your own focused intention has worked in harmony with the tools you apply and that the energy of the organ has shifted, restoring balance in your body overall.

Once I began to practice the Inner Smile and Cosmic Healing Sounds, my life was never the same. I can't tell you how special and virtually "undiscovered" these practices are, because they were under lock and key for centuries, performed exclusively by Taoist adepts who earned the right to learn them from their masters before them through supreme self-discipline and dedication. They arise out of a beautiful simplicity, inspiring us with gratitude and awe at our body's miraculous capabilities. My wonder surrounding this practice and all the closely guarded secrets Master Chia and his teachers made available to us has never waned since my first real-time experience with him. It still astounds me how our own loving intentions can heal, balance, and strengthen our bodies, down to our vital organs and our every cell.

Visiting the major organ systems of our bodies, from the heart to the reproductive organs, we will use our minds to focus our attention, bringing new awareness and energy to each, acknowledging the emotions that have been held there and infusing them with a message of compassion and empathy. Moving this stagnation out makes space for more life energy, resulting in a deep, energized calm.

The Look of Love

The look of love is what starts it all. When we are on the receiving end of a smile, we feel safe, we let our defenses down, and we open to the energy coming our way because it feels good. It sends a resounding "yes" to our parasympathetic nervous system, stimulating the relaxation response, which then catalyzes the positive chain of chemical secretions in our body that enhance our body's total systems, optimizing its overall function and health. And in the same way that it is such a powerful form of social currency, a smile is just as effective and important a tool for the cultivation of our own self-love and evolution. How many messages do you receive internally that aren't especially positive? Can you imagine how much better you would feel just by changing that internal dialogue for the better? It all starts with a smile.

It's the simple act of turning your focus inward, of giving your organs that look of love to let them know you care, that starts the magic and gets the ball rolling. And it is the combination of the look and sound of love that makes the life-changing magic happen, that triggers the cataclysmic shift in the energy inside the organ itself. Your organs feel your attention to them the same way others feel it when they receive your smile and that look in your eyes. When you look into an organ, the impact on it is not unlike the feeling you get when you call to mind a beautifully shot moment from a documentary like the BBC series *Planet Earth* or *Winged Migration*. See it now, your favorite, the scene that makes you thrill inside, shot in slow motion—a flock of birds taking wing, a kaleidoscope of butterflies erupting from their flowered nests, a herd of gazelle running across the plains . . . Looking inside your own miraculous body is felt by your body the same way, and it is a thing of beauty, no different from the captivating splendor and magnificence of the creatures in our natural world. It is the look of love that sets everything in motion in a new, life-enhancing way.

The practice of the Inner Smile asks you to develop awareness of the very act of turning your sights inward to affirm the world unseen and how vital it is to all of life, to all of *your* life. It asks you to depart from the outside world and in utter simplicity appreciate, very likely for the first time ever, what you have taken for granted for so long. It invites you to discover the untapped power you possess to heal and bolster yourself in real, pragmatic ways. Think about a smile and what it elicits in you. A genuine smile is an outward expression of what happens in your heart the minute you connect with someone. If a stranger smiles at you, it can change the entire course of your day. Why? Because it strips everything else away and in that moment reminds you of what is truly important in life—love. And love *is* your life force. Your smile—and the smiles you exchange out in the world with your fellow humans—holds more power to heal and transform than several United Nations roundtable discussions by a long shot. If everyone in the world practiced the Inner Smile, there might actually be peace in the Middle East.

Such is the nature of this and all the practices in *Waking Energy*. What you give, you receive a thousandfold, and like a beautiful waterwheel the giving and receiving never end. You are inspired to continue to explore because of the riches each venture yields. When you allow yourself to be vulnerable, go into those dark, shadowy places, and uncover the treasure, you transform what hurts into what feels good. As you start to trust in the process and come to realize that you are your own best mother and father, this deceptively simple practice will become integral to your own reparenting of yourself, teaching you that it is safe to come out and to be all that you can be. You can let go of the past, as long as you acknowledge that it happened. You can lovingly go inside to attend to all the feelings that have established residence without your conscious knowing, but with your permission, became freeloading residents. Yes, you unwittingly invited them, but as soon as you let them know that you see them (take responsibility for their tenure inside you), they miraculously and quite willingly want to move on to greener pastures, literally returning to Mother Earth, where they can become something else far more useful—fuel for the trees and flowers that give us our oxygen—our life-force fuel.

This is the gorgeous cycle of emotion-energy transformation, of alchemy. For me, even now, each time I practice and dedicate myself to the Power of Love and specifically the Inner Smile and Cosmic Healing Sounds, more and more is revealed. Each time the results confirm how the practice is integral to creating a lasting inner shift, because it cultivates gentleness and tenderness for the self. And each time I practice, the work itself reminds me to be kind to myself as I return to feelings and events. Because of this, each time I am able to go deeper, accessing yet another level of meaning and insight.

Because the nature of life presents you with experiences that reflexively echo formative ones, you revisit your own inner globe of emotions and feelings. What is it that Buddhist teacher Pema Chödrön says? "Nothing ever goes away until it has taught us what we need to know." With the ever changing and challenging landscape of life's vicissitudes, you will always be presented with more opportunities to peel away the layers from that inner globe of emotions—what I like to think of as the onion. Each time you peel another away, it makes you cry, but each time the tears are less and less painful, and they offer you the promise of ever greater freedom and wisdom. And each time you circle around and survive to tell the tale, you glean more knowledge.

You start to understand that it is we who complicate our own lives, and it is through these very practices that we can hope to evolve to a level where we can rise above the emotional fray, where it is no longer a matter of survival, but of choice, and we can embrace simplicity. Instead of suffering as we once did, now armed with new information and tools, we can "stem the tide of complexity," live more simply and with the amplified power of our consciousness, and manifest more love, gratitude, and forgiveness toward ourselves, thus attracting others who will reflect that love back to us, so that together we can beam it out into the world.

What wakes energy? Forgiveness and gratitude. Together they are wisdom. It's wisdom that leads to intelligent, self-loving choices that then give you access to the total energy package, your new self and the new world you will come to inhabit. If you follow these words of wisdom, not only will you have a strong immune system, but you will be a happier, more balanced human being, capable of traveling within and without, and it all starts with a smile and a love song.

the power of love practice

TIME OF DAY: Morning or evening

QUALITY: Yin

SUBTLE ENERGY: Stimulates and balances the meridian system and elixir fields.

BENEFITS: Deeply heals and empowers the total body at the cellular level; transforms negative emotions into positive, life-affirming energies resulting in a sense of total well-being.

PROP: Chair

The Practice:

Cosmic Healing Sound for the Lungs
Cosmic Healing Sound for the Kidneys
Cosmic Healing Sound for the Liver
Cosmic Healing Sound for the Heart
Cosmic Healing Sound for the Spleen
Cosmic Healing Sound for the Triple Warmer

Your Cosmic Courtship Ritual

The cosmic healing sounds in this practice can be used to heal six major types of organs and associated body parts and systems. Each organ has its own unique physical, mental, emotional, and spiritual associations. Meditations that incorporate these associations can be used in tandem with the Inner Smile and Cosmic Healing Sounds practice to balance and harmonize an organ when you are feeling unwell or as a preventative measure to maintain well-being. In the descriptions that precede each of the six cosmic healing sounds, you'll find the following information.

- *Mouth position:* A description of how to make the cosmic healing sound.
- *Paired organs:* Every organ is paired with one or more other organs along meridians. When you heal one, you heal the other(s). For example, the lungs are paired via their meridians with the large intestine.
- *Emotions:* Every organ is associated with certain emotions. When you heal an emotion, you heal the organ. When you heal the organ, the emotions it governs are brought back into balance.
- *Signs of imbalance:* When an organ is imbalanced, certain physical conditions emerge to indicate that healing work needs to be done.
- *Benefits:* When you bring an organ into balance, there are mental and emotional benefits.
- *Related senses:* Each organ is associated with one or more of the physical senses: sight, sound, smell, taste, and touch.
- *Element:* Each organ is associated with a different element from nature: fire, water, earth, air, or metal.
- *Sound:* Each organ resonates with a sound related to its corresponding natural element.
- *Season:* Each organ is associated with a different season of the year: winter, spring, summer, or autumn.
- *Color:* Each organ is associated with a different color.

By now you've no doubt come to understand that full integration of all the components that comprise an exercise is more important than focusing exclusively on a single aspect of it. The first time you attempt something, such as making a specific sound while holding a posture, of course you should focus intently on it to ensure that you're doing it properly. But once you feel comfortable with the main elements of the practice, start to add in other layers and aspects, such as colors and emotions, so that it can deliver its full healing potency to you. Remember, as Master Chia says, you are "rallying the troops."

Although you can do this practice anytime, I always love performing it either in the morning, to clean the energetic slate, get grounded, and set my intention to prepare for a productive and joyful day, or in the evening before bed, to clear away the energy of the day, cool the organs, recalibrate and balance my internal temperature, and prepare the body and mind for a deep, restful, rejuvenating sleep.

This beautifully simple little ritual, not unlike so many of the other practices in this book, if performed regularly, can change your life on its own—it is that immensely powerful and effective. If you perform it daily, you will significantly boost your immune system, prevent illness, and create an exceptional state of inner and outer balance. Perhaps the best news is that once you become adept at performing the different cosmic healing sounds and can move from one organ to the next in a seamless flow, you can compete the entire set in under fifteen minutes.

Finally, like anything that has to do with Waking Energy, the healing sounds follow the flow of nature: they are ordered according to the progression of the seasons. It is good to practice extra repetitions of a healing sound if you are in the season associated with it. This advice may be counterintuitive, because you would think that an organ would flourish in its own season, but it's similar to the principle in Chinese astrology that your animal year may not necessarily be the best time for you. For example, in the autumn when the lungs are vulnerable, consider performing the Cosmic Healing Sound for the Lungs sequence twice as many times as the other healing sounds, to strengthen lung chi and build resistance against bronchial issues.

If you're ever feeling an excess of a specific emotion, perform the healing sound related to the organ that governs it to balance your emotional state and restore your inner peace and equilibrium. If you feel exhausted or out of gas at work, simply practice the healing sounds for the lungs and kidneys, if you don't have time to perform them all.

Now let's explore the first cosmic healing sound.

The Practice

Cosmic Healing Sound for the Lungs: *Ssssss*

Mouth position: Semismile with tongue behind two top front teeth
Paired organ: Large intestine
Emotions: Grief, sadness, depression
Signs of imbalance: Asthma, bronchial infection
Benefits: Cultivates courage, confidence, integrity, right action
Related senses: Smell, touch
Element: Metal
Sounds: Metal bell ringing, brass Tibetan bowl singing, gong reverberating
Season: Autumn
Color: White

1. Sitting tall, rub your hands together vigorously to charge them with heaven and earth energy. Bring your hands in front of your chest at the level of your lungs with your palms open and facing you—with the fingertips pointing toward one another. Smile at your lungs, as if you were smiling at a long-lost friend, and allow the positive energy of your smile to fill and surround your lungs.
2. Close your eyes. Use your powers of creative visualization to transport yourself to a scene of snowcapped mountains surrounded by fresh green meadows and flowing springs far below. Picture the pure white

color of the snow and see the sun shining on the mountaintop, activating the powerful life-force chi of white light. Feel the energy of the mountain. Hear the sound of a metal bell ringing inside your mind. Inhale the pure, fresh, white light, inviting the energy to expand into your lungs and heal them, and allow the vibration of the bell to sound in your ears, soothing your spirit.

3. Inhale and direct your inner vision down to your lungs. Send the energy of your smile to your lungs. First, look down at your left lung and smile. Actually let your eyes move as if you were looking at your chest, but with eyes closed. Then look down at your right lung and smile. Alternate between left and right. As you do so, gently sway your body in tandem with your inner vision, rocking your body from left to right.
4. As you sway from left to right, allow your inner vision to probe the lungs more deeply, going into their lower lobes and exploring what's inside them. As you do, continue to breathe deeply and smoothly, sending healing air into your lungs.
5. Now seek out any sadness or depression that resides in the lungs. Seek out any thoughts that arise about who or what has contributed to the sadness or grief you feel. As you do this inner exploration and excavation, sway from left to right (one set) for a total of twenty-one sets. I like to think of this process as treasure hunting, because when you uncover sadness and can identify its source, you are essentially harvesting a gift that you can use for energy transformation—you can replace the emotion with courage and lightness—which translates as more energy.
6. After completing all the repetitions, raise your hands above your head, slightly in front of your forehead, and turn your palms face up toward the sky to connect with heaven energy.
7. Inhale deeply and as you exhale, turn the corners of your mouth up, forming your mouth into a smile. Place your tongue behind your front two top teeth and use the force of your exhalation to make the cosmic healing sound "*Sssssss*," like a snake hissing. As you make the snake sound, visualize any sadness, depression, grief, and upset leaving your

body like a cloudy, gray mist. Direct the energy down into the earth where it will be recycled by plants, flowers, and trees, the gifts from Mother Earth that provide us with our sustenance, precious oxygen.

Make the *Ssssss* sound three times. As you do, feel the sound begin clearing inside your lungs, mobilizing stagnant chi and any excess heat that was trapped inside the pleural sacs surrounding the lungs. Visualize your exhalations compressing the lungs and gently forcing the heat up and out of your body. See the room being made for new chi to flow in along with the fresh, cooling air that will circulate and nourish the lungs. Allow the first sound to be vocal and strong, and then the second and third times you repeat it make it subtle, and then subvocal. Internally heard, it becomes a deep inner vibration. Feel the quietude emerging from the vibration, the energy surrounding the act of breathing, rather than from using force to back up the sound. Think of why you are making the sound, and focus on integrating the qualities of the mountain scene and the sound of the bell from step 1 into your sound.

8. Once you've completed three exhalations using the *Ssssss* sound, shift your focus to the *laogong* points in your palms and use them to collect heavenly yang chi. See white light pouring down through your crown and your *laogong* points into your lungs. Do this for several rounds of breath. Then lower your arms to the front of your body, palms facing inward toward your lungs, and sense the luminescent white light radiating into your lungs and instilling you with courage, fortitude, and calm. After a breath or two, bring your hands down to rest on your knees.
9. Now resume gently rocking from side to side, and as you do smile at your lungs, inhaling deeply. As you exhale, let go, relaxing more deeply all the while and imagining you are still making the healing *Ssssss* sound. Let go of any additional excess heat and toxins. Then feel fresh, white light and bright bell energy entering your lungs, making them strong, clear, and resolute. As you inhale, see earth flowing up through your Bubbling Spring Points and leg channels and into the space that you have made by releasing the stagnant energy. Let the earth give you energy it has trans-

formed, filling you with courage, confidence, and peace. Use the positive earth energy to nourish your lungs and other organs.

10. After several breaths of smiling at your lungs and letting go of sadness and grief, perform an especially attentive search to seek out remnants of negative emotions that you can still perceive, and actively "delete" them. As you do, continue rocking gently from side to side and bring your hands up to the level of your lungs again. This time, spread your fingers apart with tips pointing at each other. Once again, turn your focus inward to look keenly at the lungs, looking left to right, back and forth, repeatedly for several breath cycles. As you are sweeping through your lungs with your eyes and your breath, literally imagine yourself pushing a "delete" key on a computer to clear your lungs of negative remnants.
11. Now, as you continue to inhale, sit taller so that you can embody the virtue of courage. With your palms still facing you at the heart and lung level, breathe in the energy of courage and righteousness or alignment with your own truth (not to be confused with self-righteousness, which speaks more to pride). Breathe in right action, positive self-satisfaction, and sincerity. Feel good inside. Tell yourself that you feel good and that you're going to feel even better.

    As you smile into your lungs, allow yourself to fill with self-love, so much that your lungs expand with your own beautiful, white inner light and the crystal-true ring of your personal bell tone. Let a deep, all-pervasive white glow emanate from your lungs and beam itself outward from your body. Acknowledge that you have created it, feel gratitude, and smile at yourself. Continue to sense the vibration of the bell inside your lungs, hear it in your mind, ringing sweetly in your ears. Rest and soak up the benefits of the work you've just done. The clean, clear, pure, powerful, white light of love will continue to heal your lungs and build your clarity, courage, and strength long after you have finished this session.
12. Repeat the above sequence of steps three to six times. In moments of respiratory-related illness, such as asthma, cough, and bronchial con-

ditions of any kind or of emotional upset from sadness, grief, or depression, repeat this sequence as many times as your instincts lead you to do.

Cosmic Healing Sound for the Kidneys: *Choooo*

Mouth position: Lips form an O shape, as if you're blowing out a candle
Paired organ: Urinary bladder
Emotion: Fear
Sign of imbalance: Lower-back pain
Benefits: Instills calm, stillness, confidence, clarity, attention, focus, willpower, purpose, good feelings; vanquishes fear, phobias, trauma
Related sense: Hearing
Element: Water
Sounds: Ocean waves crashing, a flowing stream, a downpour of rain
Season: Winter
Color: Dark blue

1. Sit tall in a chair and rub your hands together vigorously. Then bring your palms to your lower back, in the area of your kidneys, and send the energy you've generated with your hands and warmth to your kidneys and adrenal glands as you breathe deeply and smoothly. Close your eyes and imagine a soothing, deep, oceanic blue light surrounding and bathing your kidneys. Visualize and hear ocean waves washing up on shore or a gurgling brook playing over rocks. Invite the sound to soothe your ears as you listen. The ears are connected to the kidneys so they both benefit from this practice. Picture sunlight shining on the water and breathe the powerful life-force energy of the reflected rays of the sun bouncing off the water into your kidneys.
2. As you inhale, turn your inner vision toward the kidneys themselves. With your hands radiating warmth into your kidneys, smile at each one, first looking left and then right in alternation, and send the healing

energy of your intention into the kidneys. As you do so, gently sway your body in tandem with your inner vision, rocking your body from left to right. Complete twenty-one sets of looking left to right.

Tune in to your kidneys and hear what they have to say. Are they feeling depleted and in need of your attention? Is there a tender quality to the lower back, a sense of fragility or sensitivity? Your smile, the breath of your intention, and warmth from your hands is nourishing and recharging them.

3. As you look left and right, with your hands still in position over your kidneys, bring up any fear inside your body-mind and allow it to breathe. Give it space inside you, so that it can come to the surface of your consciousness and express itself fully. Then escort it out of your body-mind and send it into the earth below. As you continue your twenty-one repetitions of looking left to right, switch your focus to "deleting" fear. Acknowledge it, push the "delete" button, and then send it on its way. You have the power to "delete" anything that no longer serves a positive purpose. You have the power to release fear, to let it go completely in this very moment.
4. Now that you have started to effectively clear the fear, shift your focus. Intentionally connect to your hands on your kidneys and direct your mind to harness energy from the earth and send it into your Sea of Chi and bring energy from heaven down into your kidneys at the same time.
5. Now inhale and bring your feet and knees together, rounding your upper body forward toward your knees (creating a large C shape). Clasp your palms and press down, so that the insides of the wrists rest upon the knees.
6. Anchoring yourself by using your left hand to grab the fingers of the right, pull your spine more strongly back in opposition to your knees so that your arms are straight. Keep your eyes open and look straight ahead.
7. As you exhale, simultaneously actively draw your abdominal muscles in toward your spine and round your mouth into an O shape while you make the healing sound "*Choooo*." This deep C shape in your body conducts the vibration of the healing sound to the kidneys and lends itself

to an internal compression that expels excess heat and toxins from the fascia surrounding them.

8. As you are creating the *Choooo* sound, picture yourself sending all your fear down into the earth below, where it will be transformed and recycled. As with the other healing sounds, perform the first round of the sound audibly, and then with each subsequent repetition refine the sound until it is subvocal and exclusively internal. Your ability to subvocalize speaks to your growing ability to master the details of your practice.
9. As you inhale again, release your hold on your knees and circle your arms to either side up around your body, moving them slowly until they are overhead and turning the palms face up toward the ceiling. Throughout the movement visualize yourself collecting the azure light that surrounds your body and supercharging it with heaven chi. As your arms continue moving slowly, pass them down to the front of your body. Simultaneously, see blue light pouring in through your crown and traveling down into your Sea of Chi, where it infuses your kidneys with its healing properties.
10. Allow your hands to come to rest in front of your heart. Gather earth energy through your hands for a breath, then bring your palms down to rest on your knees. Open your legs to wider than hip-width apart and ensure that your feet are firmly planted on the floor. Direct all the earth and heaven energy you've collected into your Lower Elixir Field to replenish the kidneys.
11. Now practice your Inner Smile: rock your body from side to side and, as you do, look left to right, into one kidney and then the other, and smile at them. Visualize a deep blue light surrounding both of your kidneys and emanating from them. See this healing light grow to surround your entire body in an ocean of blue love.
12. Once again, as you continue to rock your body ever so gently from left to right, return your hands to your kidneys. With every breath you take, breathe in soothing gentle blue stillness and calm into your kidneys and exhale excess heat and fear. Hear the sound of ocean waves or a gur-

gling brook reverberating inside you, expelling excess heat and toxins from the kidneys. Invite the cooling, blue energy of water to bathe the kidneys, restoring them to the sweet, clean warmth of radiant health. Allow the new, warming energy to nurture and relax the muscles of your lower back. Smile at your kidneys, letting them know that it is safe to release, to heal, and to be restored.

13. Release any last residue of fear you may feel. Let go. Even though you're no longer actively making the *Choooo* sound now, invite the healing sound to continue to do its good work, vibrating and ushering in perfect quietude and healing stillness. Remind yourself to take this gentle quality, this stillness and calm, into your life, extending the practice and its benefits into your every moment, knowing that the next time you are overcome by fear, you can breathe it out and access the cool, soothing blue energy of the water to guide you home again.
14. Repeat the above sequence three to six times. In moments of fear and emotional duress or whenever you feel fatigued or depleted or have ringing in your ears, dizziness, or lower-back pain, repeat the sequence as many times as you feel necessary in order to restore calm, inner peace, confidence, and courage in your body-mind.

Cosmic Healing Sound for the Liver: *Shhhhh*

Mouth position: Tongue near palate to create the "*Shhhhh*" sound
Paired organ: Gallbladder
Emotion: Anger
Signs of imbalance: Rumination, impatience, restlessness
Benefits: Instills kindness; vanquishes fear
Related sense: Sight
Element: Wood
Sounds: Wooden wind chimes clacking, sticks hitting together
Season: Spring
Color: Green

1. Sitting tall on your chair, inhale and rub your hands together vigorously. With the energy you generate, place your palms slightly above your liver (just under the bottom of your right rib cage). The tips of your fingers are interlacing, and your thumbs are just along for the ride, pointing up. Once your hands are in position, inhale deeply and envision the most beautiful evergreen forest you've ever seen, replete with tall, full pine trees. Breathe in the deep, rich, refreshing scent of pine and fertile topsoil, and see the sun shining on the trees, creating a powerful, primordial bright green life force, with a light that soothes your eyes. Remember that the eyes are related to the liver, so when you soothe your eyes, you also calm the liver chi.
2. As healing warmth from your hands enters the liver, picture what your liver looks like inside your body. Scan your liver, as if you're repeatedly reading a message written on it, from left to right. Gently rock your body from side to side, moving in tandem with your inner vision, looking from left to right and exploring what lives inside the liver at this moment.
3. As you breathe, see any anger that hides inside your liver. Summon angry feelings, even if you can't immediately perceive anger in this moment; still looking left to right, continue to feel energy from your hands flowing into your liver. Once any anger has made itself known, see it (perhaps picturing the person, people, or situation that inspired the anger) and consciously breathe into the feeling. Allow yourself to continue swaying from side to side as you start to "delete" the anger you've uncovered.
4. Complete twenty-one sets of simultaneously rocking left to right, breathing, and scanning, just allowing those moments that created the feelings of anger inside you to come up in your body-mind and then be released. Breathe into these images, surrounding them with your powerful breath, and each time you feel yourself getting swept away in a current of anger, return to the moment and consciously immerse yourself in the healing light of the deep, forest-green energy and in the energy of the empowered intention to release anger that you are bringing to the moment. Each time you exhale, push the "delete" key in your

brain and in your liver, let go of anger, and send the liberated chi down into the earth below.

5. After you've completed your sets, take a deep inhalation, and as you do, interlace your fingers, inverting your palms so that they face up, and bring your arms overhead in a circle framing your head. Lean your torso slightly over to the left, with an emphasis on mobilizing the rib cage and feeling a deep stretch in the right side of your body where the liver is located.
6. Lift your head with eyes wide open and look up directly at the back of your hands. Open your eyes wide and stretch your eyeballs in their sockets to stimulate your liver chi, as you progressively stretch farther to the left, actually feeling the liver and its visceral casing stretch inside your body, both creating compression and expelling excess heat.
7. As you continue to reach the arms up to the left with energy and intention, stretching your gaze as well, press your right foot more firmly into the ground, inhale deeply, and then exhale making the liver healing sound, "*Shhhhh.*" As you do, consciously acknowledge that the sound is vibrating inside the liver, expelling excess heat and toxins, while at the same time drawing heaven chi in through your hands and sending it directly into your liver.
8. After you have completely emptied your lungs, release the clasp of your fingers, but keep your palms facing up to collect additional heaven chi through your palms. Remain here for a few rounds of breath.
9. Bring your spine back into a centered, vertical alignment and gradually circle your arms down around the sides of your body, allowing your palms to turn forward, bringing the heaven chi that you have gathered down toward the ground. At the same time see heaven chi pour through your crown and down into your liver. Finally, bring your hands to rest on the tops of your knees.
10. Resume the gentle rocking from side to side, as you breathe deep, rich, emerald-green forest energy and kindness into your liver. Relax and let go. Rock for three breath cycles, allowing your body to integrate the

energy you have just drawn down from heaven and transform it into healing green light for your liver. Continue to release anger from your body-mind into the earth.

11. Now bring your hands back in front of your liver, a few inches above it, as you did earlier in step 1, and continue rocking from side to side, once again directing your inner vision to scan the liver from left to right and delete any anger you feel. This time make a focused effort to separate angry feelings from the people and events you feel helped to create them. Add the energy of forgiveness, sensing it emanating from your hands and flowing directly into the liver. As you sway from side to side, continue to "delete" the anger. Feel the gratitude of the liver rising up to your heart to thank you for your efforts.
12. As you breathe and continue to rock from side to side, imagine the sound of wooden wind chimes vibrating inside your liver and clearing out any remaining heat or toxicity. See and feel your liver being purified and cleansed as the drying heat of anger, aggression, and frustration continues to leave your body, making space for the fresh, pure, moisture-rich, green, wood energy of the forest to grow in its place. As you consciously delete anger, feel kindness and generosity flowing into the liver and then expanding into your heart. Sense the gorgeous evergreen color of the forest surrounding your liver; it emanates from the center of the liver and radiates outward until it encircles your entire body in a magnificent glowing green halo of softness and light. Rest in this beautiful green light and imagine that you are being cradled by the forest itself, nestled like a bird among soothing, fresh green leaves. Let go now and fly.
13. Repeat the above sequence three to six times. At times when you feel especially overtaken by anger or consumed by frustration, or if you have a bitter taste in your mouth or any issues with your eyes or vision, repeat the entire sequence as many times as is necessary to feel relief and restore equanimity and balance to your liver. You may also perform the sequence multiple times if you want to detoxify the liver.

Cosmic Healing Sound for the Heart: *Hawwww*

Mouth position: Mouth wide open to create the "*Hawwww*" sound
Paired organ: Small intestine
Emotions: Hatred, impatience, cruelty
Signs of imbalance: Chest pain, palpitations, high blood pressure
Benefits: Engenders joy, honor, sincerity, patience
Related sense: Taste
Element: Fire
Sounds: Kindling igniting in a fireplace, the crackling and hissing of burning logs
Season: Summer
Color: Red

1. Sitting tall, inhale and rub your hands together vigorously. Using the energy you've just generated, bring your palms right above your heart with your left fingertips slightly overlapping your right fingertips, thumbs pointing upward. Turn your vision inward toward the heart and smile at your heart as you start to sway from left to right. Close your eyes and imagine the colors of a sunset, brilliant shades of red, orange, and pink, and breathe this vibrant light and energy into your heart.
2. As you breathe and look from left to right at your heart, scan for impatience, jealousy, and hatred. Whatever emerges, allow yourself to feel it and start to delete it, allowing your heart to ride the motion of the body from left to right in tandem with your eyes, as they explore the inner topography of your heart.
3. Complete twenty-one sets of looking left to right, breathing naturally as you do, while you consciously delete the shadow-side emotions of the heart (hatred, impatience, jealousy, and envy). With your breath, send them down into the earth below.
4. Now, as you inhale, bend your elbows and raise your palms up toward

the ceiling at the sides of your body. Then continue to circle your arms up until they are overhead, framing the top of your head.

5. Interlace your fingers and invert your palms so that they face up. Then lean your torso over to the right, with an emphasis on mobilizing the rib cage itself, feeling a deep stretch in the left side of your body, down into the heart and the pericardium, which is the heart protector, a fascial sac surrounding the heart.
6. Lift your head and with eyes open, look up directly at the back of your hands, still leaning over to the right. As you progressively stretch your arms with greater energy and emphasis, press the left foot more firmly into the ground and actually feel the heart and its visceral casing stretching inside your torso.
7. As you exhale, open your mouth, forming a large, relaxed O shape with your lips and make the healing sound "*Hawwww,*" like a whisper, with no real vocal participation behind the exhalation. Simultaneously, continue to stretch up and over to the right, compressing the pericardium around the heart, so as to expel excess heat and toxins from the heart.
8. After you have emptied your lungs completely, inhale again. As you next exhale, unclasp your hands, keeping the fingers pointing toward one another, and invite heaven chi to pour down through your crown down into your heart, bathing it in the vibrantly colored, clearing radiance of a sunset.
9. Return to sitting upright and slowly circle your arms down to shoulder height with palms facing away from you. Then continue to circle your arms to the front of your body until they come to rest with palms in front of your heart center. Radiate red light and the energy of love, joy, patience, and calm from your hands into your heart.
10. Rock from side to side, breathing the energy of love into your heart, and then radiate the infinitely powerful red light of joy outward from the heart, continuing to release impatience, jealousy, and hatred from your body-mind. As you exhale, bring your hands down to rest on your knees.

11. Continuing to rock from side to side, scan your heart from left to right while letting go of impatience, hatred, and impatience. Send these down into Mother Earth to be transformed. As you rock and breathe, forgive, forget, and let go. (There is a saying, "Forgive, but don't forget," but the truth is, you have already learned the lessons you needed to learn from your shadow-side emotions, so you can afford to forget. Let it all go. Relax and breathe.)
12. Still swaying from side to side, bring your hands together in a Prayer Position in front of your heart and continue to feel the vibration of the healing sound of the heart doing its work of expelling the last traces of excess heat from your heart. See and feel a deep, rich, ruby red and pink glow radiating from your heart and enveloping your entire being in its healing light. Breathe love right into your heart and see the energy of love filling your heart like an eternal flame, giving birth to so much joy, peace, and happiness that you can't help but smile.
13. Repeat the above sequence three to six times. When you feel moody, upset, angry, resentful, or restless, or if you are suffering physically from a sore throat, swollen gums, cold sores, or heart disease, you may repeat the entire sequence as many times as you deem necessary to support your heart and get relief.

Cosmic Healing Sound for the Spleen: *Whoooo*

Mouth position: Mouth forms an O shape to create a guttural sound that comes from the back of the throat
Paired organs: Pancreas, stomach
Emotions: Anxiety, worry, mistrust
Signs of imbalance: Digestive distress, elimination disorders
Benefits: Cultivates calm, courage, fairness, openness
Related sense: Taste
Element: Earth
Sound: Rocks and gravel crunching underfoot

Season: Late summer or early autumn
Color: Yellow

1. Sitting tall, inhale and rub your hands together vigorously. Using the energy you've generated, bring your palms right above your spleen (on the left side of your body behind the lower edge of your rib cage), with your fingertips facing in. Start to rock from side to side and turn your inner vision to look into your spleen and smile at it. Visualize the spleen being bathed in a golden, yellow light, like sunlight through stalks of wheat in a large open field at the close of a late summer day.
2. Breathe deeply and naturally as you scan the spleen from left to right with your inner vision and rock back and forth twenty-one times in all, deleting worry and anxiety on every exhalation.
3. After twenty-one sets of rocking, inhale and round your body slightly forward as you bring your arms toward one another in front of your body in a gathering motion, sweeping earth chi into your stomach and spleen on the left side of your abdomen and the pancreas on the right side of your abdomen.
4. Keeping your eyes open, exhale and press the first three fingertips of each hand gently but firmly into your spleen, on the left side of the rib cage, slightly below your sternum. Now round your torso forward into a deeper C shape, using the movement as a means to accentuate the action you are performing with your hands, pressing progressively deeper into the spleen and compressing it. Begin to make the healing sound "*Whoooo,*" like the beginning of a guttural, almost gurgling sound deep in the throat, riding into a wave that becomes a kind of deep whisper. Feel the vibrations of the sound initiating the clearing of stagnant chi.
5. Inhale to rise upright again and use your deepest abdominal muscles to actively push your fingertips out of the depression you created by pressing into your spleen.

6. Inhaling, bring your arms out to your sides, with palms facing up, and make a scooping motion in a small and gentle low arc to gather earth energy before returning to your tall, effortless, relaxed seat, where you will resume swaying from side to side.
7. You will immediately convert this fresh earth energy into the warming golden glow of healing yellow light energy. Visualize it pouring into your spleen, pancreas, and stomach through your palms, which will now come to rest right above your spleen to do their healing work of radiating courage, groundedness, openness, and fairness directly into the organ. Resume your gentle swaying motion, and breathe deeply and smoothly with your hands above your spleen.
8. Transition by placing your palms on your knees. Now as you sway, look from your spleen (left) to your pancreas (right), eyes moving in tandem with the action of your body. Use this as your opportunity to let go of worry, anxiety, and mistrust. Feel the vibration of the healing spleen sound currents continuing to reverberate throughout your stomach, spleen, and pancreas, removing any last residue of excess heat. Let it all go, sending it down to Mother Earth. Smile at your spleen, pancreas, and stomach, and enjoy the feelings of stability and peace that are riding in on the currents of soothing golden light.
9. Harness the joy you've just cultivated and with your inner vision bring it to wrap around the stomach, spleen, and pancreas. See a vibrant golden light emanating from your stomach, spleen, and pancreas.
10. As you wrap the energy of love and joy around your stomach, spleen, and pancreas, bring your hands back above your spleen and start to rock your body forward and back. Think of this as a kind of "organ love break dance." Next begin moving in a circular motion to create an inner globe of energy, folding love, joy, happiness, appreciation, openness, and trust into the orb of energy you are creating, bringing your body forward and back like a wave rolling up onto the shore and then receding. Breathe pure goodness into your stomach, spleen, and pancreas, smiling at them, and let go of any remaining anxiety, a

sheer receding echo of the emotions that were once present. Rest, let go, and relax.

11. Repeat the above sequence three to six times, as you did with the preceding organ-cleansing sequences. Increase the number of repetitions, doing as many as you deem necessary, if you are experiencing nausea, indigestion, acid reflux, intestinal distress, or constipation. You may also increase the frequency or length of your practice if you are feeling anxious or worried.

Cosmic Healing Sound for the Triple Warmer: *Heeeee*

In traditional Chinese medicine, the three elixir fields, the primary energy centers in the body, which are located in the lower, middle, and upper sections of the body and encompass, or "preside over," particular organs, when taken all together, are known as the *triple warmer.* Among other things, the triple warmer is involved in thermal regulation of the body so that each part of the body functions optimally. Its sound regulates the body's internal temperature, redistributing the excess heat that can rise to the head and heart from stress, bringing it down to warm the kidneys, which are always happy to receive any extra love and warmth they can get, thus helping you "cool off" and find calm.

Note: This exercise can be performed either sitting on a chair and leaning back with your legs extended in front of you or lying down on your back—in the qigong equivalent of *savasana* (Corpse Pose from yoga).

This cosmic healing sound does not have a set of corresponding organs, emotions, or related senses or an element, season, or color, because it encompasses the central aspect of the body.

Mouth position: Mouth forms a smile with the tongue in a semineutral position behind the lower teeth to create the "*Heeeee*" sound.

1. Sitting tall or lying down, rub your hands together vigorously and then inhale and sweep your arms out and around your body, gathering powerful, healing universal chi along the way.
2. With your palms facing you and starting at your head, exhale and make the healing sound "*Heeeee*" as your hands travel down the front of your body about three inches above the surface of your skin. Imagine that your hands are pushing a huge rolling pin as if you're rolling out a thin sheet of cookie dough, but now you are rolling excess heat from the elixir fields in your upper body down and into the elixir field in your lower body, where it will be cooled, integrated, and balanced. As your hands push the rolling pin past your head and your heart, think of cooling them with your exhalation. Intentionally move the heat from your head and heart down to your kidneys and sexual organs. Linger over your kidneys for a few seconds as you continue exhaling and making the *Heeeee* sound, feeling them warm up due to the energy that is flowing from your hands.
3. Continue moving your hands down to your upper thighs, where the energy of your intention pushes the heat you are collecting and directing through your leg channels toward your feet, warming them with new, life-enhancing energy and releasing stagnant energy as you go along. Silently repeat the following affirmation: "I am sending cold energy out through my legs and feet back down into the earth where it will be transformed."
4. Smile at your triple warmer and allow the sensation of perfect inner temperature control and balance to permeate and infuse every cell in your body. Use the energy of love and higher consciousness to charge and transform your entire subtle energy body system, sending balanced cool energy to the areas that typically overheat, such as your head and heart, and balanced warm energy to your Lower Elixir Field, which gets cold whenever it is depleted.
5. Feel the vast field of earthly yin chi underneath you. Feel the boundless field of heavenly yang chi above you. Sense that you are fully supported

and at peace, vibrating with the highest, purest energy of healing and empowerment.

6. Repeat the above sequence three to six times, using your intuition to discern your body's needs. For balancing and maintenance, perform three repetitions. During times of great stress and duress, especially if you are feeling depleted of energy or you're suffering from insomnia, perform six or more repetitions. On your final repetition, stop and rest with your hands on your belly covering your Lower Elixir Field and relish the soothing warmth and comfort of knowing that it is your own efforts that have produced the precious heart-mind elixir that is currently nurturing your kidneys and replenishing the energy of your prenatal chi.

10

moving into stillness: meditation

For years, one of my favorite things to do was to go to the Karma Triyana Dharmachakra Tibetan monastery outside of Woodstock in upstate New York. The energy there was palpable. Allegedly the Dalai Lama himself chose the spot where the temple would be built, and you could feel that it was true.

The moment I stepped onto the grounds and gazed up at the prayer flags fluttering in the wind, I was instantly transported to the Himalayas. As I walked up to the temple entrance, I applied my greatest physical control and grace to be more delicate and deliberate in my steps, to emulate the monks who seemed to float above the ground as they moved. I couldn't help feeling like an impostor when compared to these devotees who seemed to dedicate their every moment to this otherworldly, rarified way of being and pure silence.

But I would press on and find a seat in the temple, fighting the protestations of my monkey mind, allowing myself to soak up the energy from the space, convinced that it would help me cultivate patience and, if I was lucky, a taste of nirvana. So there I would sit, sometimes for up to as long as a half hour, wanting so badly to feel like a real meditator.

I've always been highly intuitive and introspective by nature, even able to enter into deeper meditative states naturally and quite easily, but I'd never succeeded in developing a consistent meditation practice. Although I had been meditating on and off for years as part of my regular yoga practice and had voraciously read a wide variety of classic and modern interpretations of Buddhist texts, I was never able to consistently sit and maintain a meditation practice that had sessions lasting more than fifteen minutes.

When I did start my day with meditation, even sitting for just ten minutes, I felt it was a great accomplishment. I always had a better day from the start, from the moment I engaged the outside world. Why? Because I'd turned my focus inward and quieted the aspects of my mind that were responsible for sapping vital energy from my inner reserves. But it wasn't until I signed up for Sarah Powers's Insight Meditation retreat at the Kripalu Center for Yoga and Health in Stockbridge, Massachusetts, that I felt as though I had really begun my meditation journey.

At Kripalu, Sarah's soothing, mellifluous voice guided us through a yin yoga practice preceding the meditations, and I came to understand that yin yoga boasted yet another extraordinary benefit. The real "end goal" of the practice was to help the body sit in meditation for long periods of time without discomfort. *Mindfulness meditation,* the style Sarah Powers taught, took the energy we harvested during the yin yoga practice and funneled it into the mind to integrate its full healing benefits.

The first day that I was asked to sit without fidgeting for an entire sixty minutes, I only made it to my usual ten minutes before I lost it (internally, that is), getting sucked into the irrational wanderings of my monkey mind. After fifteen minutes, I was entertaining a grandiose disaster fantasy in which I was convinced that I'd never make it through the meditation, or be able to get up, or maybe even walk again. My limbs had started to fall asleep, and I imagined with utter certainty that I was doing irreparable damage to the circulatory pathways in my legs. I was also convinced that the whole thing would crescendo into a massive anxiety attack, and I was obsessed with playing out, ahead of time, the terrible humiliation that would ensue. So, as soon as I felt my legs and feet going completely numb, in a panic to avoid what I believed would lead to being carried out of the room on a gurney, I uncrossed my legs. Life flooded back into my limbs within seconds, and I had what was the first of many similar realizations: that my anxiety had been the work of my mind convincing me that I couldn't continue, that I had to stop or else I would die. All in the mind. None of it real.

The good news is that before the meditation, we had prepped for this exact situation. Sarah told us that we would be tempted over and over again to move and adjust our position, but that this was really just the mind trying to take charge and convince us that we wouldn't be able to sit still. We were told that if we could focus on our breathing and recognize that different sensations, like our legs falling asleep or itching, would come and go, little by little we would become aware that we actually had the ability to handle whatever our minds and bodily sensations cooked up for us—even moments of tremendous duress that feel like life-threatening danger (yes, really, right there on your mat with just you and yourself, it can get that scary). But if you stay connected to your breath and are as faithful to it as it is to you, you live the miracle of change. You learn to welcome it and allow things to be just as they are. That allowing then becomes acceptance, which leads to calm and wisdom—on the cushion and in your life.

Despite being prepped for the experience, I had a tough time and did not feel particularly peaceful at the end of the first day's session. The next day came, and miraculously twenty minutes of meditation passed in a blink. (I cheated and peeked at the clock to monitor my progress.) The next day, a half hour passed without so much as a fidget. I was starting to actually like "finding my seat," and the effects of the practice were already proving to be profound. After six days in a row of sitting for an hour in the morning and another hour in the evening after dinner, I'd never felt so calm, so grounded, so deeply peaceful. I believe that I had my first taste of what Buddhist monks must feel: not of this earth, able to transcend it. I *was* the calm in the storm.

Coming Home

To a mind that is still the whole universe surrenders.

—Lao Tzu

It's only at night, when we venture forth into the velvety darkness that obscures sight, that we can see the stars. When we call upon the powers of our insight in the deepest, darkest recesses of the mind, illumination emerges. To access our higher mind, we must obscure distraction. Stillness is what's required for us to truly perceive this light.

Like the ancient masters, we have used our practices to achieve greater balance in our bodies, so that our minds can move beyond to dance with universal source energy—with love—our highest expression as human beings. Just as Taoist adepts have used qigong for millennia to create the immortal body with which they can leave the earth and travel to higher realms, and just as yogis have used poses to move toward enlightenment, all your journey so far has led you to this place. Now it is time for us to enter the great mother of yin, blackest night, the infinite void out of which all matter is born.

Every practice you've tried thus far has prepared you for this moment, awakening new energy and awareness, helping you to explore your limitless capacity for growth. Having stimulated, opened, and balanced your subtle energy systems, having toned and strengthened your body, and having enlivened and rejuvenated your spirit, it's time to take on another kind of challenge that will further you on your evolutionary path and yield countless rewards. On the meditation chair or cushion, all elements of the Waking Energy Way come together.

You are ready to meet your mind. You may feel like a glider plane that's been cut from its engine-run escort to fly on its own, but I'll give you some launch instructions and, trust me, you *will* be able to pilot your craft on your own when it's time. From the comfort of your meditation chair or cushion you'll meet your mind in all its uninterrupted glory. Your sole task—and mind you, it's not a small one—will be to connect to your breath and follow it as it moves in out of your body, engaging in the zenith of all the practices you've performed yet: mindfulness. As you'll soon discover, although meditation is an opportunity to tap into an extraordinary font of energy and reduce stress, it can be a challenge.

Mindfulness is the state of being fully present, one in which we can attend to the most foundational pulse we know, the breath, and in an even more focused and refined way than in our energy adventures that have led us here. Mindfulness is the personification of yin energy, a kind of artful attention replete with respect, grace, subtlety, refinement, deepest quiet, and stillness. It can help to restore you in ways that few things can.

Going Out of Your Mind

This, my friend, is what all the hoopla is about. Meet your worst enemy and best ally: your mind. After all you've experienced on your Waking Energy journey, you are well prepared for this encounter. I smile at you knowingly and with great compassion because we've all wrestled with our thoughts before. But know that every practice you've done thus far has served to mobilize and harmonize your prana in such a way that you now have the inner space and fortitude to learn to befriend your mind and get it on your side.

The mind—specifically, the notorious monkey mind—likes to undermine itself and create distractions, not just when we're seated on our meditation cushions, but when we are earnestly trying to work with it in our daily lives. The mind always tries to take us out of the present moment and embroil us in its escapades.

The solution for the mind's unilateral capriciousness is meditation. Just as *savasana* helps you to integrate the healing benefits of your yoga practice, meditation, the art of attention, deep quiet, introspection, and detachment, serves to unite all the other practices in the Waking Energy flow.

To start the journey toward enlightenment through meditation, we'll explore a mindfulness meditation practice that will bring you into a realm infused with the perfume of the Upanishads, a collection of the world's oldest Sanskrit texts on meditation and philosophy dating back to roughly 1700–1100 BCE. You'll sample a collection of simple practices here that will start you, if you are a beginner, on your insight journey. I hope they seduce you to engage in regular practice. If you are a more seasoned meditator already, you can use these meditations for inspiration and variety, allowing them to elevate you to new heights of awareness by breathing new life and dedication into your existing practice.

The rewards of meditation are incalculable. Although modern science has had quite a love affair with meditation, having studied its merit and effects for many years, so much of what goes on in the mind during meditation is still beyond human understanding and eludes even the most expert of experts in neuroscience.

Like all yin practices, meditation stimulates the parasympathetic nervous system, showing us the way to smooth inner seas by inviting ourselves to become more tranquil. Neuroscientists have proven that meditation can actually shift brain activity away from the stress-prone right frontal cortex to wave activity in the calmer left frontal cortex.

This mental shift decreases the negative effects of stress, mild depression, and anxiety. Just as you did with the Inner Smile and Cosmic Healing Sounds practices, with mindfulness meditation you'll activate the relaxation response, redirecting your energy away from the amygdala, where your brain processes fear and triggers the stress response. As a result, you'll be able to cut stress off at the pass, interrupting the negative chain of events that would affect your body adversely, before stress even has a chance to take hold of your mind and do its damage.

A true testament to our neuroplasticity, meditation is the tool that can effect some of the greatest internal reprogramming, dramatically shifting our perspective and thus increasing our capacity to grow and change our brains on a cellular level. This inner shift alone can make more energy available for productive endeavors. What engine drives these types of shifts? Your willingness and the desire to begin.

When mindfulness meditation is practiced regularly, it feels as

the moving into stillness practice

TIME OF DAY: Morning or evening

QUALITY: Yin

SUBTLE ENERGY: Activates and harmonizes the meridian, nadi, and chakra systems.

BENEFITS: Lowers blood pressure, boosts immunity, enhances brain function and concentration, balances the endocrine system, improves sleep, reduces stress, and relaxes the nervous system to instill peace and calm.

PROPS: Chair, meditation cushion, yoga block

The Practice:

Be a Tree

Blossoming Lotus

Surrender and Receive

though you've won the lottery—a windfall of physical, mental, emotional, and spiritual well-being—leading you to a higher level of mental acuity and capacity, a deeper level of relaxation, and peace of mind. Most important, mindfulness meditation opens our hearts in a way that expands our lives and those of everyone we touch.

Each of the three meditations you are about to learn, Be a Tree, Blossoming Lotus, and the Surrender and Receive, is narrated like a story. You'll take a voyage through the landscapes inside you and use tried-and-true techniques to tame your monkey mind, leading you to a place of deep stillness and peace. These visioning meditations were conceived for both the beginner and the seasoned meditator. The ultimate goal is to come to rely upon *anapanasati*, a mindfulness technique that utilizes your breath to do a complete body scan, seeking out any areas of tension and breathing into them to relax and cajole them into partnering with you to allow you to focus on your breath itself. You'll use this as your way in and your way out of each practice and use the Waking Energy meditations to rest a while longer in peaceful abidance. These visioning sessions are centerpieces for a longer meditation practice. Before you know it, you'll be immersed in a sitting practice that exceeds what you may have originally thought you were capable of, lasting up to twenty minutes or more.

I've come to treasure these three meditations as some of my finest companions over the years, sessions inspired by each and every meditation I have ever had the privilege to do in my studies with yoga teachers, mindfulness devotees, and fellow meditators. All of them can be practiced in the morning or in the evening and are also easy to incorporate into your work day. You can do a fifteen- or twenty-minute "sit" right in your office, or during your lunch hour use a meditation as a way to calm yourself before you eat, so that you digest your food better and return to work feeling refreshed. They will all calm your mind, reduce anxiety, and either enhance your mental focus for the day ahead or help you to release the stress of the day that has just ended. If performed at night, they will help you get deeper, more restful sleep.

Meditation is truly one of the few things in life that you can make your own, an opportunity to practice being in the moment, which is really the only moment we ever have. In the realm of energy, when you're in the moment, it means that you are letting go of what no longer serves you, releasing what requires your energy. Even boxes of stuff that you haven't touched or looked at in a long time demand your energy to maintain them; they are occupying real estate in your head. Likewise, holding on to negative thoughts or thoughts that don't enhance your life steals your energy. In order to earn the right to occupy that precious space, thoughts had better be worth their salt and lead to actions that manifest as positive change, gifts of health, well-being, and happiness in your life.

Meditation is a declaration of self-love that the universe recognizes. Think about it. When you clear inner space, you are sending the message out that you are ready to receive—that you are worthy, lovable, and deserving. When you clear space in your being, it's also a love song to yourself, whose vibrations echo through the ethers, across time. You open the energy gates and let positivity rush in, flooding your being and your life with new inspiration and possibility.

Now is the time. Enter into stillness, the place where you will tap into your deepest source energy yet, so quiet and reverent that you will finally able to hear the whisperings of your true heart above the noise of your mind.

Each of these meditations should last fifteen to twenty minutes, but can be extended as long as you wish.

The Practice

Be a Tree

I have always loved trees, and Be a Tree is one of the most grounding, calming, and nurturing meditations I can do. I use it on days when I feel that I have too much energy stuck in my *upper pole,* the area extending from my heart center up to my crown.

When we feel anxious, overtaxed, or overextended, we need to draw our energy down into the earth to feel anchored and calm again. Be the Tree literally helps us to root. When you embody its energy, you can weather any storm. It enables you to summon the fresh, vivifying energy of the forest, flooding your entire being with the splendors of nature and inviting negative ions, which promote health; it's especially effective as a remedy to being stuck inside for prolonged periods, breathing stale air. Be the Tree is a way to build a golden shield of protection that feeds your senses, centers and balances you, and prepares you for the day.

1. Find a comfortable cross-legged seat on a meditation cushion or yoga block and then lift and lengthen the spine, feeling as if there is a gossamer cord attached to the crown of your head that is lifting you up and extending your entire spinal column up to the sky. Deepen your abdominals, gently pulling them in and back to provide a strong central support for your torso. Relax your arms down by your sides, bringing your palms to rest on top of your knees, and close your eyes.
2. Feel your strong legs underneath your hands as they release completely into the floor, which is rising up to meet them. They are completely balanced and at ease, meeting in perfect harmony.
3. Place your right hand over your heart and your left hand on your lower belly to connect with heaven and earth for a few rounds of breath.
4. Now bring your hands together in front of your heart, uniting head and heart, and intentionally call in your spirit. Think of what you wish to manifest in this moment—not just during your practice, but in your life. Breathe into this intention. Inhale and exhale for several rounds until you intuitively know that you have come to own this intention, and then seal it by bowing your head to your heart.
5. Inhale deeply. Then, to send your intention out into the universe and acknowledge your place and your power as a part of the world and all

things, chant "*A-U-M, Ommmmm.*" Once you've finished, bathe in its healing current. Let the vibration of the sound reverberate inside your every cell, infusing your cells with the enlivening frequency of the earth's power itself.

6. Place your hands on your knees again, so that you feel even more rooted to the earth, and with eyes closed start to connect to your breath and where it lives inside your body. Perform *anapanasati:* take a tour of your body, starting with the crown, working your way down to your feet, and then returning up the back of your body to the crown, to seek out the areas of greatest sensation and send your breath into them; inhale new life into your every cell, and as you exhale let go of what you no longer need.
7. Now summon the image of your favorite tree. See it standing tall and proud. See its trunk and the portion of the roots that ride along the carpet of the earth, and imagine where the roots travel. See them extending into the rich, black soil below. Then allow your eyes to travel up to the tree's branches, its leaves, flowers, berries. Now *be* the tree, sending your strong roots down to connect with the nourishing energy of earth.
8. From the roots, rise up through the trunk of that tree and see its magnificent markings, the etchings of time recorded on its bark, and go inside, imagining its rings. See them there spiraling around the center. How many rings are there? How old is that tree? Now be the trunk of that tree, and as you breathe let your breath build you up and out expansively, like a tree that has lived for at least a few hundred years. Feel the immense and stalwart strength and solidity of your torso, your trunk. Breathe into your strength. Breathe into your rings.
9. Now lengthen the crown of your head and become the graceful bows and branches of the tree, its leaves and flowers, reaching their energy up toward the sky to receive the blessings of the sun and the showers from the clouds, the rays and droplets of precious water falling upon you, anointing your head. Feel the powerful, pulsating life force of

universal prana vibrating inside you and connecting the two poles of the world and your body, deepest yin from earth and highest, most infinite yang from the sky.

10. As you breathe, send your breath from the crown of your head down to your roots like a cleansing waterfall, sending new life and energy to every part of your body. As your breath and energy sweep down and through you, release what you no longer need into the earth below. Inhale and relax even more deeply now, as you effortlessly reach even slightly taller, lengthening your crown up to meet heaven energy, and letting Mother Earth rise up to meet you, infusing your body and soul with her healing earth energy.
11. Bring your palms together in front of your heart once again, and return to the intention that you set at the beginning of the practice.

Blossoming Lotus

Consider the Blossoming Lotus a slow dance through your chakras, the meditation equivalent of the Inner Smile practice. If there is a particular emotion out of balance, or you aren't feeling well in a specific part of your body, now that you are on intimate terms with your chakras, you can select one particular chakra to focus loving attention on until you feel a palpable energy shift and a clearing in it.

This powerful meditation opens, clears, purifies, and balances all seven chakras, bringing your attention into a sharp and loving focus. You will become suddenly aware of the brilliant spectrum of colors that glow inside you as well as each of the emotional resonances associated with the chakras, creating a kind of internal rainbow of harmony that radiates out into the world, acting as an auric shield of strength, protection, and blessings.

1. Find a comfortable seat, letting your "sit bones" sink deeply into your meditation cushion. Then lift and lengthen the spine, gently deepening your abdominals in and back, to provide a strong central support

for your torso. Relax your arms down by your sides, bringing your palms to rest on top of your knees, and close your eyes.

2. Feel your strong legs release completely into the floor, which is rising up to meet them. They are completely balanced and at ease, meeting in perfect harmony and effortlessness.
3. Bring your hands together in front of your heart, uniting head and heart, and call in your spirit. Think of what you wish to manifest in this moment, not just here in your practice, but in your life. Breathe into your intention. Inhale and exhale for several rounds until you intuitively know that you have come to own your intention, and then to seal it, bow your head to your heart.
4. Inhale deeply, and send your intention out into the universe, acknowledging your place and your power as a part of the world and all things, by chanting "A-U-M, Ommmmm." Once you've finished the sound, bathe in its healing current and let the vibration of the sound reverberate inside your every cell, infusing your cells with the enlivening frequency of the earth's power itself.
5. Bring your hands into *gyan mudra,* and with eyes closed start to connect to your breath and where it lives inside your body. Wake your inner senses with *anapanasati.* Take a tour of your body, starting with the crown and working your way down to your feet, and then returning up the back of your body to the crown. Seek out the areas of greatest sensation and send your breath into them. Inhale new life into your every cell, and as you exhale let go of what you no longer need.
6. Summon images of your seven chakras: *muladhara,* your Root Chakra, a brilliant ruby; *svadhishthana,* your Sacral Chakra, a bright orange; *manipura,* your Solar Plexus Chakra, sunshine yellow; *anahata,* your Heart Chakra, a deep emerald; *vishuddha,* your Throat Chakra, a rich turquoise; *ajna,* your Third-Eye Chakra, a deep indigo purple; and *sahasrara,* your Crown Chakra, a pure, crystalline white. See them all spinning inside you, and with your breath start to breathe into all seven, letting them know you are now present and want to speak with them.

7. Start with the first chakra. As you inhale, send your breath down into your Root Chakra and see it take on the color of your root, a brilliant, rich ruby red. At the same time, feel the higher emotional resonance of the Root Chakra merging with its inherent color. For the root, feel security, safety, and grounding. Feel your own strength and rootedness as you direct your breath into the epicenter of the chakra. As you exhale, watch your breath misting like the sea spray when an ocean wave crashes against rocks on the shore, gently expelling stagnant prana out of the chakra. As the prana exits out of the back of your spine and flows down into the earth, it resets the chakra's harmonious, natural way of being, leaving it spinning like a windmill in the wind.
8. As you inhale again, see the ruby red energy of your Root Chakra rising. Consciously draw it up your spine through the *sushumna nadi,* your central channel, like a red ribbon of cleansing energy traveling through all seven chakras until it reaches the crown and explodes with your exhalation—your very own fireworks display, releasing shimmering red light down and around your body. It becomes an aura of protective energy that falls and flows in streams like mini-waterfalls all around your body, until it is absorbed into the earth, taking with it anything that no longer serves your highest good.
9. Now repeat this same sequence in its entirety with the next five chakras, sending your breath into each one in turn, seeing its brilliant color, and then watching your breath as it becomes infused with the color and emotional resonance of the chakra.

The orange of the Sacral Chakra and its inherent creativity, joy, and enthusiasm.

The yellow of the Solar Plexus Chakra and its personal power, expansiveness, and seeds of spirituality.

The green of the Heart Chakra and its devotion, passion, and unconditional love for the self and others.

The blue of the Throat Chakra and its independence, fluid thought, and clear, empowered communication.

The indigo purple of the Third-Eye Chakra and its intuitive visioning and cosmic consciousness.

Follow the same course with each chakra, cleansing it, releasing stagnant prana from it through the spine and sending it into the earth, setting it into harmonious action, and then drawing its energy, color, and higher resonance of corresponding emotions up through the *sushumna nadi* and out through the crown.

Continue in this manner until you have awakened and worked through the first six chakras, raising the energy of each up through the spine, so that they start to communicate with one another and work as a team to bring balance and harmony to your entire body.

10. After you have brought awareness to the six chakras, see the white light of the Crown Chakra, the culmination of all seven colors, rising from your root up through the *sushumna nadi* and coming to radiate through the crown, exiting in a shimmering explosion of energy and light that showers you in waves of harmonious rainbow energy that surrounds you in a glowing cocoon of light and love.
11. Rest in your radiant cocoon of light, in your own radiance. Breathe this light and love into your heart center and third eye. Relax into its soothing sea of loving energy and know that you are supported by the earth below and heaven above, divinely protected and guided at all times.
12. Bring your palms into *anjali mudra* (Prayer Position), the hand gesture for union and peace, in front of your heart.

Surrender and Receive

Surrender and Receive inspires you to open your heart to what is—life exactly as it is—and is perhaps most representative of what we are trying to achieve with meditation in the first place. Even if you're someone who loves to clear the clutter in your home or routinely empty your closets, it's still not easy to let go of things—especially our intangible emotions. This meditation makes the notion of letting go a friendlier one, because as you clear your inner space and cultivate the courage to let go on your meditation cushion, you can then manifest the same in your life.

Just as we're not especially good at letting go, so we also don't really know how to receive. That means receiving everything from compliments and praise to love. Surrender and Receive will teach you to release what you no longer need and give yourself permission to receive your heart's desire.

When you decide to let something go, you not only create space for something new to come into your psyche and your life; your body rewards you with energy! If we return to befriending our enemies from the Inner Smile, we release ourselves from carrying the burden of what no longer serves us, and we lighten our load and make more energy available for manifesting greatness in our lives.

On a spiritual level, when you let go of what you no longer need, it's as if air traffic control has sent a "cleared for takeoff" message to your soul. You are then clear, meaning you have sufficient inner space, clarity, and proximity to your intuition, to receive sacred messages from on high—to take flight.

As we know, the mind has a tendency to glorify or regret the past and to anticipate or attach hopes and expectations to the future. Both states are unproductive and can lead to anxiety. This meditation is designed to help you release the future and the past and come into this present moment, while it also reminds you of all that you have to be thankful for, ushering in love and gratitude. On a higher level, a more spiritual plane, it also leads to a place where you can start to entertain the idea of saying goodbye to your body and your life, helping you to imagine a peaceful transition. As we move from the life we know into the unknown, we return to nature herself and what lies beyond.

1. Find your comfortable seat, letting your "sit bones" sink deeply into your meditation cushion or yoga block, and lift and lengthen the spine. Deepen your abdominals, gently pulling them in and back to provide a strong central support for your torso. Relax your arms down by your sides, bringing your palms to rest on top of your knees, and close your eyes.
2. Feel your strong legs underneath your hands as they release completely into the floor, which rises up to meet them. They are completely balanced and at ease, meeting in perfect harmony and effortlessness.
3. Bring your palms together in front of your heart into Prayer Position, uniting head and heart, and call in your spirit. Think of what you wish to manifest in this moment, not just here in your practice, but in your life. Breathe into your intention. Inhale and exhale several rounds until you intuitively know that you have come to own your intention, and then to seal it bow your head to your heart.
4. Inhale deeply, and to send your intention out into the universe, acknowledging your place and your power as a part the world and all things, chant *"A-U-M, Ommmmm."* Once you have finished the sound, bathe in its healing current and let the vibration of the sound reverberate inside your every cell, infusing your cells with the enlivening frequency of the earth's power itself.
5. Bring your hands into *gyan mudra* or the mudra that you feel best suits you and what your body needs when you are releasing something detracting from your life. Turn your palms face up.
6. With eyes closed, start to connect to your breath and where it lives inside your body. Using *anapanasati,* seek out any areas of greatest sensation and send your breath to them. Inhale new life into your every cell, and as you exhale let go of what you no longer need.
7. Now release your chosen mudra, allowing your fingers to softly open with the backs of your hands on your knees. Imagine that you are on the beach and have just scooped up a handful of sand. Watch your

hand blossom like a flower as you gently open your fingers and let sand slip through.

8. Inhale as you think of one thing that you wish to release from your life. Then, as you exhale, see it leaving your life, your body, and your mind just like the sand that has slipped through your fingers and the breath that you have released down into the earth below.
9. Inhale the new lightness in your heart that you feel when you think of the energy surrounding what you have just released from your life. Rest in this new energy you have liberated by courageously saying good-bye to something that was no longer serving your highest good. Breathe this new energy into the consciousness of your every cell and allow yourself to stay here bathing in this new light for several breaths.
10. Now breathe into your open hands and turn your attention to what you would like to usher into your life or what you would like to receive.
11. See this new energy coming in through your open hands, into your heart and into your life. Breathe the truth of this new life into your every cell. Open your heart even more to receive.
12. Shifting your focus, rub your thumb and fingers of your left hand together in small circles, as if you were sprinkling salt on a dish. In your mind, assign the past to the left hand. Think of the past and all the wonderful memories, certainly, but then also of the all-too-human regrets and disappointments, what you wish you could have done better, what you wish could have happened differently, and acknowledge the feelings that arise inside you. Feel how you are suddenly pulled out and away from yourself, whisked into times gone by, where you have no control, and allow yourself to be with the feelings that come up.
13. Now rub the thumb and the fingers of your right hand together in small circles. Assign the future to the right hand. As you do, think of all the exciting things that the future holds, bright promises and dreams coming true, and alongside the beauty see the clinging and the attachment to what you *need* to have happen, what you anticipate,

and then feel the anxiety that surely arises when you allow yourself to be pulled ahead into a space and a time that don't yet exist.

14. As you inhale, now bring the palms together into Prayer Position, bringing past and future together into the gift of the present moment, out of which greatest clarity is born—pure, clear space that you have created, perfect liberation, like the sound "*AUM*," the sound of divinity itself. Bathe in this sacred moment where you are one with your own true nature, your timeless soul essence that knows no attachment, no dissatisfaction over impermanence, no suffering, but the highest wisdom of no self and perfect, infinite transcendence, at one with all that is and ever will be.
15. Rest in this moment; open your heart and allow it to receive this clear light, the energy of infinity, true and endless love.
16. Now bring your hands into Open-Heart Mudra. As you breathe now, inhale love and exhale gratitude, remembering what you surrendered and what you ushered into your life, and feel the energy that is rising up inside and swirling around inside you from this courageous, self-loving act. Allow yourself to be swept into the currents of this profoundly healing and enlivening energy, deep inside this sweetness, softness, and light.
17. Send your breath now from the crown of your head down to your root, like a cleansing waterfall, sending new life and new energy to every part of your body. As your breath, energy sweeps down and through you, releasing what you no longer need into the earth below. Inhale and relax even more deeply now, as you effortlessly reach even slightly taller, lengthening your crown up to be anointed by the highest star and heaven energy, and letting Mother Earth rise up to meet you, infusing your body and soul with her healing pulse, a heartbeat running through your veins, flooding your heart with love.
18. With your hands in Open-Heart Mudra, return to the intention that you set at the beginning of the practice. Practice *metta,* loving-kindness, toward the self now by saying the following words: "May I

be healthy, happy, strong, safe, and free. May all beings everywhere be healthy, happy, strong, safe, and free. May the thoughts, words, and actions of my own life and my own loving heart contribute to happiness and freedom from suffering for all." Inhale love and exhale gratitude for the bounty that is your life—all that you have to be thankful for, all that you cherish and hold dear. Breathe this love and gratitude in and out for several breaths.

19. Now bring your palms to touch in Prayer Position and silently repeat, "*Namaste.* The divine in me sees and honors the divine light within me, and sees and salutes the divine light in you."
20. Bow the head to the heart, with your forehead lightly meeting your fingertips, to seal your intention. Then offer your intention to the universe, where it will be made manifest, by chanting the earth's perfect song as an act of highest love and light . . . "*A-U-M, Ommmmm.*"

Walking Meditation: The Labyrinth

Self is everywhere, shining forth from all beings, vaster than the vast, subtler than the most subtle, unreachable, yet nearer than breath, than heartbeat. Eye cannot see it, ear cannot hear it nor tongue utter it; only in deep absorption can the mind, grown pure and silent, merge with the formless truth. He who finds it is free; he has found himself; he has solved the great riddle; his heart is forever at peace. Whole, he enters the Whole. His personal self returns to its radiant, intimate, deathless source.

—*Third Mundaka Upanishad*

Although sitting is the most widely used posture for meditation, you can also take your stillness practice on the road. With walking meditation, you can move your mindfulness practice into your feet and legs, so that as your body takes on a tranquil gait, you still your mind. Your feet are moving ever so slowly and deliberately, deeply connecting to the earth, and your upper body is serenely going along for the ride on top, reaching closer to heaven, as you walk the path to the innermost you.

With its complicated, mazelike route, always returning on itself and circling around to reach the center, a labyrinth that we can walk for the purpose of prayer or meditation is a perfect representation of the voyage we have taken inside our bodies as we've integrated the wisdom of the ages. When you walk a labyrinth, you are stepping onto a clearly delineated path that offers you freedom to explore and expand, to sing your song of songs. It is through rituals such as these, acts of honoring and loving ourselves, that we can find the greatest freedom and expansion in our lives. Walking a labyrinth is what I imagine happens after death, when we get to float on a carpet of stars, the Milky Way itself, stretching out infinitely, like a diaphanous ribbon, the real-life equivalent of Stevie Wonder's song "Ribbon in the Sky."

The labyrinth is the map of life's twists and turns that, if followed like your soul's own sacred mandala, can help you find what has been seeking you. Moving beyond our own love, into the ocean of cosmic oneness energy on earth, we swim inside the sea of synchronicity itself, living into our highest purpose, a glowing embodiment of our own radiance. Like the wise adepts who came to meet themselves, moving through their timeless systems for millennia before us, we can travel across time through the labyrinth's meandering arcs, renouncing the outside world for the sake of returning to our light, to ourselves. It is the pathway home.

Somehow we are always and forever returning to the beginning when we're walking the path of the labyrinth. As we approach the doorway to the beyond, we are peering in closer to our true nature, our timeless essence, our immortal souls. Through this new way, this Waking Energy Way, we have touched our own divinity, visited the world unseen inside us that exists beyond our sight, beyond our knowing, just as we will one day merge with the world unseen that lies beyond. This is the place where we launch ourselves after dedicating ourselves to nourishing and loving these bodies that we will one day say good-bye to. It is the knowledge of this good-bye, the very real knowing that we are just "renting" these "earth suits," that we can use to inspire us to make the most of every day that we are still here. In fact, all the practices you've learned in Waking Energy will help you to do this.

Truthfully, I never actually had the patience to walk a labyrinth until recently. I used to go to Canyon Ranch in the Berkshires with my mother, and I would also bring her as my guest when I taught at Rancho La Puerta in Tecate, Mexico. Her favorite pastime was walking the labyrinth. She was by far one of the most extraordinary and fiery intellects I've ever known, and also one of the most impatient people ever. Somehow she reserved all her patience, it seemed, for walking the labyrinth. Demonstrating a kind of reserve that was truly exceptional, especially for her, whenever she stepped into the labyrinth, it was like the first moment I stepped into the temple at the Tibetan sanctuary in Woodstock, New York. It was clear that she was not only stepping onto sacred ground, but reverently into another world.

In Mexico, from day one of our arrival she would demand that I accompany her to the labyrinth. And every day that I resisted, she would ask not once, but a few times, like the bubbling, provocative child she was, with a sparkle in her eye that meant her request was more like a demand, as if to say: "You'll be sorry if you don't, because you're going to miss one of the peak experiences of your life!" Every morning at breakfast, relentlessly, all the while wearing a broad, knowing grin (knowing she was provoking me) like the little girl she was, she'd ask, "Wanna go to the labyrinth with me today?" Finally, I would submit. But even though I was captivated by the spiritual idea of it and found its arcing pathways exquisite, and even though I have always loved the kind of order it offered and embraced ritual, it inspired rebellion in me. It made me feel as though I wanted to draw outside the lines. As I watched her through my peripheral vision, gracefully gliding forward through the inner circles, the arcs and narrows, and of course her beloved spirals, it was everything I could do to stay the course and behave. Her diligence, her dedication, her solemnity and trancelike devotion to the thing, her absolute gravity made me want to fly off into space.

And that's exactly what I would do. In the middle, at a glaringly inappropriate time, in a decidedly un-Buddhist-like fashion, either when I found myself back in the very center of it or on one of its outermost circles, I would use my long legs to strategically step over the arcs and turns, to free myself in the very same way I rescued myself from that first death-defying sixty-minute sit at Kripalu.

Shortly after she passed away in July 2014, although I knew she wouldn't have wanted me to, I turned down an invitation to appear at Rancho La Puerta, convinced I couldn't survive it. Lo and behold, at a friend's recommendation, I found myself on another silent meditation retreat, just weeks afterward, at a location not more than two hours from Tecate, at the sister site to Rancho La Puerta. Walking out the front door of my casita at sunrise, I found myself the object of a cruel cosmic joke. As I was staring out at the very same mountain range and inhaling the very same intoxicating scents as in Tecate, my mother suddenly appeared before me.

Rising to my throat at rocket speed, grief wrapped me in its stranglehold, choking me. I was awash in molten hot tears—anguished. Sinking to my knees and sobbing uncontrollably, I looked up at the sky beseechingly and shouted at the top of my lungs, "I can't possibly endure this!"

Later that same day, the universe (or I should say, Mom) arranged an opportunity for me to finally complete my first walking meditation, *my labyrinth*. She was with me, smiling every step of the way, and I could hear her voice. "See, just look how exquisite! Look at that magnificent rock there, and that gorgeous, delicate little fern growing out of it. Oh my God, the spirals! And oh wow—look at you, my angel, out of all the spirals here you are the most beautiful one."

Now We May Begin

There will come a time when you believe everything is finished; that will be the beginning.

—Louis L'Amour

This may appear to be the end of our journey together, but that's just an illusion. This is actually the beginning. It may feel as though we're saying good-bye, but really this is just, "See you soon." And the most exciting part? It's the start of your solo flight. I encourage you, a baby bird being pushed out of its mama's nest to test its wings, to use nature as your guide and take flight, relishing this sacred meeting of yourself. Trust the wisdom of your body. Listen to the voice of your soul.

Now that you truly know yourself in the new way, trust is really all you need. Everything else will fall into place around you like tiny magnetized metal flecks flying toward a magnet. Believe that what you seek is seeking you. That radiant, gorgeous, loving font of boundless energy? That timeless, joyful child? That sparkling, effervescent essence? That bright light?

practice menu: seven ways in seven days

Making It Your Own

Monday (Yang)

Awaken and Play: Love Thyself
Unleash and Transform
Your Own Fountain of Youth
Empower and Flow

Tuesday (Yin)

Awaken and Play: Opening the Energy Gates
Go Deep, Open, and Energize
The Power of Love
Moving into Stillness

Wednesday (Yang)

Unleash and Transform
Empower and Flow

Thursday (Yin)

Awaken and Play: Full Practice
Go Deep, Open, and Energize
The Power of Love

Friday (Yang)

Awaken and Play: Love Thyself
Your Own Fountain of Youth
Empower and Flow

Saturday (Yin)

Awaken and Play: Opening the Energy Gates
Go Deep, Open, and Energize
The Power of Love
Moving into Stillness

Sunday (Yang)

Empower and Flow
Your Own Fountain of Youth

Acknowledgments

Waking Energy has lived inside me all my life, but the book version could never have come to pass without the integral participation of an entire team of people. Nothing is a solo endeavor. There are many people I'd like to thank.

To start, I'd like to acknowledge my incredible agent and stalwart friend, Jonathan Lyons, who has been my rock throughout this entire process. From start to finish, he has been an extraordinary support and facilitator. Without him, this book would not have seen the light of day.

Nancy Hancock, for being such a willing sport and kicking her shoes off to get down and dirty, and return to her dancing days to really experience the work the way it was meant to be so that she was properly seduced into signing up!

Libby Edelson, for taking the reins following Nancy's departure and being a stellar partner in helping Waking Energy to manifest as its current iteration.

Christine Pride, who came in and saved the day as an exceptional editing advisor and revamped the book in such a way that it was more manageable—taking it from its state as "War and Peace," and helping me to render a version that was a proper first taste for all of you who will read it and enjoy it.

To Lauri Nemetz, my talented illustrator and supporter who rendered the beautiful superimposed images that made the work spring to life off the pages.

To Chloe Crespi, photographer extraordinaire whose sensitive and discerning eye captured the essence of the movements that comprise this magnificent "way of ways."

To the many cheerleaders and lovers of Waking Energy who have patiently waited for this moment.

And finally, deepest gratitude to my beloved mother, who was a constant presence throughout the writing process, my muse from beyond.